20.00

# The
# NEURODYNAMICS
## of the
# VERTEBRAL
# SUBLUXATION

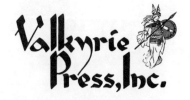

Valkyrie
Press, Inc.

International Standard Book No. 0-912760-55-9

Library of Congress Catalog Card No. 77-85117

PUBLISHED BY

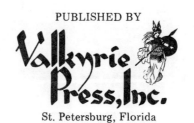

Valkyrie
Press, Inc.

St. Petersburg, Florida

# Foreword
## to First Edition

The principles and theory of spinal manipulation are presented in this volume in a new and scientific light. When one considers the heretofore unrecognized values and implications of the vertebral adjusting, it becomes evident that D. D. Palmer's chiropractic rests upon a solid foundation of neurological facts which were, of course, unknown to all investigators at the time of the discovery of chiropractic in 1895. The chiropractor need no longer undergrade his efforts in the restoration of health for lack of authentic evidence as to the validity of his approach.

Dr. Homewood is a most gifted writer. He turned his deep concern for the recognition of chiropractic by the intelligent doctor, student and public opinion-maker into a gruelling and deliberate task of explaining the complicated subject of the subluxation in an interesting and scientific manner. His appreciation for the achievements of chiropractic caused him to dig deep into the biological sciences for verification.

The author's ambition to write a chiropractic textbook, utilizing and substantiating D. D. Palmer's basic principles and fortifying them with an up-to-date neurological background, has been fully realized. Chiropractic is now dressed in modern scientific garments, but the body and soul of chiropractic remain intact. It is glorified not by empty platitudes, but by the latest findings from authentic sources. He culled much from modern works of neurology and biology to fully buttress the ideas of our founder.

Dr. Homewood worked on this volume as a man inspired, translating his inspiration into factual and meaningful words that greatly enhance our method of healing. He was motivated by a compelling drive to place chiropractic on a plane of greater appreciation by our own practitioners and of acceptance by the scientific community. In this effort, he has succeeded remarkably. His modesty predominates throughout this volume. It is the same scientific modesty that led the editors of the Medical Journal of the University of Toronto to request him to write that unusually fine and historic exposition of chiropractic for their publication.

His candor is refreshing. Of course, he did not permit himself to write an exhaustive coverage of every possible cause and modifying factor of the subluxation, but the examples given are sufficient and will awaken the imagination of the reader. The author is fully aware that a genuine science is never finished or closed. The intelligent student cannot study human behavior, biology, or any other subject without realizing that these sciences are progressing toward goals which recede as they come in sight. In the present text, therefore, the writer did not hesitate to introduce the hope that future scholars shall further advance chiropractic along its hard and lonely road of establishing itself as a worthy scientific system of comprehensive natural healing.

The mechanisms of cause and effect of the subluxation are now made sufficiently clear so that they are applicable to many situations. Here is a volume written by one of our eminent scholars that can bring chiropractic to the fore. It is high time that respect for chiropractic should come from a distinguished scholar of our own ranks.

This work takes chiropractic out of the limited field of explanation as to the causation of disease and brings it into the multiphasic situations of the etiology of disease via the subluxation. It answers why chiropractic is effective and why it is useful even when the prime cause for disease may not be found in the subluxation.

Dr. Homewood graphically describes the mechanism of the subluxation, which results in symptoms and tissue changes which lead to the neural basis of pathology. The author has used a good deal of prudent judgment in buttressing D. D. Palmer's principles with the latest biological findings. He clarifies many of the intricacies of the subluxation in relation to modern neurology.

Dr. D. D. Palmer taught us to look upon the body as a perfectly working organismic machine; that we should look to the integrated brain and nervous system as the basis for health and disease; that we must look to the body and to the mind for our total well-being; and that health comes from within. All that we needed to render chiropractic acceptable to the intelligent and unbiased mind was to correlate our founder's concept with modern neurological discoveries. Dr. Homewood has accomplished this task admirably.

Sixty-seven years later, we now have the advantage of a perspective which our founder could not possibly possess as to the relevancy of his discovery and the immensity of good that it could bring to human well-being. D. D. Palmer's key discovery was profound and history has proven the need and efficacy thereof. The basic principle he laid down is as valid now as it was then; and this volume brings it up-to-date.

HERMAN S. SCHWARTZ, D.C.
*President Emeritus, Council of Psychotherapy,*
*National Chiropractic Association.*

*Author of:*
  *"The Art of Relaxation"*
  *"Home Care of the Emotionally Ill"*
  *"Mental Health and Chiropractic"*

Dedicated to

My parents whose sacrifices made possible my education and sense of responsibility to the profession.

# *Acknowledgements*

Use of this text by nine of our chiropractic colleges and a continuing demand by practitioners in every corner of the globe dictated the necessity to edit and republish in a slightly enlarged form with the addition of an index.

Pre-eminent among the many deserving of honourable mention for the stimulus and encouragement to write the original manuscript stands Dr. Herman S. Schwartz, the author of three books listed at the end of his generous Foreword. Dr. Schwartz read, corrected, suggested and above all, through his continuing stream of letters, encouraged the completion of the original manuscript. His enthusiasm and counsel were invaluable and his "Foreword" deeply appreciated and retained for this edition.

Dr. Helmut Bittner, Former Dean, and the late Dr. Thure C. Peterson, President of the Chiropractic Institute of New York which has amalgamated with the National College, supplied valued information and encouragement.

Dr. L. M. Rogers, while Executive Secretary of the National Chiropractic Association, offered the printing facilities to produce an original paperback form, but although greatly appreciated time has proved the advantage of a hard case.

Students and graduates of the Canadian Memorial Chiropractic College, the former Lincoln Chiropractic College and the Los Angeles College of Chiropractic are deserving of credit for the stimulus to write the original and this revised edition, as well as the other effort to provide a safeguard to practice in the form of "The Chiropractor and the Law."

The bibliography has been updated in some areas, although most of the original authors have been retained, since modern authors seem to confirm the material presented.

Teachers, associates, professional friends, and students over these twenty-eight years have been responsible for the two texts written and this second edition.

Miss Lorraine Haynes, secretary to Dr. George Haynes and the author, has contributed invaluable service in the preparation of this revised edition and made it possible to accomplish the task in the face of a very short deadline period.

Dr. C. A. Pickenburg of Hoisington, Kansas, president of the American Council on Chiropractic Technique, supplied constructive criticism which has had a modifying influence in a number of areas of the text. His time, thought, and expression of helpful suggestions are deeply appreciated.

My family suffered through the neglect of the months of preparation of the original text and in this revision. Appreciation of the understanding and patience is small recompense.

To all others whose subtle influence may have received little acknowledgement appreciation is extended.

A.E.H.

# Contents

# The
# NEURODYNAMICS
# of the
# VERTEBRAL
# SUBLUXATION

## A. E. HOMEWOOD
### B.T.A., LL.B., D.P.T., D.C., N.D., F.I.C.C.

*Former President*
*Canadian Memorial Chiropractic College*
*Los Angeles College of Chiropractic*

# CHAPTER I

# Introduction

IN SEPTEMBER of 1895 Daniel David Palmer[1], a native of Port Perry, Ontario, a self-educated, erstwhile grocer in Davenport, Iowa, applied his reasoning, discovered a principle which he claimed to be as old as the vertebrata and utilized by the Egyptians, the Incas, and many other ancient civilizations, but employing a method previously unknown. By locating and correcting an anatomical disrelationship of the fourth thoracic vertebra in the spine of a Negro porter in the building in which Dr. Palmer had his office, the hearing of the gentleman was restored, after seventeen years of deafness, and a profession was born which has become second only to allopathic medicine in numbers and influence.

A controversy was that day spawned, which has raged without cessation for these 82 years, both within and from without the profession. Discussion and argument have flared and many ideas have been advanced as to the mechanism by which the disrelationship of vertebral segments and other articulations may result in widespread functional derangement and the tissue changes of disease. For half a century or more medicine of the orthodox school vehemently denied the possibility of vertebral disrelationship; the feasibility of adjusting, by hand, such a misalignment; and the likelihood of vertebral distortion interfering with neural transmission which create functional aberrations in visceral structures as a consequence.

In recent years, allopathic medicine has been "discovering" chiropractic and its literature and professional journals have been replete with references to vertebral disrelations, or subluxations, and credit given to the interference of the segmental nerves by such distortion as the cause of many and diverse symptoms, and, on occasion, medical authors have even been known to acknowledge chiropractic's prior claim to this body of important knowledge.

Dr. C. W. Weiant[2], Dean Emeritus of the former Chiropractic Institute of New York, published an entire book, entitled *Medicine and Chiropractic*, extensively quoting these medical authorities who are making the startling discoveries of the importance of the spine to the health and the well-being of the human — more than 82 years after D. D. Palmer had revealed these previously unappreciated truths, founded the chiropractic profession and signified his willingness to share his findings with all persons interested in restoring health to suffering humanity.

In his textbook, *The Science, Art and Philosophy of Chiropractic*, published in 1910, D. D. Palmer[3] wrote, "It is also a pleasure for me to observe that the medical profession are absorbing Chiropractic ideas, using its methods, as shown by their books and practice."

Controversy within the profession has been rampant over these many years. Many ideas have accumulated in chiropractic relative to the theory of the mechanism by which ill effects in the human body are produced by the articular subluxation. Despite the fact that D. D. Palmer[4] said, "Chiropractors adjust any or all of the 300 joints of the body, more particularly those of the spinal column," there have been those who condemned fellow practitioners for adjusting articulations other than those of the vertebral column, and those who looked askance at any practitioner with the temerity to adjust any and every vertebral segment found to be disrelated in preference to a dependence upon the efficacy of correction in one region only. There even has been disagreement as to the vertebra adjusted to restore the hearing of Harvey Lillard, although D. D. Palmer[5] wrote, "On September 18, 1895, Harvey Lillard called upon me. He was so deaf for seventeen years that he could not hear the noises on the street. Mr. Lillard informed me that he was in a cramped position and felt something give in his back. I replaced the displaced 4th dorsal vertebra by one move, which restored his hearing fully."

Dr. Palmer envisioned chiropractic as being part of the evolution of a health science, which had developed from the days of the priest-physician, through the allopathic, homeopathic and osteopathic forms of medicine to the discovery and development of chiropractic. In his own words[6], "As a means of relieving suffering and disease, Allopathy, Homeopathy, Osteopathy and now Chiropractic, have each, in turn, improved upon its predecessor. The latter, of all the others, is entitled to the seat of honor and distinction. But, as soon as the human mind is capable of absorbing a still more refined and advanced method and human aspiration demands it, it will be forthcoming and I hope to be the medium through which it will be delivered to the denizens of the earth."

Chiropractic came upon the scene at a time when the expansion of the United States was taking place at a rapid pace, the need for doctors was acute, and numerous proprietary medical colleges had sprung up during the early nineteenth century to "cash in" on this bonanza. These colleges were described by Arturo Castiglioni, M.D.[7] of Yale University, in his book, *History of Medicine*, as being, "a combination of lecture, quiz and cram with short sessions and few expenses, self-appointed faculties and no collegiate connections, degrees given in absentia, and even attendance not always being required."

It was not until Abraham Flexner, A.M., M.D. (honourary) backed by the funds of the Rockefeller Foundation and the Carnegie Institute, made a sweeping investigation of the medical colleges and submitted a report, "Bulletin Number Four" of the Carnegie Foundation in 1910, that a serious effort was made to clean up the education of medical physicians.

In a book, *Medical Education*, published in 1925, Flexner[8] stated in part, "Loose and shifting bands of practicing physicians, calling themselves a faculty, tried to impart, chiefly by lectures, to heterogeneous uneducated groups of students the empirical knowledge — sound and unsound — which they themselves possessed. First and last, American towns have produced over four hundred such medical schools. The teaching of medicine on these terms was, directly in cash, and indirectly in prestige, a profitable business. In time the medical profession — to its credit be it said — undertook itself to set its own house in order, and with such marked success that schools of this extreme type have within the last decade practically disappeared." But, let it be noted that there were still a few of these in operation in 1925.

In the interest of historical fact, it would have been gracious of Flexner were he to have given credit to the governments, philanthropic agencies and donors of huge endowments for the billions of dollars which made possible the correction of educational deficiencies. Organized medicine is not deserving of the glory for taking funds from their own coffers or the pockets of practicing physicians to bring into being these reforms, nor in fact for having corrected the disgraceful situation of their own free will. The reforms were enjoined upon the allopathic profession by outside powers and directed by one who had no connection with the profession.

Continuing, Flexner[9] wrote, "It was an improvement when the proprietary medical school, long suspended in mid-air, an affair of lectures, quiz, and cram, tended more or less doubtfully to settle about a hospital. In retrospect, the condition — an advance though it was — looks strange enough. Hospitals had been set up by municipalities, religious organizations, or philanthropic societies. Staffs, huge, unorganized, unpaid, unassisted, had been put in charge; appointments went variously — by political pull, by personal favor, occasionally even by merit."

In this instance credit has been given to others for the establishment of the hospitals, which are to this day built and maintained by governments, religious organizations, or philanthropic societies, and contributed to heavily by the general public; yet are claimed as the private domain of allopathic medicine, staffed and administered by allopathic practitioners, accredited by the union of allopathic practitioners, and visited only by physicians bearing the stamp of approval of the medical organization, the A.M.A.

In few, if any, areas of democratic life are the members of the public treated with such complete and utter disregard for their personal wishes, opinions or desires, as in a so-called "Public" hospital. Should the doctor of the patient's choice not be a member of the medical association, he is barred from entry and the patient must submit to the ministrations of a strange practitioner and even to a system of healing completely at variance with the desire and belief of the patient.

## Chiropractic Education

Into this chaos of so-called medical education chiropractic was born, and the practitioners of this new healing art were not backward about emulating the pattern of "education" established by the older, "orthodox," allopathic school of healing. Privately owned colleges shot up across the country for the training of chiropractors to meet the growing demand of the populace for this health service. Most of these institutions could boast of every shortcoming of which Abraham Flexner had accused the schools of medicine of possessing and perhaps a few he had overlooked in his travels.

In the words of D. D. Palmer[10] published in 1910, "I cannot remain silent when teachers and self-styled 'professors' in certain schools in which chiropractic is claimed to be taught, are so obstruce, by an overwhelming ambition to be known and heralded as authors and original thinkers that they not only teach as part of chiropractic science and philosophy, doctrines and theories which are as absurd as they are erroneous, some of whom go so far as to deny the use, if not the existence, of important organs and functions of the body, and make startling physiological discoveries, simply by boldly giving another name to functions whose existence and duties have been known by all physiologists for generations."

While chiropractic education has received a great deal of criticism from the ever loyal opposition, who conveniently forget their own not-so-ancient history, the majority of chiropractic colleges have attained a degree of educational excellence by virtually lifting themselves by their own bootstraps. While the chiropractic profession is quite willing to bask in the reflected glory and take the credit for the strides made in the educational struggle, the truth is that, like medicine, few laurels have been earned by the practitioners through sacrifice and generosity on behalf of their colleges. There have been some notable exceptions to this indictment and in very recent years the National, now American Chiropractic Assocation has made a valiant effort and stirred a segment of the practitioners to a half-hearted attempt to financially support the accredited colleges. The Canadian Memorial Chiropractic College has received support from Canadian chiropractors, but even this until 1969 had averaged a pittance per year per chiropractor.

While the amount contributed by the 25,000-odd practitioners has been a pittance in return for the ponderosity of service received, the few thousands of dollars have been a God-send to the colleges, which, unlike those of allopathic medicine, have not received the beneficence of government, philanthropies or endowments. The radical improvements in chiropractic education by ever increasing plant facilities, modern teaching methods and visual aids, as well as excellent laboratory courses, redound to the credit and bespeak the energy and enthusiasm of the educators and administrators of the institutions. Sir Winston Churchill might well have been thinking of the chiropractic educators when he made his often quoted remark, "Never was so much owed by so many to so few."

The early chiropractic colleges found, in the competition for students, that to be different was an advantage, and faculties made an effort to propound their own peculiar theories without regard for the basic teachings of D. D. Palmer and were forced to keep explanations and theories simple to meet the needs of the poorly-educated students desirous of attaining the Doctor of Chiropractic degree. Over the years, the problems of the profession have been multiplied and compounded by the perpetuation of many of the unfounded false doctrines, upon which segments of the chiropractic profession have been impaled. These harsh accusations are necessary for a realization of the difficulties faced by the profession, and an appreciation of the differences of viewpoint which exist within a relatively small profession.

In an effort to formulate a satisfactory basis for study of chiropractic principle and theory, and substantiate the rationality of chiropractic techniques for the treatment of human misery and disease, the author has leaned heavily upon the basic principles established by the founder of the science and art of chiropractic and made a diligent effort to scan the literature of biological science to cull from it the anatomical, physiological and other basic science facts which assist us in understanding the mechanisms by which chiropractic methods bring relief to suffering humanity. Certainly, no claim can be made for a complete search of the available literature, nor for any original investigation, scientific discoveries, or profession-shaking contribution of wisdom. Rather, a sincere and honest attempt is claimed for a utilization and synthesization of material from diverse sources in an effort to understand the mechanism by which the adjustive thrust of chiropractic so profoundly influences function, to share this information with all interested, and above all else, to encourage the students of this science and art to appreciate the importance of a solid foundation in the biological sciences and a new respect for the founder of their profession.

Abraham Flexner[11] might well have been writing about the chiropractic profession of the past, when he penned, "One can decry the system of those days — the inadequate preliminary requirements, the short courses, the faulty arrangement of the curriculum, the dominance of the didactic lecture, the meager appliances for demonstrative and practical instruction — but the results were better than the system."

Certainly, this writer would be the last to disparage the strides and progress made by the early members of the chiropractic profession. With the limited educational background necessitated by the circumstances of their era, they virtually performed therapeutic miracles and established the chiropractic beach-head so strongly that the most persistent efforts of organized medicine, utilizing every conceivable tactic, have not been successful in forcing this new healing art back into obscurity. This young profession, through the vision and efforts of the pioneers, spread to every state in the Union, every province of Canada, most European countries, South Africa, Australia, New Zealand, and South America. Even the countries of the Orient have had a sparse representation of this profession. Few civilized countries remain to feel the impact of the teachings of D. D. Palmer.

It is to the public detriment that too large a segment of the chiropractic profession is abdicating the role of chiropractic physician for the less demanding musculoskeletal specialization. The potency of modern drugs for iatrogenic complications and tissue damage makes it ever more imperative that the sick and suffering have an alternate school of generic medical thought that is relatively free of danger and potent as a corrective measure for a wide spectrum of disease. Spain[12] expressed the situation succinctly, "Unfortunately, therefore, iatrogenic disease can now take its place almost as an equal alongside the bacteria as an important factor in the pathogenesis of human illness."

## Original Principles

Unfortunately, the principles and theory propounded by D. D. Palmer did not meet the needs of the educators in the early days of chiropractic history and much of his teaching was either lost or distorted by the peculiar interpretations which better suited the circumstances. Therefore, it is necessary to constantly quote from the works of D. D. Palmer to establish the exact principles and separate them from the peculiar ideas and theories from the fertile brains of others. Many of these latter theories do not stand square in the light of present day knowledge, yet the teachings of D. D. Palmer will be found consistent with the facts of our present stage of intellectual insight and are likely to be found capable of withstanding investigation in the light of new knowledge yet to be discovered — for these are basic truths and principles.

It is necessary to have a theory that stands upon a firm foundation of basic science facts as we understand them today, to satisfy the enquiring mind of the college student, to defy the criticism of the skeptic and scoffer, to provide the practitioner with the confidence that he is dealing on a scientific basis with a far reaching principle, which may be applied by diverse methods to produce satisfactory and, in many instances, astounding results. It is the hope that this writing will awaken a renewed interest, especially in students, and recognition that the last word has not been written relative to the basis of chiropractic, its mechanism of health restoration and prophylactic care. Certainly, this text is not intended to be the final theory upon which chiropractic explanation will be based for posterity, but, rather, a step in the evolutionary process of understanding the basic principles enunciated by D. D. Palmer and a step closer to the truth and realization of the broadness of the principles upon which chiropractic methods were founded. If it succeeds in supplying a stimulus of this nature and kindles a new respect and interest in the teachings of the founder, the time and effort will be well spent.

With the knowledge and assurance that the basic principles of chiropractic are sound and correct, there need be no qualms regarding critical investigation of the theory. Nor can any theory, based upon the known facts of today, be expected to stand unchanged for posterity. As a clearer understanding of the functioning of the nervous system unfolds before the relentless onslaught of investigators and researchers, new knowledge will, no doubt, require the application of these acquired facts and a newer interpretation of the mechanism by which the application of chiropractic techniques accomplishes health restoration.

It may be assumed that any theory, based upon facts should be as useful for one school of chiropractic thought as another. The nervous system acts upon one set of laws and the knowledge of those laws will explain the reason for the efficaciousness of the varied methods of application of the basic principles of chiropractic. Each chiropractor may create, or modify, his methods and each technique be effective, providing it is the application of a true principle. Any theory must be of value for all or the theory is incorrect or the technique is in error in its theoretical interpretation. Since all techniques, which apply the principles of chiropractic, produce results, a common theory, which does not serve to explain all methods, must be incorrect or lacking in scope.

Be assured that the purpose of the following pages is to build a theory which may be utilized by all, and no effort will be made to favour one particular method of practice or school of chiropractic thought. Thoughts set forth are the writer's own, coloured by his educators, experience, associates, students, and writers of authority in chiropractic and the basic sciences. However, every effort to interpret the writings of neurological investigators in an unbiased manner has been made to produce an end-product in strict conformity with present knowledge and not prone to being torn asunder by criticism.

The facts that both substantiate and repudiate the chiropractic contention that structural distortion causes interference to normal nerve transmission and results in the symptoms and tissue changes of disease have been included. It is not claimed that the literature has been exhausted in this search, since the texts relating to neurology alone come off the presses faster than one man can possibly read. Nor, has it been possible to make full use of all the information on hand in this brief book, but necessity dictates the enlargement of the previous short, concentrated thesis.

# CHAPTER II

# Introduction to Third Edition

IT APPEARS APPROPRIATE that this introduction to the Third Edition should follow, rather than precede, the former Introduction. Throughout the new edition the reader will find that the thoughts expressed previously have had to be modified, since the advent of the electronic microscope, microsurgery, and more exacting techniques of biochemistry, the knowledge of the anatomy and physiology of the neural system has been tremendously expanded. Many of the thoughts, hypotheses, theories, etc., relative to the nervous system, which had stood the test of time for many years have proven erroneous. Fortunately the chiropractic hypotheses and theories previously expressed have not been found to be contradicted and minor modifications have been necessary to utilize these new facts.

It must be appreciated that research continues and that what is accepted as fact today may be supplanted by new knowledge tomorrow. Students of chiropractic must face the challenge of being ever vigilant for new findings that must be incorporated to modify the former explanation. Since chiropractic is a science, a division or school of thought of generic medicine, it must ever remain dynamic in its explanation of how its techniques modify function, maintain and restore health. Mindset and tenacious fixation on a previously satisfactory hypothesis is dogma, not science.

The necessity to maintain the status of a primary health care provider becomes greater with the ever expanding third party payment system by insurance companies and government agencies. The detractors who would exclude, and, failing that, limit chiropractic physicians become ever more desperate and vicious.

To permit chiropractic explanation of the mechanism by which the methodology produces the desired results to rest on obsolete biological "facts" is to supply the basis for justified criticism and ridicule. It is unfortunate that those "new" findings in current textbooks may be several years old and may have been contradicted or modified by later research. Regretfully, it is not possible to be up to the minute in the various areas of concern.

Modifications of the chapter on Significant Physiology of the Nervous System reflect to a considerable degree the work of Arthur Guyten, as reported in "Medical Physiology, 5th Edition." Additional findings provide a partial explanation of inhibition within the central nervous system and require some alterations in statements made in prior editions of this text.

An additional chapter has been added, Applied Embryology, as this writer experiences concern that one of the most basic and useful divisions of biological study, embryology, is almost entirely taught as an academic exercise with little or no correlation with gross anatomy, the neural system, symptoms, referred pain, viscerovisceral reflexes, etc. No textbook seems to exist to provide the extensive volume of practicality of this subject for the practitioner of any healing art, especially the chiropractic physician whose techniques are dependent upon his ability to determine and correct neural dysfunction.

No claim can be made by this author of tremendous depth of knowledge in the field of embryology, but, rather, the temerity to tackle an area of knowledge whose facts are scattered. By attempting to bring some of these facts to the attention of the reader, it is hoped that integration and understanding may result and the extensive practicality of the subject utilized.

Further, it has been the hope that this text has, over the years, acted as a stimulus, and in the future will continue to act as a stimulus to college students to appreciate the basic sciences as more than hurdles over which to jump for licensure, as chiropractic is dependent for its foundation upon these disciplines. Chiropractic is, in fact, "manipulative surgery" and requires the same detailed knowledge and attention to detail as an allopathic or osteopathic surgeon, utilizing the incision and excision methods. To be capable of influencing the nervous system for good or harm is an awesome undertaking that should be approached with respect and understanding.

# CHAPTER III

# The Antiquated Theories

UNDER THE ABOVE heading a very critical appraisal of the chiropractic theory, as tenaciously held in past years by many practitioners of
chiropractic, will be undertaken to show the necessity of revising the
explanation of the mechanism by which disease is produced by structural distortion, and to illuminate the digressions from the basic principles as taught by the founder.

In recent years, chiropractic has received more recognition from
the various government bodies, courts, compensation boards, insurance companies, etc. This recognition has been obtained through the
efforts of chiropractic leaders to bring to the attention of these
organizations the effectiveness of the application of the chiropractic
methods. In other words, clinical results have proven the truth of the
chiropractic principle to the extent that most critical and biased persons are forced to admit the benefits to be derived from the techniques used by chiropractors. Unfortunately, the explanation of the
mechanism by which results are produced has not been satisfactory
to the men of science, who have been interested in enquiring into the
theory of chiropractic. To deduce that, since the principle is true; the
application, or technique, is effective; therefore, the theory is correct;
is erroneous logic.

Chiropractic has been unmercifully criticized for having no
"scientific" proof of its hypotheses and theories other than 82 years
of clinical results, since the nervous system does not lend itself to
study under the microscope in circumstances that duplicate the in
vivo situation. Allopathic medicine prescribes acetylsalicylicacid by
the ton and many other drugs without "scientific" proof of the
mechanisms of action, but the mere clinical proof that symptoms are
abated. The latter is "science" and the former "quackery," according
to the A.M.A.

The theory of the mechanism by which the subluxation produces
nerve interference has been worded in many ways, but it may be
stated plainly as follows, "The vertebral subluxation causes pressure
upon the spinal nerve, thus shutting off the flow of nerve energy, or
Innate Intelligence, from the brain and spinal cord to the peripheral
structures and organs."

The example often utilized for the benefit of the patient of stepping on the garden hose, thereby decreasing the flow of water, has

merit for the untrained layman, but leaves much to be desired by the thoughtful chiropractic student, the critics of chiropractic who possess a knowledge of neurology, and especially neurologists who may be called to testify against chiropractic, or chiropractors, in courts of law or before legislative bodies.

Grave doubt should be immediately aroused by such a simple explanation of such an important and all-inclusive principle. Students of anatomy and physiology are well aware that there are few, if any, simple reactions within the body. Even the flexing of the forearm requires contraction of the prime movers, the relaxation of the antagonists, contraction of the fixators of the shoulder, wrist and fingers, accompanied by altered blood supply and electro-potential of the muscles. This is to say nothing of the alteration in tonus of the muscles controlling posture, the altered chemistry of the tissues, etc. An entire chapter could be devoted to the neurological changes that take place within the spinal cord, brain stem and brain, as well as the peripheral nerves to effect such a movement. It is belittling to the science of chiropractic to keep it saddled with an obsolete, simple, and naive theory — a theory very difficult to substantiate and so prone to ridicule, as well as at wide variance with the teachings of D. D. Palmer,[13] who said, "The activity of these nerves, or rather their fibres, may become excited or allayed by impingement, the result being a modification of functionating — too much or not enough action — which is disease."

Time and time again D. D. Palmer[14] wrote that the subluxation resulted in either an increase or decrease in neural activity, hence, either an increase or a decrease in function, and in exasperation wrote, "I wish that all chiropractors could take in this basic principle of our science — THAT TOO MUCH OR NOT ENOUGH ENERGY IS DISEASE."

Most of the theories have avoided the "too much" neural conduction and function, presumably because more proficiency in neurological discussion is required for such an explanation.

The interesting textbook, *The Intervertebral Foramina in Man*, by Harold Swanburg, M.D.[15] presents tables with measurements of each intervertebral foramen and each intervertebral disc. The nerves were also measured individually and the largest found to be 7 mm. in diameter. The space of the intervertebral foramen occupied by the spinal nerve varied from one-twelfth to one-third of the opening. Thus the most likely nerves to be pressed upon by a subluxated vertebra are those occupying one-third of the total space of the foramen. However, the remaining two-thirds of the space are occupied by the blood vessels, the recurrent spinal (or meningeal) nerve, very fine connective and soft, yielding adipose tissues.

It is of interest to digress to note that Burke[16] reported in his text of 1964 the discovery of the recurrent spinal or meningeal nerve under the more erudite name of the Nervus Sinu Vertebralis and states, "The existence of this immensely important nerve has apparently escaped recognition by the profession at large. It is not specifically described in any textbook, even those on anatomy and surgical anatomy."

The 23rd edition of *Anatomy of the Human Body*, Henry Gray, 1936, states on page 911: "After emerging from the intervertebral foramen, each spinal nerve gives off a small meningeal branch which re-enters the vertebral canal through the intervertebral foramen and supplies the vertebrae and their ligaments, and the blood vessels of the medulla spinalis and its membranes."

The issue of Cunningham's *Human Anatomy* used by this writer in the teaching of anatomy in 1945, contains on page 1015 the following: "Just before its division each nerve gives off a minute meningeal branch, which re-enters the vertebral canal after effecting a junction with a branch from the sympathetic trunk, and is distributed to the membranes and the vessels of the spinal cord."

In response to the harsh criticism of chiropractic by Dr. Burke, it would seem justified to enquire when and where he studied anatomy. He certainly could not have used any of the classical texts, nor read one following graduation. His is a prime example of unjustified criticism of chiropractic that reveals the abysmal ignorance of the critic. How unfortunate that he did not read page 326 or 515 of D. D. Palmer's book of 1910.

Page 326 of D.D.'s text states: "Just before their [spinal nerves] division, each nerve gives off a slender recurrent branch which re-enters the vertebral canal, after affecting a junction with a branch of the sympathetic cord, and is distributed to the spinal cord and its membranes." Page 515 adds to the description: "It, also, sends branches to the vertebrae and vertebral ligaments."

The spinal nerve in the foramen occupies the superior portion of the foramen and lies about one-eightieth of an inch from the superior pedicle. The largest spinal nerve measures 7 mm. in its superoinferior diameter, thus being 3 to 5 mm. from the pedicle which forms the inferior boundary of the foramen. It should be kept clearly in mind that the upper portion of the foramen, especially in the thoracic and lumbar regions, is formed by the inferior notch of the vertebra above, which is much deeper than the superior notch of the vertebra below, thus this upper portion of the foramen is least subject to occlusion from vertebral movement, providing the maximum protection for the spinal nerve. The most likely portion of the foramen to be narrowed by movements of the vertebrae would be that portion bounded anteriorly by the intervertebral disc and posteriorly by the articular processes.

The question must immediately arise as to the reason why many normal movements of the spine, which far exceed the range of a subluxation, do not cause pressure upon the spinal nerve. The answer lies in the understanding of the fact that the axes of movement for the vertebrae permit relatively wide ranges of movement without alteration in the sizes of the intervertebral foramina to any appreciable degree. Mennell[17] has illustrated the axes of rotation for the three areas of the vertebral column and the manner in which each type rotates through a segment of a cylinder. Neither in normal movement nor in subluxation do the surfaces of the articular processes separate, which would constitute a posterior shift of the side of the vertebral segment in question and would then cause the body of the vertebra, forming part of the anterior boundary of the foramen, to approximate the superior articular process of the vertebra, whose superior vertebral notch forms the inferior portions of the wall of the foramen. Such an eventuality would result in the spinal nerve being carried posterior with the superior vertebral segment with little likelihood of any direct osseous pressure. Should such pressure occur, it must result from contact of the superior portion of the superior articular process of the inferior vertebra upon the postero-inferior aspect of the spinal nerve.

D. D. Palmer[18] stated, "The first and second pair of cervical nerves cannot be pressed or squeezed between the occiput and atlas or in the cleft between the atlas and axis, and yet there are many diseases resulting from their displacement."

In addition to the first and second cervical nerves, all five sacral nerves and the coccygeal nerves are without true, moveable intervertebral foramina through which to escape from the vertebral canal, leaving 23 of the 31 pairs of spinal nerves subject to the effects of the old-time chiropractic theory of subluxation as a cause of pressure upon the spinal nerves. What about the other eight pairs? Also, what about the 12 pairs of cranial nerves? Certainly, no chiropractor with experience in the care of human disease would accept the contention that chiropractic technique is limited to the influence of 23 pairs of spinal nerves above mentioned. Despite this, the pinched nerve theory does not, and never has, given a reasonable explanation for the influence exerted upon all nerves. Yet, in the pages of Dr. Palmer's text attention was drawn to these nerves, which exit via foramina whose structure precludes sufficient changes in shape or size to cause pressure upon the contained nerve.

To cause an occlusion, or closing of the foramen would necessitate sufficient distortion to be classed as a partial dislocation or complete dislocation and would result in injury to the intervertebral discs and ligaments. The vertebral column is so constructed as to permit greater ranges of rotation, antiflexion, retroflexion, and lateral flexion than is to be found in the distortions called "subluxations," which do produce symptoms. Despite these wider ranges of motion normally executed, symptoms do not occur. As examples, the acrobatic dancers, the high school students in gymnasium classes, and many others too numerous to mention, undergo contortions of the spine far in excess of the distortion attended by symptoms. How can these paradoxes be explained? Certainly not by the outmoded theory of nerve pressure.

Should the injuries to the surrounding tissues, joint capsule, ligaments, intervertebral disc, etc., take place as above mentioned, adjusting the area would not, under such circumstances, result in immediate relief of pain and distress. This phenomenon often occurs in the office of each chiropractor. Also, partial dislocations would show as such on x-ray, with overhanging of articular facets, or bodies, but these findings are the exception rather than the rule, and careful measurements are required to determine the areas of disturbance. Therefore, it would seem that our subluxations are not partial dislocations. The vertebrae are then within their normal range of motion, although not functioning at their optimum.

In McDowell's[19] physiology text may be found the result of experimental pressure upon nerves, through which the conclusion was reached that pressure upon nerves does not materially alter their ability to conduct.

Best and Taylor[20] in *The Physiological Basis of Medical Practice* discuss the results of narcotizing a section of nerve, which proved that the nerve current is greatly reduced in volume or strength as it passes through the treated area but regains its original strength upon reaching the normal, untreated section beyond. Should pressure upon the nerve within the intervertebral foramen result in a decreased flow through the area, contrary to the findings of McDowell, its original strength would be regained beyond the intervertebral foramen, provided Best and Taylor are correct. The physiology textbook of Zoethout and Tuttle [21] also makes mention of similar experiments of nerve narcotization with similar findings.

Mention has been made of the nerves which leave the vertebral canal by openings other than typical intervertebral foramina. A prepared vertebral column, or skeleton, should be studied to assure the reader of the truth of the following remarks, since chiropractors should be acutely aware of the peculiarities of intervertebral foramina, the nerves passing through them, and all related structures.

The first cervical nerve is seen to have passage through the sulcus arteriae vertebralis, a notch on the superior border of the posterior arch of the atlas, bounded anteriorly by the lateral mass; superiorly, by the occiput; and posteriorly by the Posterior Atlanto-occipital Membrane.

The second cervical nerve leaves the vertebral canal between the posterior arch of the atlas above; the lamina of the axis inferiorly; the articular capsule and processes anteriorly; and the Posterior Atlanto-axial Membrane completes the foramen posteriorly.

The first four pairs of sacral nerves are found to divide into anterior and posterior primary rami within the sacral canal. The posterior divisions, or rami, leave through foramina of fixed size in the posterior surface of the sacrum, and the anterior divisions through similar openings in the anterior surface. Thus, these nerves cannot be subjected to pressure by the boundaries of bone, since these cannot approximate.

The fifth pair of sacral nerves and the coccygeal nerves are small in size and well protected, although not passing through intervertebral foramina. These two continue down in the sacral canal to pass lateralward and escape through slits bounded posteriorly by the cornua of the sacrum and coccyx and the cornual ligament; and anteriorly, by the apex of the sacrum.

Since the above foramina do not correspond to the typical and cannot cause pressure upon the corresponding nerves by alteration in size, what cognizance does the time-worn theory take of these exceptions? Very little, would seem to be the answer.

Another point of consideration is the axes of rotation of the vertebrae, which are such that the articular facets are utilized for guiding the direction of motion, rather than for weight bearing and do not separate from one another in any of the normal motions of the vertebral column. As Mennell[22] has so efficiently discussed and illustrated, the axes of rotation in the cervical region fall posterior to the spinous processes and rotation takes place by the articular facets gliding on one another, as is obvious from the arthrodial form of joint formation. Such an axis of movement assures that there will be no shift in the mass of the vertebra, but a change of facing. Such an arrangement guards against direct pressure upon the spinal cord.

The axis of rotation for each thoracic vertebra passes through the body of the segment and the articular facets are curved as a portion of a cylinder, permitting rotation to take place around a comparatively short radius.

Rotation in the lumbar area takes place around axes that fall posterior to the vertebral canal and the articular facets show by their form that they, too, are segments of a cylinder with an axis posterior to the articular cavity and have a limited range of rotation.

If the above facts are kept in mind, there should be little chance of making the mistake of thinking that the articular facets separate from one another, thereby encroaching upon the intervertebral foramina to decrease the antero-posterior diameters. On the other hand, the movements of lateral flexion and posterior flexion, or dorsiflexion, may cause a definite narrowing of the margin of the intervertebral disc, which forms a portion of anterior wall of the intervertebral foramen, thus decreasing the vertical dimension slightly. However, it would seem obvious from the facts quoted by Schwanberg that the nerve has a sufficient margin of safety, due to its occupancy, at most, of one-third of the foramen and the fact that the loose connective tissue and soft fat could accommodate for the minor degree of loss of the vertical dimension by the above forms of flexion.

From the above, it might be assumed that spinal distortion in the regions mentioned and in the manner discussed would have no effect upon the nerves and, therefore, it is useless to apply chiropractic methods to these areas. This would be a serious oversight on the part of any chiropractor and certainly not an impression which the writer wishes to leave undisputed in the minds of the readers. However, every possible objection to the chiropractic premise must be squarely faced. Criticism can best be answered, if anticipated. If justified, our theory must be altered to fit the facts, not distortion of the facts to fit the theory. While any proven fact remains at variance with our theory, no stone must be left unturned in an effort to harmonize the two. No other course is open to a science.

Textbooks on anatomy by both Piersol[23] and Donald Mainland [24] mention the possibility of slight decreases in size of the intervertebral foramina. As is to be expected, both minimize the importance of these changes in diameter. Piersol gives credit to the Ligamenta Flava, which are yellow elastic tissue, for correcting the "innumerable slight displacements."

In view of the protection offered the nerve, it would seem more likely that the thin-walled veins within the foramina would be more affected and the free flow of venous blood obstructed by subluxation than direct pressure brought to bear upon the spinal nerve. More consideration will be given this subject later.

Vertebrae are capable, in normal movements of the body, of passing through and maintaining for a time, much wider ranges of motion than are found in the ordinary subluxation. Nonetheless, the nerve does not become pinched, pain does not result, nor are any abnormal functions to be noted. The foramina would be expected to be occluded considerably in some of these positions. There must, therefore, be an additional factor, or number of factors, responsible for the wide variety of symptoms which arise from the subluxation of vertebrae.

The assumption has been made that nerve pressure does occur due to subluxation and it has been taught that this pressure inhibits the flow of nerve impulses from the brain and spinal cord to the structures supplied by the nerve in question, despite the teachings of D. D. Palmer.[25]

Each and every spinal nerve is composed of both afferent and efferent neurones, fibres conveying impulses into the spinal cord and others carrying impulses outward. If it were true that pressure could shut off the flow of nerve impulses, then there should be a decrease in the impulses reaching the spinal cord and the brain from the involved area. Thus, a degree of anaesthesia in the area of skin and a loss of proprioceptive sense from the muscles and articulations supplied by the involved nerve would result. Also, the lack of efferent nerve force should result in some degree of paralysis or weakness of the muscles supplied.

Professor Mainland[26] has pointed out in his text, *Anatomy*, the following, "Vertebral Tuberculosis will result in swelling of the nerve sheath, thus pressure upon the nerve fibres, causing pain and muscle spasm." He gives examples of appendectomies being performed when the disease was, in fact, vertebral tuberculosis. This degree of nerve pressure, which would be expected to be much greater than that caused by an ordinary subluxation, still results in stimulation rather than inhibition, as attested by the pain and active muscle contraction.

Symptoms caused by the pressure of a herniated nucleus pulposus of an intervertebral disc upon a spinal nerve trunk are known to be severe pain, muscular weakness, muscular atrophy and sensory change in the dermatome. The pressure in this instance is sufficiently severe to actually disturb nerve conductivity and thereby the tone of the muscle fibres is decreased and disturbance of the microscopic structure of the muscle follows with the lapse of time with demonstrable atrophy of the affected muscle or muscles.

Neither of the above two examples of direct nerve pressure completely fits the picture observed in cases exhibiting ordinary chiropractic subluxations.

That pressure may occur from a herniated disc, exostosis, thickening of the joint capsule, tuberculosis, collapse or compression fracture of a vertebral body is not denied, but rather, it is the intent to point out the difference in symptom pictures that ensue in contrast to the symptomatology of the true chiropractic subluxation.

The subluxation is attended by contraction of the small, segmentally developed intervertebral muscles and, in many instances, hypertonicity of the longer, more superficial muscles, thereby indicating an excess, rather than a decrease of efferent nerve impulses. D. D. Palmer[27] recognized full well that not all subluxations decreased the conduction capacity of nerves, for he wrote, "Displacement of any part of the skeletal frame may press against nerves, which are the channels of communication, intensifying or decreasing their carrying capacity, creating either too much or not enough functioning, an aberration known as disease."

Also, the tenderness found at the site of subluxation indicates a greater acuity of sensibility instead of a decrease, which would occur were the nerve unable to conduct beyond the point of pressure. There are few instances where joint and muscle sense (Proprioception) is lost as a result of subluxation, as would occur were pressure to prevent nerve conduction, as the old theory would have us believe.

D. D. Palmer[28] may be quoted to indicate that "pinched nerves" were never a figment of his imagination, "To pinch a nerve, in the vertebral foramen or elsewhere, would have a similar result as the pinching of a string of a musical instrument — paralysis of its function, by stopping its vibratory movement — its carrying capacity. For this reason, a vertebral luxation — a complete displacement, one which pinches — causes paralysis; whereas, an impingement increases tension, heat and functioning. To increase tension by impingement or otherwise, is to increase vibration and its carrying capacity, thereby increasing functional action."

## Cranial Nerves

How do vertebral subluxations pinch cranial nerves?

D. D. Palmer[29] was curious about the answer to that question, as may be attested by his words, "I very much desire to know how the 24 cranial and the nerves of the sympathetic nervous system can be adjusted, acted upon by the hands. All nerves are connected with the spinal nerves by communicating fibres. The fibres become impinged upon or pressed against by the displacement of bones."

It is a well known, proven fact that the cranial nerves have no relationship with the intervertebral foramina, but, rather, are dependent for their escape from the cranial cavity upon foramina within the anterior wall and floor of the skull. It is impossible, on an anatomical basis, to justify the disturbances to the cranial nerves by subluxations with the theory of direct nerve pressure either of the margins of vertebral foramina, or those of the foramina of the skull. How then do vertebral subluxations disturb the structures supplied by cranial nerves?

Anyone with chiropractic experience knows that the application of chiropractic methods to the spine can, and does, have marked influence upon structures supplied by cranial nerves, such as the eyes, the nose, the paranasal sinuses, etc. Is this influence only through the sympathetic system, which has its outflow from the thoracic and upper lumbar neuromeres of the spinal cord? Doesn't the cervical portion of the spinal cord have any effect upon these cranial structures?

Daniel David Palmer[30] made numerous references, throughout his book, to the inability of subluxations to "pinch" nerves or cause direct pressure upon cranial nerves to produce the adverse symptoms found in patients suffering from subluxations. When one reads his textbook, it is necessary to marvel at how far astray the teachings of chiropractic progressed from the original principles formulated by the founder. Many of the ideas propounded in the name of chiropractic were distortions of the truth as taught by D.D., while others were complete fabrications, unrelated to any of the founder's teachings. Furthermore, one cannot help but be impressed by the wisdom of this self-educated man and his intuitive insight into fundamental truths that are being discovered today by the research of such men as Hans Selye of the University of Montreal. *The Science, Art and Philosophy of Chiropractic* is commended to every chiropractor that he may acquire a new awareness of the basic principles, a new appreciation of chiropractic as a science, and a new sense of pride and appreciation for the advanced thinking of D. D. Palmer in the field of biological science. None could read this book without being impressed by the background knowledge of the author, the vision and reasoning, and the principles which even today set the pace for research in the field of health and disease.

## Cervical Cord

Before leaving the criticism of chiropractic theory to begin building an explanation, founded upon the facts of anatomical and physiological knowledge, attention is directed to the cervical portion of the spinal cord. All chiropractors apply the adjustive technique of their choice to this region with profound results in visceral structures. Looking to any of the authorities in anatomy, such as Gray,[31] Cunningham,[32] Piersol,[33] etc., it will be found clearly stated that there are no efferent fibres which supply viscera, leaving the cervical neuromeres in the eight pairs of cervical nerves. In other words, the fibres, composing each cervical spinal nerve as it leaves the vertebral canal, are somatic motor to voluntary muscles or sensory fibres from somatic and visceral structures. From this it should be appreciated that were the subluxation to cause pressure upon a cervical nerve and decrease the flow of impulses, no viscus would be affected and no visceral symptoms would result. However, it is an established fact that cervical distortion does adversely affect viscera; therefore, the simple, antique, "pinched nerve" theory cannot be correct. The answer must be more complicated.

Let us pause here to refresh the memory of the more advanced student and to clarify the picture for the novice in the field of neurology. The spinal cord is the uninterrupted downward continuation of the brain structure, composed of the fibres which form the pathways, both to and from the brain, grouped into named tracts. Each fibre is microscopic in cross-section and some are insulated by whitish, fatty material called myelin. The peripheral portion of the spinal cord is composed of these fibre tracts, completely surrounding a central gray mass, butterfly-shaped, and divided, for descriptive purposes, into two posterior gray columns and two anterior gray columns and united across the midline by the gray-commissure. All gray substance is composed of the cell bodies with which the fibre tracts make synaptic connection, either on their course from the brain downward, or from the periphery to the brain.

The spinal cord is concerned with the segmental control of the body. In other words, those structures which, during the embryological development of the individual, developed in the same region, or segment, and later migrated, continue to be supplied by nerve fibres which maintain connection with the corresponding neural segment. To illustrate this more clearly and in a more practical manner we might consider the small muscles that lie between the ribs to complete the wall of the thorax. These are the most clearly segmental muscles to be found in the body and derive their nerve supply from the cell bodies which lie in the anterior horn of the spinal segment which corresponds.

The cells in the anterior horn are found to be multipolar in type; that is, they have a number of short processes, called dendrites, which receive impulses from various sources, and a single axon which leaves the spinal cord as part of the anterior nerve root, the nerve trunk, then the anterior division or ramus, to be named Intercostal Nerve as it passes between the ribs to supply the intercostal muscles.

The afferent fibres, or sensory fibres, from these same muscles and the overlying skin return by way of the intercostal nerve, the nerve trunk, but pass as part of the posterior nerve root into the spinal cord where synaptic connections are made in the posterior horn of grey matter. The cell bodies of these sensory fibres are unipolar in shape and are located in the Posterior Nerve Root Ganglion, which may be in the intervertebral foramen or within the spinal canal. From the posterior gray horn, a short neurone may carry the impulses to the anterior horn cells, forming what is called the simple reflex arc. This latter neurone is called a connector, intercalated or internuncial neurone.

In addition to the conduction of both afferent and efferent somatic impulses, the anterior primary ramus has been joined, outside the intervertebral foramen, by postganglionic sympathetic fibres from the associated paravertebral ganglion, whose function it is to travel through the intercostal nerve to supply the blood vessels of the muscles and skin, as well as the glands of the skin and the Erector Pili muscles of the skin. This is the most clear segmental arrangement within the body and the most simple course taken by the fibres of an anterior primary division of a nerve trunk to reach the structures to be supplied.

In many instances, such as the arms and legs, the segmental tissues divide, unite together in varied combinations, forming long muscles, sheets of muscle, etc., which completely obscure the segmental formation of the structures. However, the portion of each muscle which has been derived from a particular embryological segment, retains its connections with that neuromere, or spinal cord segment, with which it was associated in development. Thus it is that long muscles derive their nerve supply from more than one segment of the spinal cord. Also, it might be kept in mind that when a muscle migrates, it still retains its neuromere connections and draws the nerve fibres out to considerable length.

An excellent example of this is the Diaphragm, which developed, in part, in the centre of the neck of the embryo, deriving its nerve supply from the 3rd, 4th and 5th cervical segments of the spinal cord. As development continued, the Diaphragm migrated downward to take its attachments in the upper lumbar and lower thoracic region, forming the floor of the thoracic cavity and the roof of the abdominal cavity. The nerve fibres, originally associated, retained their connection with the Diaphragm and with the 3rd, 4th and 5th cervical neuromeres, thus were required to greatly elongate, passing through the lower neck and the thoracic cavity, the Phrenic Nerve.

At the points of attachment the Diaphragm received contributions of tissue from the lower thoracic segments and acquired additional nerve fibres of the afferent type derived from the lower six thoracic neuromeres, but no further efferent or motor fibres.

Furthermore, it should be kept clearly in mind that the spinal cord segments are reflex centres only and do not have the ability to volitionally initiate movements or to interpret sensory impulses. Feeling, or sensation, necessitates the involvement of higher brain centres, reached from the periphery, skin, muscles, viscera, etc., by a chain of three separate neurones. Thus, a stimulus applied to the skin resulting in the sensation of pain, necessitates the adequate stimulus to disturb the special receptors in the skin, causing a change in polarity to travel as a nerve impulse along the fibre of a nerve to the unipolar cell body in the Posterior Nerve Root Ganglion. The axon of this neurone leaves the cytone to enter the spinal cord as part of the Posterior Nerve Root, then turns upward in the Tract of Lissauer, or Posterolateral Tract, for several segments before synapsing with the cells of the posterior gray horn in that portion at the tip called the Substantia Gelatinosa of Rolando. Here the first order neurone terminates and the second order neurone commences.

Prior to the following the course of the second order neurone, it would be well to bring to mind that synaptic connection may be effected with short neurones, connector neurones, which carry the impulses to the anterior horn cells and thereby result in contraction of muscle fibres in reflex response.

The axone of the second order neurone crosses over to the opposite side in the White Commissure and turns up in the Lateral Spinothalamic Tract, which continues through the remainder of the spinal cord, through the Medulla Oblongata, the Pons, and the Mid-brain to enter the Thalamus for termination by synaptic connection with the cells of this structure, which are the third order neurones. The axones of these cells leave the Thalamus as part of the Internal Capsule, become part of the Corona Radiata, then reach the Post-central Gyrus of the cerebral cortex. In this region of the cortex conscious awareness, localization and interpretation of pain take place.

Nearly every sensation experienced by the cerebral cortex requires three orders of neurones to conduct the impulse from the receptor in the periphery to the conscious area of the cortex. At each area of synaptic connection collaterals, fine branches, may make reflex connection through connector neurones with motor cells to cause some form of reflex response on the same side, the opposite side, or in segments above or below. Sherrington[34] long ago established the fact that there are few simple reflex arcs, affecting only a minute portion of a single muscle, but, rather, that the reflex response to a stimulus entering over a single fibre is plurisegmental. In other words, the response to a stimulus is not confined to one neuromere.

In addition to the somatic afferent connections above briefly discussed, it should be emphasized that these efferent impulses also play upon cells of the lateral gray horns, which are to be found in the twelve thoracic segments and the first two, three or four lumbar neuromeres. These cells are the sole out-flow of the sympathetic division of the autonomic nervous system and send their axones as part of the anterior nerve root through the nerve trunk, into the anterior primary ramus, then via a white ramus communicans to a paravertebral ganglion, in which these preganglionic, well myelinated, fibres terminate by synaptic connection with the neurones called postganglionic sympathetic fibres, whose axones are poorly myelinated and thus, gray in colour. Each white preganglionic sympathetic fibre is reported to make synaptic connection with five or more gray, postganglionic sympathetic fibres, which leave the ganglion to supply blood vessels, some smooth muscle fibres, sweat glands or internal organs. Crelin[35] credits each preganglionic fibre with synaptic connection with 100 or more postganglionic neurones. Guyton[36] makes mention that eight percent of the fibres in a somatic nerve are C-type (unmyelinated) postganglionic sympathetic fibres. Distribution through the anterior and posterior divisions of the spinal nerve trunk to all blood vessels, sweat glands, erector pili muscles of the hair. Also, some of these sympathetic fibres take part in the formation of the recurrent meningeal branch of the nerve trunk to exercise control over the vascular bed of the spinal cord, meninges, and content of the vertebral canal and even the osseous structures.

## Mechanical Pressure

It must be emphasized again that were the subluxation to cause only a mechanical pressure upon the nerve trunk as it passes through the intervertebral foramen, thereby decreasing the conduction of nerve impulses, the symptoms which would result in structures supplied by the above described thoracic and upper two, three or four lumbar nerves would be loss of somatic muscle power, loss of sensation from the skin and muscles, loss of proprioceptive sense from the muscles and articulations supplied, loss of sensation from any viscus supplied, loss of tone of smooth muscle supplied, dilatation of the blood vessels and a decrease in the excretion of perspiration. Any other symptoms could not be related to the subluxation and would not be chiropractic cases. Nothing could be further from the truth. Thus, it is imperative to look deeper for the explanation of the mechanism of the subluxation to understand the diverse symptoms that do arise from the disrelationship of vertebral segments.

The lower two or three lumbar nerves, the sacral nerves with but two exceptions, and the coccygeal nerves carry no fibres to visceral structures. Thus, pressure upon these nerves, were such possible, would not disturb visceral function. The two exceptions are the second and third, or third and fourth, sacral nerves which have, in addition to their somatic components, preganglionic parasympathetic fibres for the supply of pelvic viscera. Inasmuch as these nerves pass through foramina of fixed size in the anterior surface of the sacrum, direct pressure from the osseous margins of these foramina would be a physical impossibility. We would have to conclude on the basis of the old theory that chiropractic is not applicable to conditions indicative of disturbance of neural supply by these nerves. This, too, is fallacious.

## Sympathetic System

Attention is directed again to the chain of paravertebral sympathetic ganglia, extending from anterior to the transverse process of the atlas to the coccyx where the two chains join in a single ganglion, the Ganglion Impar, lying anterior to the coccyx. As previously discussed, the source of impulses for the cell bodies forming these ganglia is derived from the twelve thoracic neuromeres and the upper three lumbar cord segments. It must be emphasized that this is the entire outflow for the sympathetic division of the autonomic nervous system.

The superior four thoracic segments send preganglionic fibres into the ganglionic chain, some of which turn upward to travel to the Superior Cervical Ganglion, others, of course, synapse in the ganglion associated with the segment of emergence. The Middle and Inferior Cervical Ganglia receive fibres from thoracic segments slightly lower and the lower lumbar, sacral and coccygeal ganglia receive their preganglionic fibres from the lower thoracic neuromeres and the upper three lumbar neuromeres. There are, therefore, only fifteen, or sixteen, white rami communicantes on each side, composed of the preganglionic sympathetic fibres, but there are thirty-one pairs of gray rami communicantes, one for each spinal nerve. These gray rami are formed by the axons of cell bodies located in the ganglia, passing back into the spinal nerve for distribution through the anterior and posterior divisions of the spinal nerve trunk to all blood vessels, sweat glands, erector pili muscles of the hair and, also, some of these sympathetic fibres take part in the formation of the recurrent meningeal branch of the nerve trunk to exercise control over the vascular bed of the spinal cord, meninges, content of the vertebral canal, and even the osseous structures.

Other postganglionic sympathetic fibres leave the paravertebral ganglia to enter the cavities of the body to supply the blood vessels and viscera. These fibres, for the most part, follow the surface of arteries in their course. That portion of the sympathetic system concerned with the content of the abdominal cavity has an entirely different arrangement, since the preganglionic sympathetic fibres pass through the paravertebral ganglia from the fifth thoracic to the twelfth thoracic without interruption or synaptic connection, form named nerves upon emerging from these ganglia which reach prevertebral ganglia, lying relatively close to the visceral structures to be supplied. In these prevertebral ganglia the axones of the lateral horn cells of the spinal cord terminate by synaptic connection with the postganglionic neurones which complete the conduction pathway to blood vessels or viscera.

Roughly, the physiologic function of the sympathetic system may be said to be vasoconstrictor of the blood vessels, accelerator of cardiac rhythm, depressor of gastro-intestinal tone, inhibitor of gastro-intestinal secretions, motor to the sphincters of the gut, secreto-motor for the adrenal glands, secretomotor for the sweat glands. Therefore, should it be that the subluxation presses upon a thoracic nerve, or nerves, and inhibits the flow of nerve impulses, the symptoms must be, of necessity, a loss of tone in blood vessels, decreased excretion from the sweat glands, an increase in muscular tone and glandular secretion of the portion of the gastro-intestinal tract supplied, or decreased heart rate, if the heart is supplied by the involved nerves, etc. The conclusion would then be reached that a patient exhibiting the reverse of these symptoms is not a chiropractic case, since the parasympathetic contribution to these structures is by way of the Vagus, a cranial nerve not amenable to pressure from vertebral subluxation. This, from a vast store of professional experience, is known to be grossly untrue, throwing further misgivings upon a simple explanation of the mechanism of the vertebral subluxation.

The sacral nerves, which are exceptions to the general spinal nerve pattern, are the second and third or third and fourth. As previously mentioned, these two are composed of the usual somatic afferent and efferent neurones and also visceral afferent and efferent neurones of the parasympathetic division. The latter fibres are concerned with the activation of the musculature and glands of the distal portion of the colon, the urinary bladder and genitalia. Pressure upon these nerves, sufficient to decrease the neural supply to the named viscera, could only result in decreased tone in the organs and a decrease in glandular secretion. It is necessary to conclude that symptoms at variance with the pattern of inhibition are not amenable to the chiropractic techniques. Every chiropractor would take exception to such a statement and be equipped to present unequivocal proof that these visceral symptoms respond to chiropractic ministration. This should be further indication of the need for a hard, clear look at the "pinched" nerve theory.

Were the occlusion sufficient to shut off the flow of impulses from the central nervous system over the efferent fibres to somatic and splanchnic structures, the same pressure would prevent the return of afferent or sensory impulses from somatic and visceral components to the central nervous system. The erroneous conclusion must be reached by this train of thought that any structure producing direct or referred pain, or other sensory symptoms cannot do so over the nerve involved by the subluxation. Furthermore, every patient experiencing the problem of vertebral subluxation and nerve pressure should exhibit some loss of kinesthetic sense, while the fact is that such a loss of joint and muscle sensibility is rare and usually the result of disease within the central nervous system.

## Excess Nerve Supply

Throughout D. D. Palmer's[37] text, he stressed the point that most diseases are the result of too much nerve supply, rather than too little, and time after time in very strong words criticized those students of his who had distorted his teachings to a simple, though untrue, form by which the uneducated could be made to readily understand chiropractic. Utilizing only one of his statements, it may be appreciated that exasperation was his as he wrote, "I wish that all Chiropractors could take in this basic principle of our science — THAT TOO MUCH OR NOT ENOUGH ENERGY IS DISEASE."[38]

Utilizing the foot on the garden hose analogy, the chiropractor explained glibly to the patient how nerve supply was "shut off" and his particular viscus began to function in an abnormal manner, producing the unpleasant symptoms which had brought him to the office of the chiropractor. While this illustration was useful to demonstrate the idea of chiropractic to individuals who were able to cope with only the most simple aspects of anatomy and neurology, the chiropractors accepted this naive explanation as gospel truth themselves, despite the warnings of D. D. Palmer[39], "A large share of disease — all inflammatory and fever cases — are because of too much stimulus and not because it is shut off."

Such an explanation does not serve a useful or helpful purpose in the present day when laymen are familiar with much of the functioning of the human body, are kept abreast of the latest developments in biology and healing by *Readers Digest* and other popular magazines and are capable of appreciating the fallacies of the simple "pinched nerve" explanation. Therefore, it behooves chiropractors to approach the problem from the basis of science, utilizing all the available knowledge of science to substantiate the explanation of the efficacious application of chiropractic methods. Chiropractic must be based on science and must itself be a science and contribute to the general body of scientific knowledge to justify its place in the healing arts.

"There are two classes of Chiropractors, those who desire to know all they can of physiology, pathology, neurology and anatomy, and those who have aversion for intelligence, do not want to take effect into consideration, depending only upon an examination of the spinous processes," said D. D. Palmer.[40] It is essential that few fall into the latter category lest the progress of the profession come to a standstill and the dream of the founder lack substance.

## Scientific Chiropractic

Dr. Palmer[41] had this to say, "Adjusting is an Art, *not* a Science. A person may be able to adjust vertebrae, may do so without any scientific knowledge of the reason for doing so. They learn it as an art; they know how, but not why. The art of adjusting should be guided by scientific knowledge."

The following has been extracted also: "Chiropractic as a science defines the laws of life and embodies them into a system for the preservation of health. Chiropractic, also, included the art of adjusting, by hand, any or all subluxations of the 300 articulations of the human body, more particularly those of the vertebral column, so that Innate may have perfect control of the vital functions."[42]

D. D. Palmer[43] stated also, "The science and the method are entirely two different things, the method may be based on scientific principles," and then goes on to state, "The discoverer and developer of the greatest of all sciences finds but few who are willing or capable of taking in chiropractic as a science. They prefer to know it as a chance method instead of one which is scientific."[44]

His thoughts as to the composition of the science of chiropractic were expressed when he wrote, "Chiropractic is a science because it comprises the knowledge of facts concerning health and disease. This knowledge reduced to law and embodied in a system makes it a science. Knowledge of many facts concerning one subject, correlated in a system, creates a science."[45]

Furthermore, he expressed this thought: "Chiropractic is a proven fact — it is a science demonstrated by the art of adjusting. As we have become acquainted with its principles, founded upon the laws as old as the Greek prophet, we make less failures. The science can only be developed along the lines laid down by its founder."[46]

It should be clear that D. D. Palmer was a man of science and

44

anxious that his followers should be scientific and thoroughly educated. He wrote, "If we desire to reach the intellectual class we must
be educated in our profession. This should be the chiropractor's
stock-in-trade, his working capital."[47]

The founder penned the following lines: "Learn to digest that
which you take in mentally, make it of value, soak it in your system,
make it a part of yourself, develop your intellect and body by its
addition. Absorb it into your brain, use it as an instrument, an equipment to your mind."[48]

With these admonitions of the founder, D. D. Palmer, burned into
our consciousness, there should be no trepidation about critically in-
vestigating chiropractic theory and seeking answers in the allied
sciences. While at this date it may be presumptuous to refer to chiropractic as a "science," any more than allopathic medicine is a science,
it must be scientific, firmly based on known facts, willing to modify
hypotheses and theories as new facts come to light and prepared to
admit that the practice or application of this knowledge is an art
which varies with the skill, knowledge and care of the practitioner, as
is true for every branch of generic medicine.

## Intelligence

Prior to moving on to the subject of causes of subluxation, it
might be well to bring to the attention of the reader the fact that no
particular stress has been placed in this book upon two terms introduced by D. D. Palmer and accepted by the majority of chiropractors.
These are the terms "Universal Intelligence" and "Innate
Intelligence."

D. D. Palmer[49] used the term Universal Intelligence in reference
to those cosmic forces and laws which may, collectively, be called
God, or Nature, and control and regulate the universe in which we
live. In the human body a segment of this divine force, Life, is referred to as Innate Intelligence, that controlling influence over the
functions of the body from the cellular level to the integrated total
function of the body as a unit.

This force, Innate Intelligence, is accepted but not stressed, as it is
felt that all intelligent readers will accept the fact that there is "something" within the body which controls the healing process, growth,
and repair, etc. It is by no knowledge of the conscious mind that
these functions take place. No matter the number of degrees held by
the physician, he is unable to do more than approximate the ends of

a fractured bone and must depend upon the Innate Intelligence of the patient's body to effect the actual repair process. No disease has ever been cured by any practitioner of healing. He does many things to assist the healing process of the body, but in the final analysis, it is that "intelligence" within that makes the final repair and correction.

No one has a suitable, scientific explanation of this "something" within each of us so long as life lasts, which distinguishes the living from the dead. Volumes would be wasted trying to explain and prove Innate Intelligence for this is beyond the finite knowledge. It will be much more rewarding to attempt to find the mechanism by which the body functions, recognizing full well that we are not in a position to make claims for total knowledge of human function and do not have all the answers to the perplexing questions of human function in health and disease.

Since the above paragraphs were first written, an "unbiased" committee of twenty-two, thirteen of whom were allopaths or associated with allopathic institutions, quoted out of context, some of the limited references to D. D. Palmer's writings relative to the terms Universal and Innate Intelligence in an effort to disparage chiropractic in a report, "Independent Practitioners Under Medicare." The Expert Review Panel (of nine members) had five M.Ds. but not one chiropractic physician.

How "objective" this report actually was has been well covered and documented by William Trever[50] in a book entitled, *In The Public Interest.*

Despite the efforts of these committees, working under HEW Secretary Cohen, and the wide distribution of the report by the AMA, Congress was not unduly impressed, as demonstrated by the inclusion of chiropractic under Medicare coverage for senior citizens.

A term, such as homeostasis, used by physiologists to convey the similar meaning of the cell, tissue or body's attempt to maintain a stable condition without the ability to explain exactly the entire mechanism, is considered to be "scientific," but a term to express much the same idea, coined by D. D. Palmer in the late 1800's, is "cultish."

Any attempt to reduce to explainable realities the terms ego, id, libido, even consciousness, awareness, life, etc., runs headlong into difficulties.

Coining more erudite terms may help to confuse and hide present ignorance, but the fact remains that there is much for which science cannot provide, at present, a sound explanation. Ignorance has been rolled back a substantial distance since 1895 when D. D. Palmer used the term Innate Intelligence, but there remains much of the function of the individual cell, organ or body that defies sound explanation and must be covered in the generality by a blanket term, such as homeostasis or innate intelligence.

The chiropractic profession need make no apology for the use of a descriptive phrase that is explanatory of the mechanisms for which there are no factual data at the moment. However, there can be no excuse for the failure to seek and utilize known facts, depending upon the term Innate Intelligence as an excuse for intellectual laziness.

On the other hand, those who labour under the misapprehension that all functions of the human body, are explainable by biochemical reasoning are doomed to a rude awakening, as Kervran[51] has illustrated. Nitrogen and oxygen can be made to combine by man under very high temperature and pressure, but "Living organisms do the same at room temperature." The "know-how" to perform much more complex reactions than this within the living tissues that defy the best scientists with all the paraphenalia is certainly an expression of an inborn wisdom, or Innate Intelligence for lack of a more factual or descriptive explanation.

# CHAPTER IV

# General Causes of Subluxation

A SUBLUXATION IN the chiropractic sense is not a partial dislocation (less than a luxation), but an alteration of the normal anatomical or physiological relationships, or dynamics, of contiguous structures. Biochemical, biomechanical, pathophysiological, radiological, subjective and objective symptoms, and other manifestations demand attention, investigation and consideration in depth by every chiropractic physician.

Consideration of the causes of subluxation is best commenced by looking to the founder of the science of chiropractic to determine his opinion. In the pages of *The Science, Art and Philosophy of Chiropractic* is to be found the following: "The determining causes of disease are traumatism, poison and autosuggestion,"[52] and again on another page, "As may be seen in the article on spasm, disease may be caused by injuries, or poisons or from the mind."[53]

His opinion of the mechanism by which these factors cause the subluxations may be found in a number of passages throughout his textbook but are clearly and concisely stated in his discussion relative to poisons, "Poisons act on sensory nerves; these affect motor nerves, which, in turn, draw vertebrae out of alignment."[54]

It must be added that Dr. Palmer was not so naive as to think that the motor nerves draw the vertebrae out of alignment by their own direct action, but, rather, through the stimulation of muscle which is directly attached to the osseous structure and whose function it is to move the bone.

## Irritation

The writer had the privilege of studying under one of the oustanding chiropractic educators, the late Dr. H. G. Beatty of Denver, Colorado, who had reworded D. D. Palmer's statement and thought as to the cause of disease. Dr. Beatty[55] taught that the cause of all disease is irritation. The term "irritation" encompasses all forms of stress and strain to which the human is heir. Irritation of a mechanical, chemical, or mental nature, alone or in any percentage of combination, may be sufficient to overcome the normal resistance of the body, cause structural distortion, or subluxations, which interfere with normal transmission of nerve force; somatic or visceral structures show disturbances of function, with symptoms and tissue changes of disease. The pattern of disease, cause and course may be briefly stated thus:—

Hereditary weakness and the traumatic history of the body, as well as the degree of emotional stability, will determine in large measure the site of structural distortion under stress. Another factor, of course, is the concentration of stress upon a particular limited area. The variable condition of splanchnic structures supplied by a common neuromere may be an additional determining factor as to the locale of greatest disturbance in response to a subluxation.

It should be appreciated that not all irritation produces structural distortion. The irritation must be severe enough to overcome the natural resistance. A very simple example might do much to clarify this point. A table is built to bear weight and can support several hundred pounds, but there is a limit, after which one more pound would cause the legs to buckle and break loose from the table top. The quality of wood and its construction are determinants as to the load capacity. So with the human, there is much constitutional variation between individuals as to the stress load that may be borne before resistance is overcome and distortion occurs. One person may undergo an adverse reaction to a stress and become ill, while an equal stress may have little appreciable effect upon another.

Not all persons, who are subjected to the stress of pathogenic micro-organisms, develop the associated disease syndrome. Nor do all persons subjected to identical emotional stresses show symptoms of neuroses or psychoses. Each has his own breaking point. Mechanical trauma may bruise one person, while an equal force fractures a bone in another.

The foresight and depth of understanding of great chiropractic educators such as Dr. D. D. Palmer and Dr. Homer G. Beatty, have recently been substantiated by the careful, painstaking research of Dr. Hans Selye[56] of the University of Montreal, whose word "Stress" expresses similar connotation as "Irritation" as used by the chiropractic scholars above quoted.

Needless to say, Dr. Selye's book *Stress* has not been written to substantiate the teaching of chiropractic. Perhaps the author of *Stress* did not even know of the existence of chiropractic or its theories. Dr. Selye's work has been concerned primarily with the influence of stress upon the endocrine glands and their resultant disturbance of bodily function. To date, he has not utilized the nervous system to the fullest in the explanation of how stress produces the adverse influence upon ductless glands, causing them to produce the manifold tissue changes and functional disturbances observed. It is hoped that with the resources at his disposal his attention will be directed toward the nervous system in its relation to stress and disease. Dr. Selye may be said to have investigated the "physiology" of stress, while the chiropractic profession has concerned itself with the "anatomy" of stress.

## Environment

It has been unquestionably established that all changes in the external environment cause changes in the internal functioning of the individual. This has been clearly stated by W. Sachs[57] in his book, *The Vegetative Nervous System.*

As an example, changes in temperature of the room may cause very definite changes in function. First, if the room becomes cold, there will be a contraction of the blood vessels of the skin to prevent the loss of heat from the blood, and the blood will be directed into deeper structures to maintain body heat at the normal level. If this constriction of blood vessels is not sufficient to maintain the normal heat level, then shivering commences, which is the rapid contraction of the somatic muscles. Muscular contraction produces heat as a by-product and is one of the most important sources of caloric energy to maintain the temperature of the body under normal or adverse circumstances. Guyton[58] mentions that an environmental temperature change of fifty degrees is necessary for a one degree alteration in human body temperature, demonstrating the efficiency of the temperature regulation mechanism.

The redistribution of the blood from the surface of the human to the deeper structures is under the control of the sympathetic portion of the autonomic nervous system, while the contraction of somatic muscle is under the control of the cerebro-spinal nervous system. While these two systems are separated for descriptive purposes and understanding, there is little justification for a complete, arbitrary separation of the nervous system into compartments, for it is, in truth, a functional unit, highly organized and integrated.

Not only is the structure of the body disturbed by such a condition as cold, but the individual feels this as a definite sensation, which is not pleasant. The ability to feel is a function of higher brain centres, as previously discussed briefly, and has a definite influence upon the emotion and thinking processes of the individual. Thus, higher brain activity may be demonstrated as our victim of cold seeks a blanket, a warm coat, or turns up the thermostat to provide more heat. Such activity requires the function of levels above the spinal cord, in contrast to the spinal cord control over the calibre of the blood vessels, and even in this example higher neural levels, especially the hypothalamus, are likely participants. However, this treatise must remain simplistic, since attempting to thoroughly trace each neural connection would do nothing but confuse the issue and lose the reader in a welter of trivia.

It should be emphasized that the body is a unit of structure and function and that the nervous system is that correlating and co-ordinating system of the entire body which keeps functions in harmony, produces the efficient response to changes in environment, or governs the reactions to irritation or stress, to result in the altered functions and tissue changes, called disease.

F. M. Pottenger[59] draws attention to the interrelation between somatic and visceral functions as follows: "There is a continuous stream of impulses received by the sensory somatic nerves which are transferred to the connector neurons of the sympathetic system and expressed as reflexes in the internal viscera."

It should be appreciated that the changes in external environment which impinge upon the somatic structures result not only in responses of these somatic structures but also in harmonious alteration of the functions of splanchnic organs. Furthermore, the condition and function of the internal organs reflect in the somatic division of the human structure.

The nervous system plays as important a role in the process of disease as it does in the processes of health, or physiological function. It is through the nervous system that the multitude of irritations, which have been classified under the three general headings of mechanical, chemical, and mental, have their effects upon the body, both somatic and visceral divisions. It is the nervous system that is responsible for the greater proportion of effects in response to any of the irritants which overcome resistance to produce distortion. The distortion of structure adds irritation to the nervous system to result in further ill-effects in the form of changed function of somatic and splanchnic components. Such a structural distortion, or subluxation, may serve as the determinant of the structure or viscus that manifests the symptoms and tissue changes of disease and pathology.

### Hereditary Influences

The chiropractor is not unmindful of the part heredity plays in providing the individual with the characteristic familial body type, passed from generation to generation, each type with its own peculiar structural weakness. Joel E. Goldthwait[60] states this proposition in these words: "Individuals of different body types show different susceptibility to various diseases. The pattern of the body is inherited and depends upon the body type of the ancestors."

The short, rotund individual shows an increased lumbar lordosis with its consequent lumbosacral weakness. Thus, a heavy lift is likely to result in a lumbosacral strain with its attendant muscular and ligamentous damage. From these damaged tissues noxious nerve impulses will arise which are carried by neurones through the posterior nerve roots into the spinal cord, where synaptic connections are made with efferent neurones, resulting in contraction of muscles in "splinting" action to protect the involved area from further injury. This is in accordance with Hilton's Law,[61] which states that the muscles that move the joint are supplied by the same segments of the spinal cord which supply afferent fibres to the joint. The greater the number of afferent impulses, the greater the action of "splinting," thus, the more widespread is the muscular contraction.

These contractions also follow Pflüger's Law of Reflex Action,[62] "If the stimulus received by a sensory nerve extends to a motor nerve of the opposite side, contraction occurs only from the corresponding muscles, and if the contraction is unequal from the two sides, the stronger contraction always takes place on the side which is stimulated." Hence, a vertebra may be fixed in a relatively normal facing by bilateral muscle contraction of approximately equal degree, or be rotated, laterally flexed, or both, by the unequal contraction of muscles of the two sides. This patient then exhibits a subluxation, or fixation, with afferent impulses arising from the contracted muscles and injured articulation which tend to perpetuate the distortion, establishing a vicious cycle, which can best be interrupted by chiropractic or other manipulative methods. Some fixations, of course, correct themselves through rest and relaxation or by accidental twisting which restores movement and normalizes muscle tone.

The tall, slender individual is likely to injure the thoraco-lumbar area by a similar lift, since this is a weaker area of his spine and prone to distortion under mechanical stress of the nature cited. While the individual with a better build, stronger muscles, and a higher degree of physical fitness may make a similar lift without adverse effects upon his structure.

## Developmental Anomalies

Other inherent factors must be considered in arriving at an understanding of the spinal predilection to injury or distortion. Developmental abnormalities of vertebrae may be present in the spine without symptoms until well into adult life and then under varied conditions and minor stress serious disturbances occur with protracted incapacitation. An example of this type of structural weakness is to be found in the sagittal facing of the facets between the 5th lumbar vertebra and the sacrum, which normally are in the coronal plane and transmit a degree of body weight to the facets of the sacrum. Sagittal facing results in weakness of the lumbo-sacral junction, which may give way under stress with the result that one, or both sides of the 5th lumbar may be forced anterior with serious damage to the joint capsule.

Another form of developmental abnormality is the potential spondylolisthesis, in which there has been failure of the posterior arch of the vertebra to ossify with the centrum. Such a condition may be quiescent for many years to suddenly become a severe problem when a lift, or other form of mechanical stress causes centrum to separate from the posterior arch and shift anterior. Many other anomalous formations are to be found in the vertebral column, each weakening the area of their location and making the region distortion-prone under stress. Spina Bifida, the failure of the posterior arch to close in the formation of a spinous process, sacralization or lumbarization of lumbosacral segments, hemivertebrae, abnormally long transverse processes, etc., result in changes in leverage for the contracting muscles. This unusual and unequal muscle pull may have serious detrimental influences upon the associated articulations and lay the foundation for distortion by minimal stress situations. Many additional examples might well be mentioned.

## Contributory Posture

Faulty posture adds an additional form of mechanical stress and weakness to the structure, thereby allowing comparatively minor irritations or stresses to overcome the resistance to produce distortion which may interfere with normal nerve transmission with the resultant tissue changes of disease. Faulty posture has its insidious effects upon the articulations of the vertebral column and as Lowman[63] has stated part of the problem, "it ages the vertebral joints more rapidly than would otherwise be the case."

A very high percentage of men and women show evidence of serious postural faults. Nor is this indictment true only of adults. It is a serious castigation of North American civilization to learn that 57.9% of children under six years of age are unable to pass tests for posture, physical fitness and strength, as compared to an 8% failure rate for European children, as demonstrated, brought into focus and concern by Kraus and Weber.[64] The rate of rejects of young men, supposedly in the prime of life, who have been called for military service is a further blot upon our health record and way of life.

President J. F. Kennedy,[65] speaking at a banquet, pointed out that it was necessary to call seven young men for examination in order to obtain two physically and mentally fit for military service. World Health Organization statistics show that the infant death rate in the U.S.A. ranks eleventh among countries surveyed and the male life expectancy in 1965 was 65.6 years, a decline from 70.2 years in 1961, and the U.S.A. stands in twenty-first place, despite the boasts of the finest standard of living and health care. These few facts should make us eager to re-appraise our system of life and health care.

While the general remarks relative to the predisposing factors which establish the areas of weakness have been associated with mechanical forms of stress, these same elements provide the fertile fields of predilection for subluxations, fixations, or gross distortion, when stress of a mental or chemical nature is brought to bear.

In subsequent chapters detailed consideration of the mechanism by which mechanical, chemical and mental stress overcomes the natural resistance to produce structural distortion, interference with the nervous system and the ensuing functional changes in splanchnic structures, symptoms and tissue changes of disease, will lead to a clearer understanding of the rationality of chiropractic reasoning. It must be appreciated that only a few examples can be utilized to establish the basic principles and the reader is expected to apply the established explanation to any given situation.

While the forms of stress have been compartmentalized for ease of discussion, it must be accentuated that the subluxations of the average patient are the result of summing the stress factors, mechanical, chemical and psychological.

# CHAPTER V

# Mechanical Causes

THERE ARE MANY subdivisions of mechanical irritation, such as falls, strains from lifting, postural stresses, occupational distortions, automobile accidents, etc., too numerous to list. The site of the actual subluxation is likely to be pre-ordained by the structural weakness of the individual vertebral column, by reason of the heredity, anomalies, past history of injury, postural, occupational, or recreational abuses which may have produced frank trauma or merely microtraumata which tend to summate, or by mechanical force being concentrated upon a localized area. The primary weaknesses are dependent upon the heriditary characteristics of the individual, the sites of transition from one spinal curve to another, and the general distortion present in the column, as well as the postural stresses present over a long period of time. Previous injury may have established a predilection for another traumatic experience of the same locale. It might be mentioned that the tensions of an emotional nature and muscular contractions due to chemical irritation within the body also play their part in establishing the susceptible region for the occurrence of a subluxation.

The first consideration of mechanical causes of subluxation will be that of posture and its varied effects upon the human structure. In normal good posture, seen in health and efficiency, the gravity line should pass through the body in such a manner that it falls between the feet approximately 5.8 cms. anterior to the medial malleoli of the ankles, according to the calculations of Scott.[66] Around this gravity line the body weight should be equally distributed for proper balance and efficient action. In other words, there should be an equal amount of weight posterior to the gravity line as anterior to it and the weight on either side of this line should be equal.

A simple method of visualizing this gravity line is to imagine the body being divided equally by a median sagittal plane and by a coronal plane at right angles to the first. The junction of these two planes would be the Gravity Line. The body should be divided into four quarters of equal weight by these two planes. Since the human is not symmetrical, it should be appreciated that the gravity line does not pass through the body of every vertebra. Rather, in the ideal state, it passes through the adontoid of the Axis, the body of the seventh cervical, the bodies of the tenth, eleventh and twelfth thoracics, the body of the fifth lumbar and the antero-superior portion of the sacrum. The Centre of Gravity of the vertical human body has been estimated by Scott to be a point 2-3 cms. anterior to the second sacral segment.

A spine is said to be "compensated" when the distribution of weight around the gravity line remains normal despite increases in the depth of the antero-posterior curves or primary curves, or opposing scoliotic curves.

It is to be appreciated that such changes in the vertebral column with adequate compensation may result in no adverse functioning, productive of symptoms, but are not ideal and establish a pattern for distortion with a lesser degree of stress than would be required to cause a similar problem in an ideal spine. Furthermore, it is not the compensated spines that the chiropractor sees in his office. When the spine fails to compensate for basic distortion, weight distribution becomes abnormal, excess energy is required to maintain the vertical biped posture, the nervous system is disturbed in its function and symptoms develop.

## Weight Distribution

Proper weight distribution of the body is extremely important for the human, who, from an engineering point of view, is very poorly constructed for stability or static existence. However, the human is not designed for static function, but is a dynamic mechanism. Man is built for motion and it has been truly said that motion is life. The peculiar architecture of human form makes it possible to overcome inertia with the minimum of effort. While the upright biped posture has a preponderance of advantage from the functional point of view, there are many inherent structural weaknesses which provide the background for most of the diseases to which man is heir. It may be said that the upright position is not an unmixed blessing.

The human architectural plan might well be likened to three pyramids stacked one upon another with the head and neck forming the upper pyramid, with the apex of this pyramid in the centre of the base of the second, comprising shoulders and trunk. The apex of the latter would be the fifth lumbar vertebra, sitting upon the base of the sacrum which, in turn, is the central portion of the base of the third pyramid, embracing the pelvis and the lower extremities. The apex of this inferior pyramid is bifurcated to form the legs and feet.

Johnston[67] is deserving of the credit for this concept and Feldenkrais[68] utilized a similar explanation. Such an explanation is ideally suited to the visualization of the problems of weight distribution, body balance and postural assessment.

The upright position is maintained by virtue of osseous locks, ligaments and the tone or active contraction of muscles. The muscles act as guy wires and are continually adjusting the flexible column, the spine, to compensate for the alterations of weight distribution that take place with every movement of the structure. Only by redistributing the weight around the Gravity Line can the upright position be maintained. Should the mass of the body shift in such a manner that the greater percentage moves beyond the base formed by the feet, the body will fall. Any inequality of weight distribution around the gravity line necessitates the continued action of muscle with an energy drain. Thus, the poorer the weight distribution, the more faulty the body mechanics and the greater the depletion of energy and the more disturbed the function is likely to become.

As the years advance there is a tendency for the adult to utilize the muscles of his back to a lesser degree, locking his knees in a position of relative dorsi-flexion to the point that many exhibit the "sabre-leg" distortion. Such a position of the knees forces the pelvis to shift anteriorly, which requires compensation in the superimposed vertebral column, as described by Willard Carver[69] and H. G. Beatty.[70]

The lumbar anterior curve becomes shorter, the apex of the curve moves down from the third lumbar to either the fourth or the fifth lumbar vertebra; the thoracic posterior curve acquires additional vertebrae at both the lumbar and cervical extremities; and the cervical curve decreases in the number of vertebrae in its formation, with the apex moving superiorly. There is no change in depth of the curves due to this basic distortion of anterior shifting of the pelvis.

Accompanying the anterior shift of the pelvis, in most instances, is to be found an anterior nodding of the pelvis which does require an increase in depth of the antero-posterior curves to balance the weight of the body over the base. Now, there is a short deep lumbar lordosis, a long increased thoracic kyphosis, and a short deep cervical lordosis. There is also a tendency to lean backward from the lumbo-sacral junction, or as Dr. Lyman C. Johnston,[71] Research Director for the Canadian Memorial Chiropractic College, so aptly states, "These people try to lie down, while standing up."

Such a posture results in the head and neck projecting still further forward much like a turtle. As the head and neck are carried forward and inferiorly, the leverage for the anterior cervical muscles is disturbed and the thorax is no longer efficiently supported. The thorax flattens from anterior to posterior and the leverage for the abdominal muscles is lost, as the chest droops to approximate the pelvis. The lower abdomen bulges into that unseemly "pot," common to middle age, and the support for the pelvis is decreased, permitting further anterior nodding. While such a picture is all too common in the middle-aged and senior citizens, it is frequently observed in the young adult and even the teen-aged group.

The posture above described requires little active function on the part of the postvertebral musculature. Since one of the laws of life is, "Use it, or lose it," these muscles show a loss of normal tone, even the atrophy of disuse, and later the fibrotic change and shortening associated with many of the chronic sufferers from low back distress, which is in accord with Davis' Law.[72]

Dr. Johnston found, in assessing many hundreds of cases of low back discomfort, 67% carried an excess of their body weight posterior to the normal gravity line. Such a posture causes the weight to be shifted from the bodies of the lumbar vertebrae posteriorly to be transmitted by means of the articular facets and even from one spinous process to the one below — a condition never intended by the design. Structural change, as a result of the stress of faulty weight distribution, is common in the form of exostoses, cartilaginous change, and fibrotic changes of muscle previously mentioned.

The fifth lumbar is particularly prone to suffer from the evils of altered weight transmission, since the entire weight of head, neck, shoulder girdle, upper extremities and trunk must be transmitted by the fifth lumbar vertebra to the sacrum. It is small wonder that a high percentage of the population experiences low back discomfort, even to the point of incapacitation.

The osseous structures are not solely affected. The intervertebral fibrocartilaginous discs are placed at a mechanical disadvantage, especially the disc between fifth lumbar and sacrum. The posterior edge is compressed and the entire disc assumes an unnatural wedge-shape, the Posterior Longitudinal Ligament is made lax in this region, and the disc is likely to show change in its composition.

Nor is the lower lumbar area the only region to show ill-effects. Each portion of the spine is likely to demonstrate structural change as a direct consequence of faulty posture. The thoracic region will show the signs of stress along the anterior borders of vertebral bodies and intervertebral discs, while the cervical vertebrae show the greater stress in the posterior components. Such stress causes irritation to nerve endings in the capsules of the articulations of the facets, the intervertebral discs, the ligamentous structures, the tissues pinched between spinous processes, and those tissues put under tension by the abnormal, long continued, faulty posture.

Using the articulation of the fifth lumbar vertebra with the sacrum as the example, noxious impulses are traced into the spinal cord by way of afferent nerve fibres, whose unipolar cytons are located in the posterior nerve root ganglia. Upon entering the spinal cord, these fibres make synaptic connection by means of collateral branches which leave the main fibre at an approximate right angle with connector neurones, whose cell bodies assist in the formation of the posterior horn of gray matter. The axone, itself, divides into ascending and descending branches, which travel superiorly or inferiorly through a variable number of neuromeres, giving off in each segment collateral fibres for additional synaptic connection with intercalated neurones. In *Functional Neuro-anatomy* is to be found this statement relative to these collaterals by W. J. S. Krieg,[73] which is confirmed by the other neurological authorities, "Along their course the longitudinally-running fibres send off numerous collaterals at right angles. The collaterals are most numerous at levels near the one at which they enter and decrease at greater distances. In general they run ventrally to synapse with the nerve cells of all parts of the gray matter."

Sir Charles Sherrington[74] points out, "For each efferent root there exists in immediate proximity to its own place of entrance in the cord (e.g., in its own segment) a reflex motor path of as low a threshold and of as high potency as any open to it anywhere. Further, in response to excitation even approximately minimal in intensity, a single afferent root, or a single filament of a single root, evokes a spinal discharge of centrifugal impulses through more than one efferent root, i.e., the discharge is plurisegmental."

If the irritation is not very severe, the afferent fibres may make synaptic connection and stimulate only those motor cells having control over the segmental postvertebral muscles, resulting in mere hypertonia of the said muscles. Should the noxious stimulation to the receptor end-organs be severe, there may be very marked contraction of the longer muscles supplied by a variable number of neuromeres both superior and inferior to the segment of entrance of the afferent fibres, and the individual shows marked distortion. Furthermore, it should be noted that the strongest contraction of muscle is likely to be found on the same side as the source of noxious stimuli, which is in accord with Pflüger's Law,[75] which states, "When the excitation of a sensory nerve elicits reflex action involving both halves of the body, and the action is unequal on the two sides, the side of stronger contractions is always that homonymous with the seat of application of the stimulus."

## Autonomic Involvement

It is not difficult to realize that the descending branches of these afferent fibres pass caudally in the spinal cord from the level of entrance of the fifth lumbar segment into the sacral neuromeres, containing lateral horns of gray matter composed of preganglionic parasympathetic cell bodies, which supply the viscera of the pelvic cavity, the descending colon, sigmoid colon, rectum, urinary bladder, prostate gland of the male, ovaries and uterus in the female. The lumbosacral problem may well be complicated by additional symptoms of dysfunction of one, or more, of the pelvic viscera. Such disturbance adds to the stream of afferent impulses returning to the spinal cord and may compound the problem of postvertebral muscular contraction by instituting visceromotor reflexes.

The ascending branches of the afferent fibres under discussion reach the upper lumbar and lower thoracic segments of the cord, in which collaterals may well make synaptic connection with the lateral horn cells of the sympathetic system, which are the preganglionic fibres over which the vastomotor control of the blood vessels of the pelvic viscera is exerted, as well as the blood vessels of the somatic structures in the region of the fifth lumbar vertebra. These sympathetic fibres control the blood vessels of the skin and the excretory activity of the sudoriferous glands of the lower back and the lower extremities. Symptoms of disturbed function of any of these structures supplied by the sympathetic neurones of this level of the cord should then be considered as complications of the picture.

The above serves to illustrate the importance of posture and its relation to health and disease. However, the examples are legion. Subsequent chapters will detail the mechanism of the subluxation's role in disease with the neurological facts offered in substantive evidence for the contentions of the chiropractic profession.

## Basic Distortion

Attention is next directed to the conditions resulting from a unilateral short leg, a fallen longitudinal arch of one foot, or a sacroiliac subluxation of a unilateral nature. Any of these and many other factors may result in the base of the sacrum being tipped to one side, or lower on one side than the other. Such a basic distortion is usually accompanied by a degree of rotation with the sacrum being relatively anterior on the side of inferiority. The sacrum might then be said to be tipped right and rotated left, as a concrete example. Such a sacral distortion would cause an inanimate column to slant to the same side, the right, and face left as a unit, like the Leaning Tower of Pisa. Such is not the case for the dynamic human spine, which compensates by redistributing the body weight by a series of lateral curves, called scolioses.

Using Willard Carver[76] and Homer G. Beatty[77] as the authorities, it will be found that through the action of the musculature, the lumbar area is pulled back and toward the left with the third lumbar crossing the Gravity Line and being the transition from the right scoliosis, which includes the sacrum and fourth and fifth lumbars with the apex of the scoliosis at the lumbo-sacral junction, to a left scoliosis with the twelfth thoracic as the apex and the transition at the eighth and seventh thoracic vertebrae above.

The spine above this level forms a right scoliosis with the apex at the fourth thoracic. The first thoracic and seventh cervical vertebrae cross the Gravity Line with the formation of a left scoliosis in the cervical region, having the apex at the fourth cervical and the final transition at the occipito-atlanto-axial junction. This would leave the head tipped slightly to the right so the Axis rotates a little to the left and the Atlas a little to the right to bring the eyes to a horizontal plane and looking forward.

The rotation of the sacrum to face slightly to the left requires compensatory changes of the superimposed spinal segments. The fifth lumbar is rotated right and the fourth also, but to a lesser degree, while the third lumbar, the transition, faces almost directly anterior. Left rotation begins at the second lumbar to increase progressively to the apex at the twelfth thoracic and above this level decreases until the transition is again reached at the seventh and eighth thoracic segments which face anterior. Right rotation increases to the apex at the fourth thoracic vertebra and decreases above this level until the transition at the first thoracic and seventh cervical segments are reached and these face anterior. Again left rotation is found increasing to the level of the apex of the scoliosis at the fourth cervical and decreasing above this level. The atlas is required to rotate slightly right to make the final compensation.

Should such compensatory distortion occur, there will be normal function without symptoms, although these compensatory rotatory scolioses do add to the structural stress and predispose the vertebral column to distortion under degrees of stress that would not normally overcome the resistance of the structure.

Johnston,[78] whose detailed study of posture and development of the Panoramic Double Plumb-line Posturometer, led him to an ability to assess an individual's postural faults in relation to his personal, ideal gravity line. Through painstaking and ingenious experimentation he demonstrated that the compensated spine took on the appearance of a spiral in the third dimension and the uncompensated spine appeared as a Z at a 45° angle from the sagital plane. While present x-ray techniques do not permit the viewing of the spine in a vertical direction, the application of drafting and engineering techniques permit the spine to be plotted from A-P and lateral views to reveal the third dimension, thereby providing the concept of the total spinal contour within the body.

Accentuation must be placed upon the realization that "compensation," the distribution of weight in proper proportion around the Gravity Line, does not result in symptoms and physiological disturbance, hence many spines show gross distortion but their owners enjoy a degree of health that is nothing short of amazing. It is the uncompensated distortions, often of a seemingly insignificant degree, which result in functional derangements and unpleasant symptoms. It is this latter group that is to be found in the offices of the chiropractic profession and the former group which is used in an attempt to discredit chiropractic by those who have little appreciation of body mechanics or the compensatory ability of the human.

The group of basic distortions and compensatory effects discussed are anterior shifting of the sacrum or pelvis, anterior nodding of these basic segments, lateral tipping and rotation of the sacrum or pelvis as an entity. Such conditions are not considered ideal and should be corrected. At times it may be necessary to resort to the aid of mechanical means to accomplish this correction, e.g., the use of a lift to equalize leg lengths, etc.

One other basic distortion should receive consideration prior to moving into another area of mechanical stress and that is the unilateral narrowness of the base. This problem is primarily due to developmental peculiarity, the sacrum being narrower on one side than the other, or the neck of the femur shorter on one side, or one innominate smaller than the other. Without compensation, such a condition would result in half of the body weight being transmitted to a narrow base with a loss of stability. The compensatory reaction of the spine is to form a long "C-curve" from base to occiput, thereby resulting in the Gravity Line falling through the actual centre of the base rather than through the anatomical centre as marked on the surface by the median sacral crest.

In an instance where the right side of the sacrum, pelvis, or neck of the femur is of smaller dimension than the left, there would be a long, left scoliosis. No attempt should be made to correct this scoliosis because the basic cause cannot be removed. Increase in the scoliosis or decrease in the curve is a loss of compensation with attending disturbance. Unless the basic distortion is amenable to correction, no interference with the compensatory symmetry of the vertebral column should be attempted. Deviations from compensation are productive of distress and deserving of correction, as are the subluxations and fixations which occur within the gross compensatory mechanism.

## Predisposition

Emphasis should be directed to the likelihood of subluxations to occur at the apices and transitions of the compensatory distortions. Thus, mechanical stress brought to bear upon an area of the spine is likely to produce a local distortion at the vertebral segment which is an apex or a transition within the compensatory opposed rotatory scioloses.

Carrying this thought further, it should be noted that even in the normal anteroposterior curves the third lumbar, seventh and eighth thoracics, and fourth cervical are apices of the curves, while the lumbo-sacral articulation, twelfth thoracic, first thoracic and seventh cervical are the transition regions. Referring back to the discussion on the compensatory rotatory scolioses, it should be apparent that rotational stress and apex stress are added at the lumbo-sacral joint to the transitional stress of the anteroposterior curves.

The third lumbar is the apex of the anterior curve and the transition of the scoliotic curves. The twelfth thoracic is the apex of a scoliosis with the greatest degree of rotational stress and is the transition from the normal anterior lumbar curve to the posterior thoracic curve. This vertebra is also of a transitional type, being neither a true thoracic, nor a true lumbar vertebra in structure. It is little wonder that this vertebra is so frequently subluxated. D. D. Palmer[79] recognized this fact and wrote: "In the dorsal region, I fully agree with Macdonald that the twelfth segment is the one most frequently displaced."

The seventh and eighth thoracic vertebrae form the apex of the thoracic kyphosis and are the transition from the left to the right scolioses in the thoracic region, thus, another region of frequent subluxation.

The fourth thoracic segment is the apex of the right scoliosis with the maximum of rotation, but does not suffer from additional stress because of its position in the primary curve.

The seventh cervical and first thoracic segments form the transition from the thoracic kyphosis to the cervical lordosis and also are the transition for a right scoliosis in the upper thoracic region to the left scoliosis in the cervical area.

The stress upon the fourth cervical vertebra is a combination, due to it being the apex of the anterior cervical primary curve and the apex of the cervical scoliosis with a maximum of rotation of any vertebra in this lateral curve.

The suboccipital region has in addition to the stresses of compensatory distortion, being the final area of compensation, structural peculiarities which permit greater ranges of motion at the expense of stability.

The above brief outline indicates that the most structurally weak areas, making them subluxation-prone, are the occipito-atlanto-axial complex, fourth cervical, seventh cervical and the first thoracic, seventh and eighth thoracics, twelfth thoracic, third lumbar, and lumbosacral regions. These portions of the vertebral column should be given special consideration by the chiropractor.

Prior to moving into another area of consideration, it must be reiterated that few patients, consulting chiropractors, show the patterns of compensation. Wide deviation from these compensatory examples is the rule in cases with frank symptom complexes and the tissue changes of disease. Furthermore, a sick patient may show a relatively straight spine which takes on the compensatory curves as the symptoms disappear, resulting in an x-ray visualization that may appear worse to those not familiar with compensation. It may then be essential to correct the basic distortion, if possible, and aid the body to compensate for this improved base of support by normalizing muscle tone, ligamentous length and intervertebral disc shape. Here lies the reason for the necessity of the repetitive adjustive care of the spine over an extended period of time. Chiropractic adjustive application is not the mere stacking of the osseous structures into a nice symmetrical column.

## Trauma

Under the general heading of mechanical irritation, our attention should now be turned to the subluxations that are produced by direct force to the spinal column itself, such as falls, strains from lifting, accidents of all types, etc., which bring sufficient force to bear upon localized areas that the resistance is overcome and distortion occurs. The sites of the actual subluxations may be preordained by hereditary weakness of the vertebral column, or such factors as briefly enumerated in the preceding paragraphs. As has been emphasized, lifting a heavy object may result in strains of the articulations of the vertebral column, especially in those regions under the greatest mechanical stress from hereditary weakness, developmental abnormality, postural and occupational peculiarities, or compensatory stress.

Having injured the holding elements of the articulation, noxious impulses begin to bombard the associated neuromeres and involve the efferent neurone-pools to create the peripheral postvertebral muscle tension and fixation of vertebral segments in accordance with Hilton's Law,[80] previously quoted. The subsequent disturbance to visceral structures created by such a disrelationship receives consideration in a future chapter.

The occupation of the individual may have developed the postvertebral muscles in a bilaterally asymmetrical manner, one side being more strong than the other. In such an instance, were it conceivable to imagine the neuromeres being bombarded by afferent impulses from the two sides of equal intensity, the side boasting the strongest muscular development would demonstrate the actual structural distortion. Hence, a relatively minor bilateral mechanical irritation could result in a subluxation or distortion of an area.

The lack of use of the postvertebral musculature from sedentary occupations and non-participating recreational pursuits creates weak postvertebral muscles and lays the foundation for injury of the articulations by minimal stress of a mechanical nature. The office worker, who does little more physical activity during his working day than lift a heavy mug of coffee to his lips at coffee-break and spends his evenings in his private "Lazy-boy" before the television, attempts to be a farmer on Saturday morning in his fifty-by-seventy-five feet of back yard. One of two things is likely to happen. One, he lifts a bag of fertilizer, using his arms and back, twists to set it in another location, and falls to his knees in mortal agony. He has strained his lumbosacral region or created a sacroiliac subluxation.

If he is fortunate and avoids such an injury, he works like a Trojan with perspiration dripping from his every pore until exhausted, then sits in the shade with a cold breeze playing across his damp back while he imbibes a bottle of cold beer. The poor muscles, which have not experienced such activity since the previous spring and are not conditioned by an adequate blood supply to endure extended activity, suddenly go into spasm and the would-be gardener limps into the house in misery to be laid low for several days. Bilateral inequality of muscle development may result in very pronounced subluxations and gross distortion as a corollary of the muscle spasm. The very least that is likely to transpire for a weekend gardener, such as mentioned, is the muscle tension, stiffness and soreness experienced for a number of days after an interlude with Nature.

The hero with the sacroiliac subluxation may experience no agonizing pain at the time, but in a variable period of time may develop pain which radiates into the groin and superior portion of the medial thigh. This may not be associated in any way with the sacroiliac, but the self-diagnosis of hernia, inguinal strain, etc., may be considered and the professional diagnosis by those not prone to consider structure important might be similar with the additional investigation for renal calculus, ureteritis, and so forth. The mechanics of such a symptom complex are that as the sacroiliac subluxation occurs, the innominate on the involved side is forced to assume a position of relative posterior nodding and slight flaring. This disrelation places unusual tension upon the Ilio-lumbar Ligament, which has attachment to the inner margin of the crest of the ilium on a limited area anterior to the Posterior Superior Iliac Spine and from there passes superiorly and medially to attach to the transverse processes of the fifth and fourth lumbar vertebrae. Under this form of irritation, noxious afferent impulses travel into the twelfth thoracic and first lumbar neuromeres to result in referred pain being interpreted by the brain as arising in the regions above mentioned.

Applying deep pressure to the iliac attachment of the ligament, to its "trigger point," may increase the pain and, combined with the structural disrelationship observed, establish the diagnosis. Correction of the sacroiliac subluxation should remove the cause of the distress.

Hackett[81] considers that many of the symptoms arising from the Ilio-lumbar Ligament are the result of ligamentous relaxation or stretching and has devised a technique of injecting an irritant into the ligament to cause the proliferation of fibrous tissue, thereby strengthening the ligament and eliminating the symptoms. There may be instances of chronic sacroiliac subluxation when the ligament has been seriously over-extended that the chiropractor would appreciate the need to refer such a patient to an orthopaedic practitioner for such supportive measures. However, in the majority of cases the osseous correction is sufficient to free the patient from further distress.

Not all sacroiliac subluxations produce symptoms as outlined in the above paragraph. Another painful condition may occur as a consequence of the stress brought to bear upon the posterior and anterior sacroiliac ligaments with the pain referred to the postero-lateral aspect of the buttock, thigh and leg in a pattern atypical to sciatica. Sciatica is frequently a result of sacroiliac distortion, also.

Such painful experiences of the sacroiliac region have a two-fold ill-effect upon the superimposed osseous structure. The first is the necessity of the vertebral column to accommodate for the basic distortion of the sacrum being disrelated to the innominate and the second is the response of the body to pain.

The pain may well cause the "splinting" action on the part of muscles, as previously discussed, and the patient favours the area, thereby accentuating distortion. Such factors may result in added stress being brought to bear upon regions of the spine at still higher levels, making them subluxation-prone to minor forms of added stress.

## Stress from Furniture

The manufacturers of furniture, automobile seats, and most other forms of accommodation for the seated position of the human have mistakenly assumed that softness and comfort are synonymous. They go blandly along making instruments of torture for the vertebral columns of the unsuspecting public, who have been motivated to buy by the application of the sales techniques of the merchandising psychologists, the languishing bevy of Hollywood pulchritude in negligee apparently enjoying their ease on one of the torture racks manufactured by Who-Dun-It and Sons. Colours, patterns and the ever-present desire to keep up with, and out-do, the neighbours has trapped most families into the purchase of the over-stuffed furniture and all manner of chairs, divans, love seats, kitchen and office furniture with eye appeal but no spine support. Fahrni[82] in his investigation of backache and their causes came to similar conclusions that the softer seats are a greater menace than firm ones.

A particularly insidious and inevitable evil has reached almost every vertebral column through the medium of the automobile seat, in which the average person is forced to spend a considerable percentage of his life. The tremendous increase in time spent in the seated position since grandfather's day would indicate the wisdom of improving the conveniences for such a position. Such has not been the case; there has been an inexorable and infamous decline in the support offered human structure.

The one ineptitude common to most forms of seating devices is the lack of support afforded the lumbar area of the vertebral column. Each montrosity may have its evils compounded by other shortcomings, but space dictates the need for dealing with the common denominator only and leaving the other iniquities to the reasoning of the reader.

Seated in a furniture manufacturer's dream of softness the postvertebral muscles are deluded by the feeling that their job has been taken over and it is safe to relax. The structure sinks back into the luxury and folds anteriorly as the lumbar area receives little or no support, almost reversing its normal primary curve.

The postvertebral musculature, unaccustomed as it is to physical activity, is content to relax and stretch under this habitual sitting posture. In accord with Davis' Law,[83] the postvertebral musculature tends to elongate and lose tone, while the iliopsoas, other flexors of the thigh and the iliotibial tract tend to shorten. Upon standing, the pelvis anterior nods and the primary curves of the column are accentuated.

With the retrogression of the spine to its embryonic form of a relatively uniform dorsal curve from sacrum to occiput, the thorax flattens, the tone of the abdominal muscles decreases and the abdomen bulges, while the Diaphragm finds itself at a severe mechanical disadvantage. Adequate respiration and venous return from the abdominal and pelvic content, as well as from the lower extremities are hampered. The individual also looks as though he were trying to sleep in a Navy hammock in the vertical position, lacking both dignity and comfort.

This gross anterior flexion of the trunk compresses the anterior

borders of the intervertebral discs and the posterior borders are tractioned correspondingly, as is the Posterior Longitudinal Ligament
and the postvertebral structures, such as the Supraspinous Ligament,
the Interspinous Ligaments, the postvertebral muscles, and perhaps,
even the articular capsules of the articulations between the processes.
Receptor nerve endings in these structures are stimulated and commence the bombardment of the spinal cord segments with afferent
impulses to result in the feeling of discomfort and the necessity of
repeated squirming movements to seek relief. A protracted session in
such an instrument of torture may result in the individual experiencing difficulty to attain the upright position.

The castigation levelled at the over-stuffed furniture may be
directed with even greater vehemence to the automobile and aero-
plane seats with added criticism for the manner in which many slant
from front to back with the anterior margin cutting into the driver's
thigh, interfering with circulation and nerve supply to the extremity,
especially the right leg with its constant trapped position on the
accelerator. The vertebral column is relatively unprotected, due to
the relaxation of the postvertebral muscles and in this vulnerable
state is subjected to hour after hour of vibration, jars, bumps and
joggles. The amazing thing is not that so many persons, who are
forced to spend long hours behind the steering wheel of a car, suffer
low backache and sciatica, but that more are not virtual invalids.
Thousands of car drivers have the good sense to purchase a spinal
support in the form of a contrivance to be placed on the car seat,
none of which have been found ideal, but are a tremendous improvement over the manufacturers' contribution.

The interference to respiration and circulation presents a very
serious hazard to the motoring public. With the interference to respiration comes a rapid onset of fatigue, since muscles and neural
tissues are affected. With fatigue comes disturbance to the normal
sensory appreciation and the reflex response to such afferent stimuli.
A fatigued driver becomes accident prone and a menace on the road.
The failure of the Diaphragm to function through its normal range,
due to faulty posture in the sitting position, throws an added load on
the heart as a consequence of the failure of the venous blood to be
propelled to the right side of the heart by the increased intra-abdominal pressure and relative negative pressure in the thorax. The Diaphragm should elongate and decrease the diameter of the Inferior
Vena Cava with each expiration, thereby further aiding in the propulsion of the contained blood.

It may, therefore, be no coincidence that the rate of heart failure and of other cardiac diseases has rapidly increased with the use of the automobile. British researchers found that coronary heart disease occurs more than twice as frequently among those physically inactive than in their active counterparts. British bus drivers proved to be far more susceptible to coronary heart disease than conductors, who climbed the stairs of the double-decker buses innumerable times per working day.

Interference to circulation of the brain may disturb its function and compound the problem of anoxia. Goldthwait[84] discusses the symptoms resulting from circulatory disturbances of a relatively minor nature in these words: "The abnormalities that may be found, if carefully looked for, are increased irritability, decreased alertness, decrease in the rapidity and skill with which volitional acts are performed, decreased activity of sensation, abnormal flushing and blanching of parts, and increased sensibility to changes in temperature."

While this writer made an attempt to bring the dangers of the automobile seat to the attention of car manufacturers, after a modest research project of x-raying subjects seated in the driver's seat of a number of makes of cars, little consideration was given and no likely improvement is to be expected, until the masses demand a seat that combines comfort and support.

## Trauma to Extremities

Attention is next directed to the mechanical injuries of somatic tissues at a distance from the spine, such as the lower extremity. While a sprained ankle is to be used as the example of the mechanism by which an injury to a peripheral joint may create a subluxation of the spinal segments related, it must be stressed that this is one example only and that the mechanism must be extended by the reader to encompass all forms of mechanical trauma of sufficient magnitude to any of the articulations.

The medial portion of the joint capsule of the right ankle is sprained. The resulting pain is experienced by the brain, but the strong afferent impulses, returning first to the spinal cord segments, have the ability to radiate to the anterior horn cells to produce the "splinting" of the muscles which move the ankle joint in accordance with Hilton's Law.[85] This muscle contraction, in response to the mechanical irritation or stress, occurs through the mediation of the nervous system only. The attendant swelling, which perpetuates the pain, is of two-fold origin: one a neural response, and the other a local response to the histamine-like substances liberated by the injured tissue.

The afferent fibres enter the neuromeres of efferent supply to the muscles which move the articulation. Connector neurones carry the impulses to the anterior horn of gray matter where synaptic connections are made with the neurones which motivate the muscles mentioned, but also an irradiation or "spill-over" takes place to the anterior horn cells which activate the postvertebral muscles of the region. In conformity with Pflüger's Law,[86] the strongest contraction occurs on the side of the source of afferent stimulation, or the side of the injured ankle. The vertebrae, to which these muscle fibres are attached, may then be pulled into an abnormal facing, or a limitation of movement within the normal range may occur, either being a subluxation.

F. M. Pottenger[87] also states that intra- and inter-segmental reflexes usually occur on the same side of the cord as the afferent fibres enter.

Sherrington[88] stated the law in more ornate language, "Broadly speaking, the degree of reflex spinal intimacy between afferent and efferent spinal roots varies directly as their segmental proximity."

Sir Charles emphasized that the extent of the reflex response increases with the increase in intensity of the stimulus. Thus, the more irritation caused by the injury, the greater will be the field of spread within the spinal cord and, therefore, the greater the number of muscles affected to produce "splinting," both in the extremity and the spine.

Furthermore, Sherrington[89] has this to say: "Further, in response to excitation even approximately minimal in intensity to a single afferent root, or a single filament of the single root, evokes a spinal discharge of centrifugal impulses through more than one efferent root, i.e., the discharge is plurisegmental."

The response to the stimulus is in accord with the All-or-None Law.[90] As the stimulus increases in intensity, more efferent neurones respond, causing more muscular fibres to contract, rather than stronger contraction taking place by the originally activated muscle fibres. The more severe the sprain, the more widespread the muscular response, including those of the postvertebral group.

## Summary

Summarizing the mechanical causes of subluxation, fixation, or gross distortion, it must be said that local injury by strain or sprain is one of the major factors. Faulty posture and occupational habits; gross distortions, such as scolioses, exaggerated lordoses and kyphoses; hereditary asymmetries and anomalies are additional factors of importance, which predispose to subluxation and are instrumental in determining the likely site of local disrelation. The mechanical causes of subluxation are appreciated as being almost innumerable, yet to these must be added the chemical and mental causes.

# CHAPTER VI

# Chemical Causes of Subluxation

CONSIDERATION IN THIS chapter will be directed to another classification of irritation or stress, which may overcome tissue resistance, produce structural distortion, interference to normal nerve transmission, and the symptoms and tissue changes of disease, namely noxious chemical factors.

In at least forty places in his textbook, D. D. Palmer[91] mentions the importance of chemical irritants or poisons as causative elements in the production of subluxations. One illustration is utilized from his writings: "The poison, acting on certain nerves, irritates their structure. They in turn contract muscles which draw vertebrae out of alignment, thereby impinging upon nerves which go to and affect certain portions of the body."

In the pages which follow it is hoped to demonstrate the complexities of the mechanism by which the human body responds to chemical irritation and substantiate the statement so succinctly embodying a fundamental truth. Unfortunately, the truth of D. D. Palmer's contention would seem to have been long overlooked or ignored by the majority of chiropractors and has, certainly, never permeated the consciousness of other healers. This is another example of the intuitive insight of an intellectual giant of his day, whose basic principles have been neglected, perhaps because they were cloaked in voluminous verbiage of criticism of the practitioners and teachers of chiropractic of the era.

This author is not unmindful of local adverse effects of the chemical irritants to be discussed, although apparently ignoring, or at best minimizing these changes, to follow through to the vertebral column. However, the problem at hand is to paint a word visualization of the mechanisms by which subluxations are produced by causes often ignored in chiropractic literature and to leave the reader to the study of local tissue changes from the excellent works of pathologists and diagnosticians, with whom it would be presumptive to compete.

Pottenger[92] pointed out that every viscus and tissue may send afferent stimuli to the central nervous system which, when sufficiently potent, may cause reflex somatic reaction. Again in the same text Pottenger[93] brought out clearly the fact that each viscus sends its afferent impulses back to the neuromere with which it was embryologically associated and finds, "Reflex motor paths of as low a threshhold and of as high a potency as any open to it anywhere."

Other neurologists confirm Pottenger's[94] contention that each viscus is capable of producing skeletal muscle reflex contraction and a myriad of other responses, some of which receive consideration later in this book.

It has been proven that all visceral structures are equipped with afferent nerve fibres which convey to the central nervous system information relative to the state of the splanchnic structure. Furthermore, the somatic structures are profoundly affected by the condition of, and the afferent neural impulses transmitted from, splanchnic structures.

Albert Kuntz[95] states: "Both visceral and somatic afferent neurons effect reflex connections with preganglionic visceral efferent neurons and, consequently, are functionally related to the autonomic nerves. Afferent neurons which terminate in the central nervous system may not be regarded as constituents of the automatic nerves, however, since both somatic and visceral afferents also effect reflex connections with somatic efferent neurons."

This statement crystallizes two points: one, the afferent fibres from visceral structures do have reflex association with the efferent neurones of somatic muscle; second, the disagreement between neurological authorities as to whether the afferent fibres from viscera should be classified as visceral afferents or somatic afferents, since they are indistinguishable from somatic fibres of the afferent type and the location of their cell bodies and the point of entrance into the spinal cord is the same as that of somatic fibres. Thus, it becomes a purely academic question of little practical import. Throughout the remainder of this text the term "visceral afferent" will be utilized to designate those afferent neurones conducting impulses from the visceral structures to the central nervous system.

It is essential to appreciate the fact that sensory impulses from somatic structures, such as skin, mucles, joint capsules, ligaments, etc., influence the splanchnic efferent outflow to the organs and that the afferent impulses from the visceral structures influence the efferent nerve supply to the somatic structures.

## Mechanism of Fixation

With the above facts refreshed, attention is turned to the point in question, the mechanism by which chemical irritants may produce a vertebral subluxation. Using the stomach, the most abused viscus, as our example, it is assumed that some irritant is ingested, such as strong alkali or acid, faulty food combinations, etc. The afferent nerve endings of the stomach wall are stimulated by the irritant, causing impulses to be transmitted to the fifth to the ninth thoracic neuromeres, especially to the right halves of the seventh and eighth segments, according to A. T. Rasmussen.[96]

The authorities would agree that in these segments synaptic connection would be effected with the anterior horn cells of the same side predominantly with reflex muscular contraction resulting in the upper portion of the Rectus Abdominus, the External and Internal Obliquus Abdomini, and the Transversus Abdominus muscles. These contractions have been noted by diagnosticians and are to be found mentioned in texts dealing with the subject of stomach disease. In addition, there would be increased contraction of the postvertebral muscles supplied by the posterior primary rami of the corresponding nerves, especially the right seventh and eighth thoracic nerves. Thus, the deep postvertebral muscles are likely to present the greatest noticeable hypertonicity, as demonstrable by palpation. The unequal degree of tonicity on the two sides of the vertebral column may limit the normal range of motion or hold one or more segments of the vertebral column in a position unnatural to the resting state, called by chiropractors — a subluxation.

To enlarge upon the above, it must be brought to mind that all viscera are equipped with special receptor end-organs capable of excitation by an adequate stimulus to result in nerve impulses being transmitted by way of myelinated afferent neurones, constituting a portion of the Celiac Plexus and the Greater Splanchnic Nerve, which reach the paravertebral sympathetic ganglia, through which the fibres pass without synaptic connection, then assist in the formation of White Rami Communicantes of the appropriate thoracic nerves, to travel through the Posterior Nerve Roots to the unipolar cell bodies located in the Posterior Nerve Root Ganglia. The axones of these unipolar cells continue through the posterior nerve root to enter the spinal cord.

Albert Kuntz[97] quoted Foster Geigel's writings of 1933, in which the latter emphasized that afferent fibres make synaptic connection with intercalated neurones which connect, or synapse with, the dendrites of lateral horn and anterior horn cells of the appropriate segment of entrance. In response to this afferent source of stimulation the efferent neurones must conduct impulses centrifugally, for the Law of Gravity: "What goes up, must come down," may be paraphrased to apply to the central nervous system, "What goes in, must come out." To every adequate stimulus there must be a response in either somatic or visceral structure. Neural impulses are not just stored in the brain and spinal cord. The response to a stimulus may occur in a distant structure or in a subtle way, but it occurs.

Plutchik,[98] writing in his section of the anthology, *Mental Health and Chiropractic*, edited by Herman S. Schwartz, D.C., stated this principle in these words: "The energy of the neural impulses, set up by chronic muscular activity must be handled in some way or other, and will be expressed either by bodily restlessness, stereotyped movements, tics, increasing tension in other muscles, such as the heart and capillary system, or increased activity in the glandular and secretory systems."

As established by such authorities as Sir Charles Sherrington,[99] the response to such afferent stimulation is likely to be plurisegmental, thus, in the case in question, results in increased tonus of the abdominal musculature, as well as the postvertebral musculature. The axones of the cell bodies in the anterior gray horns may be traced through the Anterior Nerve Root, the nerve trunk, through the Posterior Primary Ramus of the thoracic nerve to the postvertebral muscles. The greatest hypertonicity would be noted in the deep, segmental muscles, such as the Rotatores and portions of the Multifidus. The longer muscles, composed of portions of the myotomes of a number of segments, would be involved also and may, or may not, be readily noted. In many cases local distortion of the vertebral column in the form of scoliosis, or the straightening of a scoliosis, may occur due to the pull of the longer postvertebral muscles, while the segmental muscles produce the disrelations of adjacent vertebrae, the subluxations.

H. Kamieth,[100] writing in the orthopaedic journal of Germany in 1958 and quoted in the journal of the American Medical Association, November 15, 1958, reported under the title, "Pathogenetic Importance of the Thoracic Portion of the Vertebral Column," that of 100 patients with stomach and duodenal ulcers, proven by roentgenography, 86% had scoliosis of the thoracic area of the spine. Sixty of these patients had a right scoliosis, twenty-one had a left scoliosis and five showed an S-shaped scoliosis. He stated: "The percentile distribution of right-sided and left-sided scolioses coincided with the percentages of duodenal and gastric ulcers."

Seventy-two had duodenal ulcers, twenty-three had gastric ulcers, and five had both gastric and duodenal ulcers. Furthermore, he had established that eighty-three percent had postvertebral muscle spasticity, and ninety percent showed pathological changes of the intervertebral discs.

This writer would hazard the guess that had these patients been examined by a chiropractor with a knowledge of basic distortion and compensation, it would have been found that in the remaining fourteen percent, a scoliosis of a compensatory nature had been straightened, thus, in fact one hundred percent of the cases had associated vertebral column manifestations of their visceral problem.

At this point it must be emphasized that the present chapter deals with the causes of subluxation and kindred vertebral distortion and future chapters deal with the mechanisms by which the spinal disrelations produce the visceral changes, both functional and pathological. Once established, the ulcerous condition continues to bombard the neuromeres with afferent impulses which by synaptic connection with the efferent neurones continue the muscle hypertonicity of the postvertebral group and maintain the scoliosis and subluxations. This is the rationale for the use of the bland diet during the correction of the spinal contribution to the symptomatic picture of the disease process.

Which came first, the spinal distortion or the peptic ulcer, is a matter of individuality among patients, but experience would seem to bear out the fact that all sufferers from peptic ulcer do show alterations of the vertebral column. During the period of vertebral correction, it is essential to minimize the irritation to the peptic mucosa of roughage, condiments, faulty food combinations, etc., that the least possible visceromotor reflex be active twenty-four hours per day, while the doctor of chiropractic is available only two or three times per week to reduce the hypertonicity of postvertebral muscles, adjust the subluxations and normalize the neural supply.

## Cervical Involvement

While the thoracic area from the fifth to the ninth vertebrae has received the considered attention of this writing, it must be borne in mind that the stomach also has afferent fibres of the Vagus (Xth Cranial) Nerve conducting impulses back to the Medulla Oblongata. Through intimate connections within the brain stem and the superior portion of the spinal cord, the irritation from the gastro-intestinal tract may be reflected in changes in the superior cervical segments of the vertebral column, and vice versa.

The experiences of chiropractors would indicate that some of the peptic ulcer cases have an upper cervical problem, rather than a mid-thoracic one. No derogation of the importance of the subluxation as a causative factor is intended, but each, cause and effect, must be considered separately. Furthermore, there is a need to stress the removal of the basic causes of vertebral subluxations and not develop mind set on the subluxation as a be-all and end-all.

For every subluxation there is a cause and there may be a continuing factor of causative nature which perpetuates the subluxation and makes the correction of this abnormality difficult, requiring repeated chiropractic ministrations of adjustive force. Here lies the true reason for patients being required to return several times each week for a number of weeks to have their spine adjusted. Were it not for the vicious cycle of afferent-efferent impulses, the problem would be one of pure mechanics, freeing the vertebra that it might once again take part in the normal range of motion within the functional requirements of the spine in health. Muscles could be persuaded to relax under the skilled hands of the chiropractor and would not return to their hypertonic state were it not for the bombardment of the spinal cord by afferent impulses from the splanchnic structures, showing pathological change, and the tissues under stress in the environs of the subluxation.

Should certain foods be a source of irritation to the gastro-intestinal tract, they must be eliminated from the diet. As D. D. Palmer[101] so aptly worded it: "In proportion as the ingesta induces irritation, it becomes a poison and ceases to be food. That which is food to one may be a poison to another. When that which is food for one person impairs the functions of another, it becomes a poison to that other."

Further, he states: "From baby in the high chair to grandma in the rocker, the axial bones are as liable to be displaced by noxious substances which enter the system in our food and drink or by inhalation as they are by accident direct."[102]

## Constipation

Another nearly universal gastro-intestinal problem, constipation, should be considered to further direct the attention of the reader to the import of visceral irritations as factors in the causation of subluxations and more gross vertebral distortions.

The putrefactive end-products and the mechanical pressure of the fecal material within the colon irritate the receptor nerve-endings, thereby bombarding the associated spinal cord segments with afferent impulses, which result in muscular response and subluxations in the lower thoracic and upper lumbar areas, as well as predisposing to sacroiliac subluxation, due to asymmetrical hypertonicity of the post-vertebral muscles supplied from these neuromeres. Alverez[103] of Mayo Clinic fame and author of several outstanding textbooks relative to gastro-enterology, reported experiments in which the colons of normal young people were thoroughly cleansed and then the rectums packed with sterile gauze with the resultant symptoms of constipation and so-called auto-intoxication.

Certainly, these findings indicate that the symptom complex of constipation is neurogenic, rather than toxic. Needless to say, Alverez did not investigate the ill-effects upon the spine and its musculature by the irritation produced by sterile gauze packing of the rectum.

Toxicity is a factor in constipation, as the urinalysis establishes. The presence of indican in the urine has long been considered as a certain indication of the absorption of toxins from the colon, but in the light of investigations, such as those of Dr. Alverez, may be considered as a failure of the body to rid itself of end-products of metabolism. In either event, the noxious material in the blood stream circulates to the central nervous system and has a deleterious effect, changing its irritability. With an increased irritability the response to afferent stimuli becomes more pronounced, the hypertonicity of muscles increased and the likelihood of subluxation more certain.

## Respiratory Irritations

Not only is the gastro-intestinal tract the offender in producing subluxations, due to chemical irritation, but the respiratory tract may be cited for its contribution to structural distortion by way of the body response to chemical irritants to the mucosa. The same may be said for any of the other visceral structures, but these are not as prone to irritation from external sources as are the respiratory and gastro-intestinal tracts.

Any form of irritating gas, or solid material, taken into the respiratory tract may stimulate the receptor nerve-endings in the sensitive mucous membrane, causing afferent impulses to travel over the myelinated nerve fibres, which pass through the paravertebral ganglia associated with the first four thoracic nerves especially, through the White Rami Communicantes, the nerve trunks, the Posterior Nerve Roots, to their cell bodies in the Posterior Nerve Root Ganglia. From the cytones, the impulses are transmitted over the axone portion of the nerve fibre to enter the spinal cord as a portion of the Posterior Nerve Root.

The respiratory system demonstrates not only visceromotor reflexes from the neuromeres receiving the afferent impulses, but in addition the structures supplied by mid-cervical segments may be involved in the muscular response. Quoting F. M. Pottenger's[104] text, "It is further evident that reflexes occur between the sympathetics and spinal nerves, not only in the segment of the cord which receives the afferent, sensory impulse from the viscus, but also in segments removed, the cell bodies receiving the impulse and those causing the reflex action being connected either by collateral branches of the afferent fibre or by intercalated neurons. This is true of the pulmonary reflex in which the afferent impulse enters the cord by way of the posterior roots of the upper six thoracic nerves, but the reflex is mediated in the mid-cervical segments of the cord."

This leads us to an appreciation of the fact that the subluxations may be found in the upper thoracic segments or in the mid-cervical portion of the vertebral column. It must be mentioned that there are also afferent fibres of the Vagus Nerve distributed to the respiratory tract, but the visceromotor response is less dominant in the spine than that of the pathways above considered. When such response does occur, it is the suboccipital segments that are involved.

Irritations to the mucosal lining of the nasal cavity and paranasal sinuses stimulate the receptor end-organs of the Trigeminal Nerve, the fifth cranial nerve, according to Gray,[105] Cunningham[106] and other authorities on the subject. There are afferent fibres, whose cytones are located in the posterior nerve root ganglia of the upper thoracic nerves, distributed to the same tissues.

The afferent fibres of the Trigeminal Nerve follow a devious path to reach their unipolar cell bodies located in the Gasserian Ganglion on the sensory root of the nerve trunk, which rests on the anterior portion of the petrous portion of the temporal bone within the cranial cavity. The sensory root of the Trigeminal nerve, composed of the axones of the unipolar cells above mentioned, enters the lateral surface of the Pons. Within the Pons the afferent fibres separate into three main groups to make synaptic connection with the cells of three distinct nuclei.

The group of fibres, with which there is present concern, turn inferiorly as components of the Spinal Tract of the Trigeminal Nerve to make synaptic connection with the cells of the Nucleus of the Spinal Tract, which is first distinguishable in the lower portion of the

80

Medulla Oblongata and is continuous inferiorly with the Substantia Gelatinosa of Rolando of the gray matter of the spinal cord, according to Kreig[107] and other standard authorities.

A second portion of this same nucleus, continuous with the Substantia Spongiosus of the spinal cord, lies more medial and extends to a higher level of the Medulla, reaching the lowest portion of the Pons. The two sections of the nucleus have distinct functions and are composed of cells of differing shape and staining qualities. That portion, which is of present concern, is the Gelatinosus and receives the impulses which, when transmitted to the appropriate cortical area, result in the sensation of pain, while the Spongiosus portion receives the impulses that eventually result in the sensation of touch, a sensation unlikely to arise in the paranasal sinuses.

Those afferent fibres of the Trigeminal Nerve which reach the anterior portion of the nasal mucosa, by way of the Nasociliary branch of the Ophthalmic division of the fifth cranial nerve, may extend down the neuraxis to the level of the second cervical neuromere prior to making synaptic connection with the cells of the Substantia Gelatinosus. Kreig,[108] Gray[109] and other authorities have noted that the fibres of pain, carried by the Ophthalmic division, extend to the above mentioned level of the cord. Those of the Maxillary division terminate in the nucleus just short of the first cervical segment, while those of the Mandibular division are confined to the upper portion of the nucleus.

It is appreciated, of course, that the neurones, whose cell bodies form the Substantia Gelatinosus, are the second order of neurones on the pathway of pain conduction and terminate in the Thalamus by synapsing with the third order neurones, whose axones reach the Postcentral Gyrus of the cerebral cortex, the conscious centre of appreciation and interpretation of sensations of this nature. However, it must be reiterated that these first order neurones may, either by collaterals or connector neurones, stimulate the anterior horn cells of the segments within which they make synaptic connection, second and first cervical neuromeres, thereby resulting in a state of hypertonicity of the muscles supplied. The possibilities of subluxations of the occipito-atlantal, atlanto-axial, or axio-third cervical articulations must be obvious to the chiropractic student.

Furthermore, it must be mentioned that there is very real likelihood that connector neurones from the more superior portions of the Nucleus of the Spinal Tract of the Trigeminal Nerve descend into the upper cervical neuromeres to make synaptic connection with the motor cells of the anterior horns. In this event the afferent fibres, which supply the remainder of the mucosa of the nasal passages and paranasal sinuses and are derived from the Maxillary division of the fifth cranial nerve, may disrupt the normal tone of the musculature supplied by these upper cervical segments of the spinal cord, and contribute a fair share to the causative irritation resulting in subluxation.

It must not be overlooked that there are also afferent fibres distributed to the same mucosa, whose cell bodies are located in the posterior nerve root ganglia of the upper thoracic spinal nerves. The course of these fibres is even more circuitous, commencing from the receptor nerve-endings in the mucous membrane and following the path of the postganglionic sympathetic fibres. These sensory fibres assist in the formation of the carotid plexus, reach the Superior Cervical Sympathetic Ganglion, travel down the ganglionated chain, compose a portion of the White Rami Communicantes of the superior four or more thoracic nerves. They pass through the nerve trunk and assist in the formation of the posterior nerve root to enter the spinal cord and make synaptic connection with the cells of the gray matter. Their unipolar cell bodies are indistinguishable from those of the somatic afferent fibres in the Posterior Nerve Root Ganglion and their potency of influence upon the anterior and posterior gray horn cells is of equality with the somatic afferents. Such a source of irritation can effect synaptic connection, either through collateral fibres or connector neurones with the motor cells of control of the postvertebral muscle fibres supplied by the neuromeres under present discussion. An upper thoracic subluxation of the spine is a very real possibility and even probability.

## Micro-organisms as Stressors

Chiropractors are frequently accused of "not believing in germs." Such a statement is far removed from fact. Having devoted several hundreds of hours to the study of Bacteriology and peered through the microscope at all manner of micro-organisms, no chiropractor would be so obtuse as to deny the existence of micro-organisms, or even the ultra-microscopic factors, called viruses. The allopathic practitioner places his emphasis and bases his method of treatment upon the micro-organism as being "the" cause of a wide spectrum of disease, while the chiropractor gives greater credit to the condition of the host, the potential patient, than to the germs. This latter contention is receiving justification in these recent years from authorities in bacteriology, neurology, and other biological sciences. In a future chapter, the mechanism by which the subluxation establishes the suitable condition for the growth and reproduction of micro-organisms in the tissues of the human will receive more extensive elaboration.

Providing that the state of the tissue is conducive to the life and reproduction of germs, the exogenous toxins produced by such minute forms of life may become an active irritation to the receptor nerve-endings of the tissue, resulting in a stream of impulses being transmitted over afferent fibres to the spinal cord segment, to stimulate efferent neurones and result in hypertonicity of post-vertebral muscle in the manner described in greater detail previously.

That the environment is of prime importance to the micro-organism is borne out by A. D. Speransky,[110] who wrote, "The microbe perishes in the normal tissues, even in the immediate vicinity of the pathologically altered parts where it is able to maintain itself, as long as this vicinity retains its normal biochemical, and hence functional, state. If the first changes, which were the cause of the tissue dystrophy, prove to be temporary and gradually pass away, then the tissue alterations also disappear and the microbe disappears along with them. No special form of immunity is required for this."

Again Speransky[111] is quoted: "Contact with the meningiococcus is not sufficient by itself for the development of the disease. Some other process takes place in advance, preparing the situation in which the interaction of the macro-organism and micro-organism will subsequently take place."

Albert Kuntz[112] has stated: "Under ordinary physiological conditions, infective organisms are present on the skin and mucous membranes, but, due to the local resistance, infection does not take place. Prolonged ischemia tends to reduce the local resistance and favors infection. This is well illustrated in infections of the upper respiratory passages following exposures to low temperature or drafts."

Gordienko,[113] et al, demonstrate that antibodies are not formed by direct contact of the antigen with tissues nor by chemical mediators, but require the mediation of the neural system. The chiropractic physician concerns himself with an effort to maintain the optimum function of the nervous system that the body may best respond to the stresses of environment, including pathogenic micro-organisms. Thus, an efficient neural system is likely to cause the production of appropriate antibodies to meet the threat posed by this form of ubiquitous stressor.

That micro-organisms play a part in the disease process receives the concurrence of chiropractors; that micro-organisms are always "the" cause of such diseases is categorically denied.

It must be appreciated that the problem of disease is one of immense complication. Disease is the reaction of the body, through the nervous system, to adverse environmental, external and internal, factors and is not the simple invasion by an evil spirit, germs, or curse of the gods. As D. D. Palmer[114] has stated the case, "Students of Chiropractic should constantly remember that disease is not a thing, but a condition. It is an abnormal performance of certain morphological alterations of the body. Agencies and conditions which the body cannot adapt itself to, sway the capacities of energy above or below, inducing the functional abberations and structural alterations known as disease."

D. D. Palmer[115] admonishes chiropractors as follows: "Impingements, poisons and intense thinking, auto-suggestion, unrelieved change of thought, insufficient rest and sleep, increase or decrease the momentum of impulses. In the study of pathology we should look to the etiological factors which, by their exciting or debilitating effects, retard or liberate stored up energy, resulting in abnormal functioning and morbid structure."

It is unfortunate that allopathic physicians have not appreciated the nervous system in its correlating and integrating functions in health and disease. The disregard for detrimental irritation of the neural system has led to a plethora of adverse side effects, many of which are life threatening. Despite their good intentions in the words of Spain,[116] "Unfortunately, therefore, iatrogenic disease can now take its place almost as an equal alongside bacteria as an important factor in the pathogenesis of human illness."

Fortunately, while chiropractic may not be a panacea, properly administered it does no harm and is likely to provide, at least, palliation.

## Contributory Factors

Prior to leaving this consideration of chemical irritants, including micro-organisms, as causative factors in the production of subluxation, it should be brought to mind that a lesser stress of this nature may be required, if the afferent impulses are returning to areas of the spinal cord being bombarded by the impulses from sources under mechanical forms of irritation. To produce a clearer visualization of this contention a practical, though hypothetical, example will serve to illustrate the statement.

An individual has a basic distortion which required the four opposed rotatory scolioses in compensation, thus placing the fourth cervical vertebra as the apex of the cervical scoliosis, with the stress of being deviated furthest from the gravity line and expressing the greatest degree of rotation of any of the vertebrae in the particular scoliosis. Furthermore, the patient has poor posture with an anterior nodded pelvis, creating a compensatory deeper anterior curve of the cervical portion of the spine, increasing the mechanical stress upon the fourth cervical vertebra which is the apex of this lordosis. Being a heavy cigarette smoker, the mucous membrane of the bronchial tree has been irritated by the chemical components of the smoke and afferent impulses are coursing back to the spinal cord to enter the upper thoracic neuromeres, but, as quoted from Pottenger[117] previously, the mid-cervical segments are intimately involved in the reflex response to this latter form of irritation. To these may now be added the afferent impulses arising from the nasal mucosa in response to the chemical irritation of the tissue by micro-organisms.

The stimuli are conducted over the fibres of the Trigeminal Nerve, as discussed previously, and through connectors, descending neurones add to the stimulation of the efferent, or motor cells in the mid-cervical segments to the degree sufficient to cause contraction of postvertebral muscle fibres, resulting in the subluxation of the fourth cervical vertebral segment.

Any one source of irritation may not be sufficient to create the degree of muscular contraction necessary for the production of a subluxation, but, by the process of summation of afferent stimuli, the effector mechanism is activated with the result that a local distortion occurs, the subluxation or fixation.

## Neural Chemistry

Attention must next be directed to the importance of the chemistry of the nervous system itself in determining the response to stimuli aroused by all forms of mechanical, chemical and mental stress. This subject is deserving of an entire volume. The best that can be done in this text is to utilize examples to stimulate the thinking and enquiry of the reader.

This author can do no more nor less than confess an abysmal ignorance of the intricacies of modern chemistry and a mere extrapolation of the wisdom of others has been necessary.

The irritability of the central nervous system is characterized by inconstancy and is a variable which, in a measure, characterises individuals. There are the languid and the volatile personalities. The majority are a mixture between the extremes, but under varying circumstances fluctuate toward one extreme or the other. This variation in irritability is, in large measure, dependent upon the biochemical components of the neurones and intercellular fluid which bathes them, as well as the toxic endogenous and exogenous products which may influence the degree of normality of these units of structure of the nervous system.

Pottenger[118] states, "Neurones may be injured in many ways. Certain poisons may alter their stability; they may be injured by chemical or mechanical action; by severe or persistent stimuli which act peripherally upon their corresponding segmental afferent neurons as is shown so plainly in pulmonary tuberculosis or by malnutrition."

In *Body and Mature Behaviour* by M. Feldenkrais[119] is to be found this statement in support of the contention of variable irritability: "The excitability of the nervous tissue depends very closely on the chemical composition of the irrigating blood and the hormones present, its pH, salt content, etc."

In *Physiological Psychology*, G. L. Freeman[120] said: "Just as vigilance may be lowered by toxic substances in the blood, so the presence of chemicals which act as excitants will raise vigilance. This is the principle which lies behind the giving of stimulants such as coffee, the action of adrenalin and other hormones. The effectiveness of food or warm milk as a sedative is probably due to the shifting of large quantities of blood containing chemical excitants from the brain to the digestive organs, the vigilance of brain centers thereby being lowered."

E. M. Abrahamson and A. W. Pezet[121] in their textbook, *Body, Mind and Sugar*, discuss at length the importance of the optimum quantity of glucose being available to the central nervous system to maintain stable function and the erratic response of the nervous system in cases of hyperinsulinism with a low blood sugar level.

Wyke[122] has demonstrated that, if oxidation of glucose is reduced for any reason, the nervous system's response to the narcotic effects of anaesthesia is increased and "any variation in the rate of oxidation of glucose in neurones will alter their excitability."

Normal function and optimum response to afferent impulses is dependent in large measure on adequate nutrition, which includes oxygen, and the elimination of the end-products of metabolism from the central nervous system. Best and Taylor[123] state that 0.7 cu.mm. of oxygen is required for each gram of resting neural tissue, and an additional 0.25 cu.mm. is essential for each gram during activity. A decrease in the oxygen supplied to the brain or spinal cord has deleterious results upon the ability to respond in a correct manner to stimuli and there is a progressive loss of excitability.

Glucose and thiamine are as essential to normal neural function as is oxygen, and Wyke[124] has stated that 70-74 mg. per 100 ml. meets the usual needs of neural tissue and capable of supplying the 5 mg. per 100 g. per minute required by the brain. Further, that 3.5 ml. per 100 g. per minute of oxygen is required by the cerebral cortex, but only 0.13 ml. per 100 g. per minute for active peripheral nerve fibres, which is almost twenty-seven times less oxygen than necessary for the cerebral cortex.

In a future chapter, an effort will be made to show the mechanics by which the subluxation may contribute to this process of anoxia of neuromeres. The lack of oxygen to the central nervous system may be due to local causes or general causative factors. The former could be illustrated by local vasospasm, occurring in some area of supply to the central nervous system, while the latter would be illustrated by anemia, failure of respiration or circulation.

Anoxia of the central nervous system, brain or spinal cord, modifies the response of the body to stress and, hence, must be considered in the problem of subluxation. As Freeman[125] says, "Body sway, critical flicker frequency, retinal perimetry, mental addition and motor coordination are all adversely effected by anoxic conditions."

Fatigue, either of the body as a whole or of specific neural pathways, may also modify the response to irritation and predispose to subluxation. As neurones commence to show the disturbances from fatigue, Matzke and Foltz[126] have demonstrated chromotolysis occurs, the cells enlarge and the nuclei become eccentric. In the early stages of fatigue the irritability of the neural tissue is marked and as the detrimental influence of fatigue continues, there may be a marked loss of the capacity of the neurones to respond to stimulation and finally irreversible structural damage with consequent functional loss. In the state of accentuated responsiveness, the external afferent stimuli need to be less pronounced to result in the motor discharge that causes postvertebral muscle contraction and the disrelation of vertebral segments in the form of a subluxation or fixation.

## Need for Total Consideration

The Doctor of Chiropractic, of necessity, must take cognizance of the patient's nutrition, elimination, degree of fatigue, general hygiene, exercise and employment habits, as well as being concerned about the posture and specific physiological activity of the vertebral column. The irritations, to which the structure is subjected, result in responses that are markedly modified by the general condition of health and degree of irritability of the patient's nervous system at the moment of application. It is for this reason that an individual may have lifted a given weight hundreds of times per day over a number of years in his occupation, but, under general conditions of fatigue, toxicity from the end-products of metabolism, faulty nutritional intake, over-indulgence, etc., the same mechanical stress produces a severe, incapacitating subluxation.

It is difficult to apportion the responsibility between the mechanical stress and the chemical irritants to his central nervous system. Furthermore, the locus of subluxation is likely to be determined by the many factors brought to the attention of the reader in previous pages. Nor, are these all of the possibilities to be considered. The following chapter deals with the contribution of the mental irritants to the problem of subluxation. No consideration of a subluxation can be complete without taking heed of the three forms of external stress, mechanical, chemical and mental, and the biochemical state and degree of irritability of the central nervous system itself.

This chapter has merely touched upon the chemical factors involved and it is hoped that the reader will be constrained to delve more deeply into the problem and acquire a deeper appreciation of the complexity of the cause and effect of the subluxation.

For these many years, the subluxation has been discussed as a simple mechanical problem by the average chiropractor, and scoffed at by men of science as a machination of naive, pseudo-practitioners of healing. The stature of the chiropractic profession demands that the subluxation be divested of its simplicity and clothed in the physiological and anatomical facts, that permit it to stand unashamedly in the marketplace, the courtroom, the legislative chambers, or in the dissection laboratory of pure science.

CHAPTER VII

# Mental Causes of Subluxation

THIS CHAPTER WILL deal with the mechanism by which psychic stress may contribute to or cause the body's response in the form of a vertebral subluxation. The writer is attempting to awaken interest in the teachings of D. D. Palmer[127] who wrote: "The determining causes of disease are traumatism, poison and auto-suggestion." And again another example of his admonitions: "These luxations are caused by direct traumatism, poisons, or auto-suggestion."

There are numerous other references by D. D. Palmer to the importance of the mind as a causative factor in the production of subluxations and generalized vertebral distortion. Unfortunately, the chiropractic profession failed to appreciate the depth of insight of the founder and did not emphasize this causative area. Of late, the chiropractic profession, or a segment of it, has been taking an interest in courses which stress the spiritual and mental approach to the problems of disease. Unfortunately, these would seem to de-emphasize, or fail entirely to appreciate, the mechanism by which the emotional stress manifests itself in somatic disturbances, or disease, through the distress of function of the vertebral column, known as subluxation.

While it is not the purpose of the writer to derogate practitioners of other forms of healing, it is of the utmost concern to awaken an appreciation in the minds of doctors of chiropractic for the heritage left by D. D. Palmer, which provides the basis for the most complete understanding of the patient as a unit of structure and function yet to be devised by man to this date. Nor is this to be assumed to indicate a concurrence with the total writings of the founder of this profession. Basic principles have been gleaned from the welter of random thoughts, criticism of others, and ideas of the turn of the century which cannot be justified by present knowledge. Out of 985 pages, approximately 69 quotations of a couple of lines each have been utilized to punctuate this text, and 69 is not a high percentage of a bibliography of over 500 references. Without apology to the critics of chiropractic it is reiterated that these fundamental principles, supplied by D. D. Palmer, provide a skeleton for the biological facts which make scientific chiropractic one of the most comprehensive schools of generic medicine yet devised.

Many ingenious approaches to the health problems have been

thought out carefully, but none seems to be as all-encompassing as the teachings of D. D. Palmer. The chiropractor needs to experience no twinge of inferiority as he views the mottled array of theories. The founder of the science of chiropractic appreciated the working of Universal Intelligence (God); the function of Innate Intelligence (Soul, Spirit or Spark of Life) within each, which he recognized as a minute segment of Universal; and the fundamental causes of interference to the planned expression of that Innate Intelligence in the form of Mental, Chemical and/or Mechanical Stresses, which create the structural distortions that interfere with nerve supply and thereby result in altered function to the point of demonstrable cellular changes, known as pathology.

The above paragraph was quoted by the committee under HEW Secretary Cohen[128] in its effort to derogate chiropractic, but in no instance was any ability demonstrated to understand the neurological mechanisms explained in later chapters to justify this statement of fact. Had attention been directed to the writings of Kervran[129] the gentlemen of the committee might have avoided mindset on the fallacy that allopathic medicine has all and the only answers to the restoration of health, for he states: "The greatest men of science now recognize that neither the chemistry nor the physics of inert matter is integrally applicable to living matter."

While the phenomena of life and functions of living matter have been unravelled to a very marked degree by scientists working with lavish expenditures of tax dollars, there remains much that is yet inexplicable, as Kervran[130] stated: "It will be widely demonstrated that there are other biological phenomena unexplainable by the movements of the electrons — that is, by chemistry or physico-chemistry — because of a frequent incompatibility between biology and these sciences."

While it may be unpopular in this "enlightened age" to acknowledge that there is or may be a power and wisdom greater than that of the most learned scientists, chiropractic physicians do not suffer from this egomania and acknowledge that they do not have a panacea nor the total knowledge of health and disease. Recognizing the multiform stress of environment upon the total human structure, the doctor of chiropractic seeks to normalize the neurological and anatomical responses to such disease-producing factors, recognizing that in instances other branches of generic medicine may be required for specialized skill and knowledge. The total patient and his welfare should be the first concern of any would-be physician. The chiropractic physician does possess the skill and knowledge to correct the majority of anatomical distortions which disturb neural function, producing dysfunction or disease.

As Dr. C. A. Pinkenburg kindly pointed out, Thomas Sydenham (1624-1689) called "the healing powers of nature"; Haller (1709-1777) named it "vital force"; A. T. Still, the "father" of osteopathy, referred to this healing and regulating phenomenon of the body as "divine essence"; while D. D. Palmer coined the phrase "innate intelligence" to express this manifestation for which the best minds of this enlightened age have no explanation, although much has been learned about the mechanisms of the body since D. D. Palmer's day and Innate Intelligence has been pushed into a smaller area. The day may come when scientists have unravelled all of the mysteries of the human body and there will be no need for terms such as Innate Intelligence, Ego, Libido, Homeostasis, etc., to hide ignorance.

The adjusting of each and every articulation of the human frame was stressed by Dr. Palmer[131] in a number of places in his text, as follows: "It is, or should be, the business of the Chiropractor to restore to normal position any displaced portion of the bony framework . . ."

What more could any doctor require of his science? What more has science, metaphysics, or religion to offer the conscientious would-be healer?

The failure to appreciate the teachings of D. D. Palmer has created many fallacies, deficiencies, partial truths, discontent, bickering and, above all, feelings of inferiority within the ranks of the profession. A return to the basic principles, as enunciated by the founder, would remedy many of the problems.


## Psychosomatics

In recent years, a whole new specialty has grown up in allopathic medicine, called Psychosomatic Medicine. As is prevalent in most specialties, the practitioners of this segment of healing cannot see the woods for the trees, and have become so engrossed with the mind as a cause of physical disturbance that they overlook the remainder of the patient and fail to appreciate that disturbances of the body have a deranging influence upon the mind. A structural problem, brought about by a mechanical or chemical cause, may so disturb the mental balance of the individual that he is no longer capable of coping with the emotional stresses of his environment.

Dr. Herman S. Swartz[132] discussed an essential phase of this disturbing relationship of the subluxation to the Psyche in an article in the year 1954 and it is doubtful that a better enunciation of the problem could be written than the direct quotation, which follows: "The art of restoring disrelated skeletal and/or muscular tissue to its normal design is psychosomatic, per se, because it corrects and removes the faulty structure or subluxations responsible for the nerve irritations affecting a particular organ or gland. Every nerve infringement within the vertebral column is an incipient pathological state involving some concurrent psychic infringement. This initial "malformation" may readily lead to a true psychosomatic condition if the patient centrally superimposes upon this localized neural irritation evoking specific regional pain the additional generalized or widely distributed weight of fear in any one of its protean forms. Thus increased by a remoter reinforcement from another power area or energy source, the pain is necessarily paralleled by a corresponding growth in fear, worry, and anxiety, and the slow nibbling away of the sufferer's psyche goes on apace.

"In this fashion, a minor subluxation can turn into a full-flowered psychic upset if the patient uses his unalleviated discomfort (1) to escape reality; (2) to avoid his obligations to himself and others; (3) to "get even" with some superior, associate, or family member; (4) to interpret his pain as divine punishment for some offense, etc. If, as is so commonly the case when sedatives are administered, the pain is deadened by medication, then the mental faculties are benumbed in some degree with the further result that temporary personality deterioration ensues, normal confidence and poise are destroyed, and childhood fears, frustrations, and feelings of guilt and rejection become prominent to such an extent that the initially uncomplicated "winding base" goes unrecognized by both doctor and patient. In this way a simple fall, blow, or other injury eliciting some anatomical distortion can grow into a full-bodied neurosis or psychosis. Conversely, correcting the distortion brings relief, recovery, and cure in enough cases to demonstrate that chiropractic, per se, is beneficial to the mentally disturbed, whether used alone or in conjunction with auxilliary psychological aids."

Guyton[133] deals with the influence of the hypothalamus and reticular activating system as parts of the neurological mechanism of psychosomatic illness. He discusses three routes by which the adverse effects of increased activity of the hypothalamus may occur: (1) through motor nerves to the skeletal muscles; (2) through the sympathetic and parasympathetic divisions of the automatic system; (3) through pituitary hormonal secretion. No attempt is made to follow the neural pathways.

The doctor of chiropractic must maintain an objective point of view and not be carried to extremes by either the psychosomatic or somatopsychic approach. Both are important. In one case the emphasis may be required on the former, while in another instance the latter is the secret to unravelling a complex health problem. However, the doctor of chiropractic should be acutely cognizant of the importance of structure in every health problem and be astute enough to appreciate that his adjustive ministrations are indicated in each instance. If mental stress is the basic cause, structural distortion precedes, or is a concomitant of every disease and is deserving of his skill and knowledge. If mechanical disrelation has upset the affective mechanism and disturbed the ability of the mind to cope with emotional stress, it is crystal clear that correction of the physical is of paramount importance. Thus, the chiropractor should not hesitate to utilize the purely adjustive techniques in every instance, but may find it advantageous to employ methods to directly influence the psyche.

The influence of the mental state upon the somatic structure is emphasized by W. Sachs[134] in his textbook, wherein attention is called to the buoyant posture and movements indicative of pleasant emotions: while grief results in drooping and slowness of movements.

Lowman and Young[135] have taken cognizance of the effect of body type and posture upon psychological functioning, pointing out that the lithe, esthetic or ectomorphic type tends to greater postural problems and emotional instability. Further, recognition is indicated of the interdependence of the physical and mental traits, also that good structural relationship and posture are not to be found in the psychotic.

Every emotion has its counterpart in the posture assumed. Should an emotion, such as despondency, be persistent, the somatic counterpart may result in changes of muscular tension with attendant osseous distortion and visceral disrelation which are more or less permanent. It has been well established also that the mental state disturbs function of splanchnic structures through psychovisceral reflexes. Hence, through the mechanism of the visceromotor reflex the related vertebral segments may become fixated or subluxated.

## Somatopsychic

In the textbook, *Body and Mature Behaviour*, the author M. Feldenkrais[136] states: "In all neurotic states we find anxiety, nausea, giddiness, muscular tension, digestive and breathing troubles and sexual disorders of some sort. So long as there is no improvement in these troubles there is no improvement in the general state — and vice versa. Muscular tension and anxiety are invariably so closely interwoven in all states of emotional disorder that it is difficult to see how any real advancement towards clearer understanding of the nature of cures is possible without greater knowledge of the phenomenon of anxiety."

Indicative of Feldenkrais',[137] appreciation of the interweaving of mind and body is the following quotation: "With a proper technique it is possible to analyze a personality solely by a study of his muscular behaviour, in the same way, and with the same results as by an analysis of his mental processes alone."

Fahrni[138] makes the statement: "An individual's posture is in fact his attempt to present himself to the world in the most acceptable light possible." This may not be true, if accepted literally, since the posture assumed may be one of belligerence or submissiveness and selfpity which are not "acceptable" in normal circles of society.

These are not revelations to the observant chiropractor who has astonished patients by enquiring relative to their emotional problem, after having palpated the muscular tensions that point like accusing fingers towards the psychological source of stress. It is necessary, of course, to understand the patterns of muscular tension created by the adverse emotions and to distinguish them from the muscular contractions produced by other sources of irritation.

Fear has a characteristic somatic manifestation which is recognized by everyone. The muscular tone has been modified by the emotion to present a definite posture and thus a definite appearance. Worry, anxiety, anger, etc., are other emotions whose characteristic postures are known to the layman, as well as to the doctor. It is not necessary, to be versed in psychology or other phase of healing to be able to recognize these postural and muscle tension patterns. Everyone is able to determine at a glance when a friend is happy, angry, despondent, etc.

As Feldenkrais[139] has brought out clearly, there are three phases to take into consideration: the appreciation of the stimulus to receptor nerve endings, called perception; the appreciation and integration of the stimulus in terms of the state of the nervous system at that moment, which is sensation; and the reaction of the body and mind, or the psychosomatic aspect. There are no sensations without emotional and somatic overtones. Alexander Lowen, M.D.,[140] contributing to the anthology, *Chiropractic and Mental Health,* by Herman S. Schwartz, states: "There is no neurotic problem which does not manifest itself in every aspect of the individual's function." It could be stated also that the term "somatic," in this instance, must not be confined to its usual limited meaning of the locomotor apparatus, but must be broadened to include the visceral components of the body. The concern of the moment will be with the reactions of the true somatic portion of the body, especially the voluntary or striated muscles, but an attempt will be made to show the mechanisms by which these disturbances contribute to and perpetuate the psychovisceral reflexes, resulting from the emotional stress.

## Psychogenic Subluxations

It must be admitted that the majority of the body's responses to emotion are gross and it is, therefore, difficult to demonstrate single subluxations of the vertebral column as a direct result of emotional trauma only. However, the reader will have little difficulty appreciating that even generalized muscular tension of a psychogenic nature superimposed upon the insult of irritation caused by other, previously discussed forms of stress, could be conceived to be the "straw that broke the camel's back," creating localized subluxations in the regions of the spine under greatest total strain. The available authorities will substantiate the psychovisceral reflexes which upset the normal functioning of the splanchnic structures and by tracing the visceromotor reflexes to the embryologically associated spinal cord segments and thence to the postvertebral musculature local subluxations are well within the realm of possibility and probability.

Perhaps the one best known reaction of the body to emotional stress is the upper cervical postvertebral tension and the headache occasioned by worry, prolonged concentration, or the stress of a protracted meeting in a supercharged atmosphere of unpleasant emotion and cigarette smoke. Not only is much tension found in the suboccipital area but can be demonstrated in the muscles of mastication, especially the Temporalis, in which hypertonicity and frank tenderness may be readily demonstrated by palpation. The Diaphragm is another revealing source of information of the muscular response of the body to emotional stress. Chronic hypertonicity of this vital muscle may be demonstrated in a very high percentage of the population.

One deep inspiration will reveal Diaphragmatic hypertonicity to the experienced observer. If the lower thorax does not lift freely, expand laterally and anteriorly, and the subcostal angle does not become markedly obtuse, there is Diaphragmatic tension. Palpation of the sternal, costal and crural origins of the muscle fibres will reveal tenderness and knots of tension. This exploratory palpation may meet with resistance from the muscles of the anterior and lateral abdominal wall, which are very frequently the victims of associated tension and are unable to relax when the individual lies supine. This tension is readily observable for the relaxation of the abdominal muscles should result in a marked depression of the epigastrium, delineating clearly the borders of the subcostal, or substernal, angle. The tension in this region of the body is, with few exceptions, a direct reflection of emotional disturbance of an unpleasant nature.

Retracing our steps to the brain, the centre for emotion, it is well to appreciate that the human has but two basic, inherited fears with which he is equipped at birth. These are the fear of falling and the fear of a loud noise. The first is associated with the semicircular canals and the Vestibular division of the Auditory Nerve, while the latter is related to the stimuli received from the cochlea by way of the Cochlear division of the Auditory Nerve. All other fears are acquired.

By adult life, fear, worry and anxiety have been well learned and the reasons for such conditioned reflexes seem to increase in numbers with the advancement of civilization. Primitive man had reason to fear personal injury from predatory animals, including other men, and, no doubt, the fear of losing stature and respect in his family and tribe. Modern man has accumulated and produced a multitude of reasons for fear. He must protect himself from mechanical monsters, rather than animals; must avoid the more subtle injuries inflicted by others as they seek to best him in business and social competition; must protect his position, his social status, his family love and respect, his ability to provide the luxuries in keeping with the standard set by his neighbours, etc.

Man has never been bombarded with knowledge of the workings of his own mind and body, with emphasis upon the dire calamities that lurk around every corner in the form of disease, to the comparable degree of the present. Man has never been better informed of every pestilence, earthquake, tornado, or other caprice of nature, occurring in any and every nook and cranny of the globe. Man has never known such awesome weapons of war and never been kept more cognizant of each whim and notion of the leader of each opposing nation.

Added to all such stress and an infinite variety of others, statistics are utilized to the extreme to keep him aware of the slender thread of sanity that separates him from his less fortunate friends confined in mental institutions. There is little cause for speculation as to the reasons why modern man, with his tremendous advances in knowledge and technological skill, is a composite of fear, worry and anxiety.

Into primitive man was built the simple "fight-flight" mechanism, which demanded expression of fear in musculo-skeletal activity, the adequate response to the stimulus. By the use of muscles, the stimulus, which caused the unpleasant emotion of fear, was utilized and dissipated with little residual tension to disturb the smooth, harmonious function of his somatic and visceral components.

Civilized man is prevented by the mores and ethics of society from responding to the emotion of fear in a muscular manner and an innumerable number of the causes cannot be adequately handled by such a response. How does one fight the threat of an atomic bomb; or where can one take refuge, if he were to flee from cancer? Yet, man still has that "fight-flight" mechanism built into his body, demanding an adequate response to the stimulus that has aroused the emotion of fear.

Every physiology textbook explains in detail the subtle alterations in function that take place as components of this "fight-flight" response. Unable to express in action his reaction to this emotion, residual tension of somatic muscles and altered function of visceral structures become the curse of civilized man. With long continued tension of somatic muscle comes structural alteration. The muscles become noticeably "stringy" to the experienced palpating fingers. Chronic hypertonicity with increased and uneven pressure of articular surfaces causes alteration in form and texture of bone, cartilage and ligaments.

This persistent residual tension and alteration in physiological function is reflected back through the afferent components of the nervous system to give rise to the feelings of anxiety, which are prevalent in the vast majority of neurotic states. Anxiety, then, is the body's continued fear-response long after the cause of fear has disappeared.

The original stimulus that aroused the emotion of fear results in a complex body response, of which sudden inspiration by Diaphragmatic contraction, assisted by other somatic muscles, is merely a small segment of the reaction. The entire "fight-flight" mechanism has been thoroughly discussed in the standard physiology texts and needs no complete repetition in this treatise.

Attention is here directed to some of the chief alterations in function, as the body responds to this unpleasant emotion. Tachycardia, rise in blood pressure, slowing of gastro-intestinal movement, the conversion of glycogen to glucose, etc., are a few of the complex reactions. More important to our subject is the fact that the Thalamus is considered to be the emotional centre and from this important relay centre impulses are distributed to many areas of the central nervous system, viz. to the cerebral cortex for conscious awareness, interpretation, association, integration, etc.; to the Corpus Striatum for distribution through the Extrapyramidal System to the Reticular Formation of the brain stem, which, in turn, exercises an inhibitory effect upon the final common motor pathways of control over the antigravity muscles.

Consequent to this inhibitory influence, the body takes on a degree of flexion that is reminiscent of the embryonic position of the body within the protection of the uterus. It is little surprise that anxiety, the expression of chronic fear without immediate cause, has a detrimental influence upon posture and the individual assumes a characteristic arrangement of his structural components. Since anxiety is a facet of neurosis and is also an expression of somatic retrogression toward the embryonic stage of development, it is consistent with the emotional retrogression of the neurotic toward a more infantile mental reaction to the environmental stresses.

Such gross structural and postural reactions to psychogenic stress may be superimposed upon a body bordering upon the breaking point from mechanical or chemical irritations and thus serve to be the final factor in overcoming the resistance of structure, with resultant structural distortion of sufficient degree to warrant the name "subluxation." Or, the emotional stress may lay the background of structural disturbance against which the mechanical and chemical noxious influences play and aid in the determination of the area of the vertebral column that will succumb to the distorting influence of these more selective forms of irritation.

Curtis, Jacobson and Marcus[141] discuss in detail the extensive areas of the central nervous system concerned with emotion and illustrate the circuitry of the afferent and efferent impulses concerned, giving the pathway from hypothalamus to the spinal sympathetic and parasympathetic outflows. The influence via the sympathetics upon the production of epinephrine and norepinephrine by the adrenal medulla with subsequent responses in vascular tissues and release of glucose by the liver is explained. These neural disturbances add an additional dimension to the matter at hand.

## Diaphragm

In an instance of Diaphragmatic hypertonicity, consequent to an unpleasant emotion, afferent impulses will return to the spinal cord from the Diaphragm, entering bilaterally via the posterior nerve roots of the seventh to the twelfth thoracic segments. Intrasegmental synaptic connection may be made with the motor neurones of supply to the segmentally associated postvertebral muscles, thereby increasing their tone and the bilateral pull upon the posterior arches. The crura of the Diaphragm tend to pull forward on the twelfth thoracic and superior two or three lumbar vertebrae, while the post-vertebral muscles tend to approximate the posterior arches of the lower thoracic segments. Especially when coupled with hypertension of the Psoas Major muscles, a local lordosis of the thoraco-lumbar junction may be found. From previous discussion, it should be appreciated that this is an inherently weak area of the vertebral column, as the twelfth thoracic is developmentally a transitional vertebra; this is the transition from the lumbar lordosis to the thoracic kyphosis and the twelfth thoracic is likely to be the apex of a compensatory rotatory scoliosis even in the relatively healthy individual. It is one of the most common areas of subluxation, recognized as such by D. D. Palmer.[142]

The afferent impulses from a contracted Diaphragm may have many other important adverse influences in addition to the disturbance of somatic structure. The medulla of the adrenal glands is supplied by direct preganglionic sympathetic fibres from the lateral horn cells of the fifth to the ninth thoracic neuromeres without having made synaptic connection in any paravertebral or prevertebral sympathetic ganglion. The noxious impulses from the Diaphragmatic contraction may thus stimulate these important sympathetic neurones, especially within the neuromeres of thoracic seven, eight and nine. Increased norepinephrine and epinephrine production is accompanied by tachycardia, rise in blood pressure, slowing of intestinal movements, the conversion of glycogen to glucose, with a rise in blood sugar level. Adrenalin also exercises a stimulatory influence upon the thyroid gland and the secretion of thyroxin compounds the symptom complex.

It will be noted that the symptoms enumerated above are common to most "nervous" states, to anxiety and neurotic disturbances. The chiropractor, willing to take time to release the hypertonicity of the Diaphragm, will be rewarded by increased somatic correction and the alleviation of many of the associated symptoms in short order.

The flattening of the Diaphragm, attendant upon hypertonicity, presses the abdominal viscera inferiorly, increasing the intra-abdominal pressure. The contraction of this important septum between thorax and abdomen also pulls the lower thoracic components, ribs and costal cartilages, inward, further decreasing the capacity of the upper abdomen and forcing viscera inferiorly, both through lack of support and by virtue of the increased pressure. The thorax, in such instances, is flattened, due, in a large measure, to the tendency to assume a more flexed posture as a direct concomitant of the emotional state. Such drooping of the thorax approximates the origins and insertions of the musculature of the abdominal wall, allowing the excess intra-abdominal pressure to bulge the wall anteriorly. This increased prominence is most noticeable in the lower portion, immediately superior to the pubis, with flattening of the upper abdomen. The concentration of splanchnic structures in the lower abdominal cavity, visceroptosis, adds a mechanical and vascular handicap to ptosed abdominal organs as well as the pelvic viscera, upon which they rest.

The Diaphragm, in accordance with the findings of Joe E. Goldthwait,[143] and the consensus of opinion of anatomists, serves as a "second heart," in that its normal action should materially aid in the venous return from the lower extremities, pelvic and abdominal viscera. The wall of the Inferior Vena Cava is intimately related to the margins of the Diaphragmatic hiatus, through which it passes from the abdominal cavity to the thorax and right atrium of the heart. As the Diaphragm contracts and descends, it pulls the Inferior Vena Cava open, materially dilating the lumen of this vein, at the same time increasing the intra-abdominal pressure to propel the venous blood from viscera and lower extremities into the enlarged vein. As the Diaphragm relaxes and ascends, the Inferior Vena Cava is tractioned superiorly, elongated and narrowed, thereby increasing the intraluminal pressure and hastening the blood superiorly into the right atrium of the heart, and the return inferiorly is prevented by venous valves.

No single muscle would seem to be as important to the structural and functional integrity of the human as the Diaphragm, and none other is more adversely influenced by the emotional stresses of life.

## Psychovisceral Reflexes

The psychovisceral reflexes might well receive some consideration at this point to illustrate a more circuitous route in the production of vertebral subluxations.

Boyd[144] has established the possibility of emotional stress occasioning peptic ulcers and Hans Selye[145] has shown that gastric sites of mucosal erosion are the rule in the "Alarm Reaction" to most stressors, including emotional stress, in those members of society who are aggressive and willing to fight, while those prone to flight from the unpleasant situations demonstrate a gastric muscosa that is pale and flattened.

Once established, the ulcerative condition of the gastric mucosa, as an example, would begin bombarding the sixth to the ninth thoracic neuromeres with noxious impulses, especially the right halves of neuromeres seven and eight, according to Rasmussen.[146] The somatic reaction, or visceromotor reflex, expresses itself in hypertonicity of the superior portion of the right abdominal musculature and hypertonicity of the postvertebral muscles of the same side. Subluxation is to be found in this region of the vertebral column and frequently gross distortion in the form of scoliosis.

Kamieth[147] was quoted from his report of research in Munich, Germany, in which 100 patients with peptic ulcers, proven by radiography, demonstrated scolioses of the thoracic spine involving T.6-9 and 90% intervertebral disc changes.

Again, it must be accentuated that the noxious impulses from the hypertonicized Diaphragm return to thoracic segments seven to twelve and in neuromeres seven, eight and nine there could be expected a summation of impulses to stimulate the motor neurones, thereby producing increased tonus of muscles supplied by those segments. Reverting back to previous discussion of the compensatory spinal distortions, it should be recalled that the seventh and eighth thoracic vertebrae are the transition area for the opposed rotatory scolioses and are the apex of the normal thoracic kyphosis. Such stresses may be minor in themselves, but the summation of noxious impulses from a number of sources becomes sufficient to produce a degree of postvertebral muscle hypertonicity consistent with the limitation of segmental movement or frank distortion, which may be considered to be a subluxation. This disrelation and disturbance of segmental function becomes a source of further irritation and either aggravates or perpetuates the problem.

Wilhelm Reich[148] has explained the tendency of those, whose mental and emotional attitudes toward the procreative function have been adversely disturbed, to show a retraction of the external genitalia by an anterior nodding of the pelvis. As discussed in a prior chapter, such pelvic abnormality of relationship to the gravity line necessitates compensatory redistribution of the superimposed body weight around the gravity line, resulting in accentuation of the depths of the primary and secondary curves of the vertebral column. The lumbar and cervical curves would become more lordotic and the thoracic curve more kyphotic, adding stress at the transition areas and the apices of the sinuosities. Feldenkrais[149] and others have stressed that disorders of sexual function, disturbances of breathing, and gastro-intestinal function, as well as anxiety and muscular tension are concomitances of the neurotic status.

## Summary

This brief and sketchy presentation of some examples of the psychogenic stresses as causative agents in the mechanism of subluxation production is hoped to be a stimulus to chiropractic students and chiropractors to delve more deeply into the psychology of the human, look with renewed respect upon the founder of the profession, D. D. Palmer, and heed the exhortations of Dr. Herman S. Schwartz,[150] President Emeritus of the National Council on Psychotherapy, who has for many years attempted to interest the chiropractic profession in a deeper understanding of the functioning of the human mind, the symptom complexes that the mind may produce, and the inestimable value of the correction of somatic disrelations to the normalization of mentation.

Prior to moving into another phase of the problem of subluxation, it is essential to mention that the majority of subluxations and gross distortions of the vertebral column are the result of summation of a number of causative factors. Perhaps the only subluxations that have a single cause are those resulting from traumatic experiences, such as falls, car accidents, etc. Most patients have been subjected to stressors of all three general classes, mechanical, chemical and mental, before sufficient irritation attains the ability to overcome the structural resistance and produces a distortion of a degree worthy of the name "Subluxation."

Furthermore, it is unjustifiable to brand a patient as being neurotic or excuse his symptoms with the convenient diagnosis of "nerves" until the subluxations and somatic distortions have been corrected. In the words of Mennell,[151] "Not until every possible physical cause has been explored are we justified in putting 'functional' as a sole diagnosis: cure the physical basis on which the functional element is built up and the neurasthenic element will usually take care of itself and disappear."

# CHAPTER VIII

# Variability of Response

IN THE FOLLOWING few pages attention will be directed to the modifying influences, which determine the susceptibility of an individual to react to the mechanical, chemical and psychological irritations of his environment by the development of subluxations. There are many and varied predisposing factors which establish the suitable circumstances against which a relatively innocuous irritation results in a pronounced vertebral distortion in one individual, while another of comparable size and physical development may withstand much more severe stress without demonstrable structural disrelation. Furthermore, the same person may be subjected to identical stressors at different times and have no untoward effects time after time, then suffer severe subluxation on another occasion.

Stanley Cobb[152] says, "Brains in different human beings are not alike; their individual history since birth has changed them so that they react differently to the same insults, whether traumatic, neoplastic, degenerative, inflammatory or emotional."

The average, experienced chiropractor has had instances where a patient, engaged in heavy manual labour for years without a history of injury or noticeable adverse results, stoops over to pick up a light object only to suffer an incapacitating lumbo-sacral, or sacroiliac subluxation.

The same general principle is seen to apply in the matter of resistance to infection. Certainly, it is well recognized that all persons exposed to pathogenic micro-organisms and viruses do not develop the symptom manifestations of the disease with which these organisms are associated. An individual may be exposed on one occasion to the influence of pathogenic germs and have no symptom, or sign, of a disease following the established incubation period, but on a later occasion may have a similar exposure, even of lesser degree, and proceed to develop the textbook picture of the disease complex. The Russian scientists appear to have shown conclusively that the parasympathetic system, especially the Vagus nerve, is responsible for the increase in agglutinins and leukocytes, while Gordienko[153] et al report also that the sympathetic stimulation results in leukopaenia. It may be reasoned that any stress that causes the body to sway to the sympatheticly dominated side from the ideal homeostatic state, decreases the resistance of the individual to pathogenic micro-organisms.

The reasons are legion. No two persons are identical in structure, or function, and no individual is the same from hour to hour. The nervous system of each is being conditioned by each new experience, occurring against a background of historical conditioning, some of which is hereditary, but most has been acquired since birth. Thus, the nervous system varies in its irritability from hour to hour and new patterns of neural integration are constantly being established, while previous patterns are being canalized and made less resistant to the passage of neural impulses.

Heredity provides a peculiar backdrop that is as individualistic as fingerprints, if not more so. Each member of the human race has inherited a nervous system with a variable degree of irritability and an ability to organize itself upon stimulation into innumerable patterns of synaptic configurations. A few basic instincts have been inherited, as have the mechanisms for control, regulation and integration of the visceral components, in keeping with the changes of internal and external environment. The degree of stimulation necessary to set activity and response into motion varies considerably. Thus, one person has a nervous system which responds to minor stimuli, while his brother may require much stronger stimuli to cause a reaction. The efficiency with which a nervous system copes with environmental change also varies between persons and in the same individual at different periods of time. The ease with which people are capable of learning new activities and benefiting from the experience of others is not fixed and constant and elaborate tests have been devised to measure and compare this Intelligence Quotient.

"The variations in the sensibility of nerves is past our comprehension. There are no two of us who sense alike. We differ in the make-up of our tissues, and in our likes and dislikes," said D. D. Palmer.[154] While Boyd[155] has stated that, "man's biochemistry, is as individual as his fingerprints," which is not difficult to appreciate when the same author has estimated that there are 70,000 billion cells forming a human and each is a minute chemistry laboratory.

The nervous system lacks stability of irritability, varying with the internal environment of its cells, the chemistry of its cytones, the degree of fatigue, exogenous and endogenous toxins, nutritional status and oxygenation, to mention but a few of the modifying influences.

## Disease

In the words of Dr. Abrahamson[156] in his work, *Body, Mind and Sugar*, ". . . if we recognize this multifaceted complexion of life, we do not fall into the errors of today's faddists and cultists who ascribe all human ills to this or that cause."

It is unrealistic and deceitful for the antagonists of the chiropractic profession to attempt to label this branch of the healing art with the designation of "cult," since D. D. Palmer[157] recognized and expounded upon the manifold causes of structural distortion and went so far as to say: "The cause of all diseases are not in the spine, more especially when defined by the word 'primary.' Quite a large percent have their origin from concussion and pressure on the brain, because of blows on the skull, or an indirect force transmitted to the base. . ."

While the doctor of chiropractic recognizes disease as a change of structure and function, rather than the addition or deletion of something, he recognizes the causes as being almost beyond number and that the response of each body is individualistic to the irritants or stressors and dependent, in the main, upon the irritability of the nervous system at the moment of application of the stimulus. Nor does he lack appreciation for the local tissue conditions, whose response to nerve stimuli is modified by the history, chemistry and environment of the moment.

Looking first to the factors that modify the response of the nervous system to environmental stresses, a few examples from the multitude may serve to indicate the importance of the present condition of irritability as a determinant of the response that is to be expected.

## Toxemia

As F. M. Pottenger[158] has illustrated, generalized toxemia augments the excitability of the entire nervous system, more particularly the sympathetic division of the autonomic portion. Should an individual, suffering from toxemia as a concomitant of poor eliminative function of the emunctories, be exposed to a minor mechanical trauma at the lumbo-sacral articulation, the afferent impulses, originating at the site of injury, would encounter less resistance at synaptic connections within the spinal cord segments, thereby producing an exaggerated motor response and muscular contraction beyond the degree justified by the severity of the damage. Such contraction could well produce the movement of a vertebra out of normal relationship to those contiguous of sufficient magnitude to be classed as a subluxation, or fixation, and, in turn, add afferent bombardment upon the neuromere, perpetuating the problem or increasing the disrelation and extending the results of noxious stimulation.

In order to maintain a balanced consideration it must be added that metabolites or other sources of adverse chemistry of the extra-cellular fluid of the neural system may have opposite effects upon the function of the nervous system. Excess of the acid radicles or outright acidosis depress the function to varying degrees. Guyton[159] states that should the pH of the blood fall below 7.0 disorientation and later, coma result. He makes the point, also, that alkalosis causes overexcitability of the neural system, both peripheral and central, with the peripheral subdivision showing adverse effects first. Muscle tetany is one of the important symptoms of alkalosis. The pronounced conditions of acidosis and alkalosis are seldom seen in ambulatory practice.

It would be propitious to draw attention, once again, to the fact that, as Matzke and Foltz[160] and other neurologists over an extended period have emphasized, each afferent fibre upon entering the spinal cord divides into an ascending and descending branch, each of which travels through a number of neuromeres, giving off collaterals in each segment through which it passes. Matzke and Foltz[161] consider that the proprius, septomarginal, interfascicularis fasciculi and comma bundle are such groups of the limbs of ascending and descending afferent root fibres. Each collateral has the potentiality of eliciting reflex somatic motor and sympathetic responses. With the altered irritability of the entire nervous system, due to toxemia, the synaptic resistance is decreased and afferent impulses become more potent in creating more widespread responses at higher and lower levels than normally receptive to their influence. The local segmental response is increased also.

Sir Charles Sherrington[162] in his dissertation has expressed the fact that, even under normal conditions of irritability, the motor pools of final common motor pathways for specific somatic muscles have a variable resistance to the afferent impulses entering the cord over a specific sensory fibre. It would be anticipated that, under conditions of accentuated general irritability, this selectivity would continue to manifest itself and could be changed only by additional forms of irritation concentrated upon the pools of greater resistance to increase their irritability, thereby reducing the threshhold resistance to a degree permissive of reaction of the motor pools in a manner and combination out of keeping with the normal pattern of response.

With the altered irritability of the entire nervous system, due to toxemia, the synaptic resistance is decreased and afferent impulses become more potent in creating widespread responses at higher or lower levels than normally receptive to their influence. Should additional irritating factors exist, such as distortion of the vertebral column, irritations in embryologically associated visceral structures, etc., the somatic reflex response may be at an unexpected level, as well as of unanticipated severity at the expected level.

For purposes of illustration, an example may be best utilized to make the above abundantly clear. The afferent impulses from the strained tissues in the lumbo-sacral region, returning through sensory fibres of the fifth lumbar nerve and posterior nerve root, travel over collaterals in the fifth lumbar neuromere and each segment through which the ascending division of the sensory axon may pass on its course cephalad for a variable number of segments.

As Sherrington[163] has explained and other authorities have confirmed, these collaterals are most numerous and potent in the segment of entrance and become more scattered and less potent the further the ascending, or descending, branch travels from the point of entrance into the spinal cord. In the instance in question, all neural components are more irritable than normal because of the generalized toxemia, but at the third lumbar neuromere there is added the irritation of the stress of this vertebral segment being the transition between a right rotatory scoliosis in the lower lumbar area and a left rotatory scoliosis in the upper lumbar and lower thoracic regions. Also, the third lumbar experiences the stress of being the apex of the lumbar lordosis. Our present example shows a subluxation of the third vertebra in response to a relatively minor mechanical stressor centred at the junction between fifth lumbar and sacrum, because of the summation of irritation, each inadequate to produce the necessary degree of muscular contraction, despite the generalized hyperirritability of the nervous system. Such peculiar responses of any region of the vertebral column are by no means rare and hold no element of mystery for the chiropractor versed in neurology and the mechanisms of basic distortion and compensation.

Toxemia has the less dramatic effect of making the patient more pain sensitive than usual. Pottenger[164] has illustrated the increased susceptibility of the patient with lung or intestinal disease to viscerosensory reflexes, or referred pain, in the presence of toxemia. The same may be said for the patient with a somatic disturbance, such as arthritis, sprains, or subluxations. Considering the latter, it may be appreciated that many people have subluxations of vertebral segments without conscious awareness of the structural problem until toxemia, or other modifying influences, reduce the synaptic resistance of the neural pathways to that degree necessary for the transmission of neural impulses from the locus of distortion to the higher brain centre, the postcentral gyrus of the cerebral cortex, where the stream of impulses are interpreted as pain or discomfort in the involved spinal area. Such developments often bring the person to the office of a chiropractor with the expectation that, since they have just become aware of the disturbance, it should be corrected in one or two visits, little appreciating that the problem is chronic and multifaceted.

It is agreed by physiologists that the structural units, the neurones, of the nervous system are living, functioning cellular organisms, requiring nutrition, oxygen and efficient elimination for their normal function. G. L. Freeman[165] has quoted the experiments of Tashiro, who demonstrated the metabolism of the neural tissues, showing that an increase in oxygen consumption and an increase in carbon dioxide production occurs with activity of these cells. Other investigators demonstrated that neurones produce a minute amount of heat as a result of their metabolic processes. Furthermore, the chromidial inclusions, called Nissl bodies or granules, demonstrated by Minckler[166] to be accumulations of the ribosomes on the endoplasmic reticulum to the degree that identification with the light microscope has been possible, undergo alteration in size and distribution with neural activity and must be replenished during the periods of rest from the intercellular fluids surrounding the cells. Further, the same author provides the information that each ribosome is approximately 180 A units in diameter, contains about 50% RNA and protein synthesis occurs on the surface.

## Anoxia

It may be appreciated that any disturbance of either the oxygen or nutritional supply will have a deleterious result upon the function of the nervous system and hence alter its response to the stressors of the environment. Freeman[167] has mentioned that the neural tissues require glucose for their metabolism, but an excess, as in diabetes mellitis, results in a marked decrease in irritability and a marked decrease in the functional activity.

Another authority of later contribution, Curtis[168] has demonstrated the dependence of neurones upon a continuous optimum supply of oxygen and glucose.

Abrahamson[169] gives convincing evidence of the greatly increased irritability and erratic behaviour of the nervous system, due to hypoglycemia attendant upon hyperinsulinism resulting from a diet high in carbohydrates and coffee, but low in protein and fats.

It is to be appreciated that the case experiencing a depression of neural irritability would respond less to environmental irritations than the hyperirritable person. In the former, the stressors would have to be stronger, or more numerous, to result in the degree of muscular contraction necessary to produce a vertebral fixation or subluxation, while relatively minor noxious stimuli could be responsible for pronounced subluxations in that person of irritable neural disposition.

Anoxia plays an important role in disturbing the smooth, harmonious function of the nervous system. It has been well established that anoxia may be of four major classes: lack of oxygen in the inspired lung content; inability of the blood to transport oxygen in sufficient quantities, as in anaemic conditions; deficiency in quantity of blood reaching the tissues, ischemia; or, congestive, as a result of stagnation and the slowing of blood flow through the tissues. The depletion of oxygen supply below the normal requirements has an adverse influence upon the neurones of the central nervous system and G. L. Freeman[170] emphasizes that the cerebral gray matter, or mass of cytones, is very sensitive to anoxia and furthermore, that the higher brain functions appear to be disturbed first by anoxia. Physiologists have demonstrated the irreparable damage to neural cell bodies of the brain occasioned by complete anoxia for more than three minutes. Anoxia results in a variable degree of chromatolysis of the Nissl granules with attendant progressive failure of function.

That acute anoxemias of sudden onset may result in convulsions has been pointed out by Alpers.[171]

H. W. Magoun and Ruth Rhines[172] report in their writings the experiments of Harreveld, Marmont and Harreveld which demonstrated that anoxia has a selectivity injurious effect upon the neurones of the spinal cord, disturbing the intercalated neurones to the point of dissolution with little, or no, adverse effect upon the anterior horn cells and their afferent fibres from the posterior nerve roots. They showed that such selective disturbance sets free the anterior horn cells from the inhibitory influence of higher neural centres, resulting in spasticity.

Cobb[173] makes mention of the variation of the vascularity of the brain in accordance with the oxygen requirements. Thus, "white matter has from 200 to 300 mm. of capillary length per cubic millimeter of brain substance, while gray matter has from 600 to 1000 mm." Further, this author has computed from the experimentation of others that 1400 grams of human brain would receive blood at the rate of 700 cc. per minute, or one quarter of the volume displaced by the left ventricle of the heart each minute, although the brain is a mere one-fiftieth of the entire weight of the body. These figures graphically demonstrate the importance of a constant supply of arterial blood to the central nervous system to maintain functional integrity. Thus, any factor that modifies the blood supply, modifies the function and the response to environmental change.

In the words of M. Feldenkrais,[174] "The excitability of the nervous tissue depends very closely on the chemical composition of the irrigating blood and the hormones present, its pH, salt content, etc."

Not only is the quantity of blood important to the nervous tissue, but the quality is of equal import. Disturbance of one, or the other, is equally detrimental to function. Venous drainage is an additional factor that must be adequate to maintain normal neural function. If the detritus of cellular metabolism is not efficiently removed by the venous flow, the cells become intoxicated with their endogenous metabolites, materially altering their functional capacity and their response to stimulation.

## Fatigue

Fatigue plays an important role in disturbing the excitability of the nervous system and modifying its response to the stimuli received from the environment. Albert Kuntz[175] quotes the experimentations of Vas, Lambert and Mann in the latter part of the last century, in which they, working separately, demonstrated the enlargement of neural cytones, the migration of the chromidial substance to the periphery of the cells, then a gradual decrease in size of the cytones as fatigue commenced and chromatolysis was demonstrated as fatigue increased.

Pottenger[176] and the standard physiologists have demonstrated that the effects of injury, including fatigue, is first, an increased excitability of the affected neurones, followed by disruption of function as the progressive disturbance of the structural components of the nervous system, the neurones, undergo alteration with associated change in function to the point of complete loss of functional ability and irreparable loss of integrity. A mild degree of general fatigue increases the irritability of the person and is readily noted by the change in emotional tone, a disposition that becomes more irrascible than is in keeping with the usual character of the individual. Slight affront results in violent reaction. So, too, slight noxious stimulation may result in violent muscle contraction and osseous distortion out of proportion to the degree of physical, chemical or mental stress.

Guyton[177] discusses the fatigue of synaptic connections and points out that presynaptic terminals of nerve fibres store excitatory transmitter chemical for about 10,000 normal transmissions, which could be used up in a few seconds. In such instances the reflex effect would quickly dwindle and a decrease in activity would result. However, he goes on to mention that prolonged stimulation over days may result in an increase in the number of presynaptic terminals with alteration in size and shape. This alteration may permit activity across the synapse by a lesser stimulus.

These serve but to direct the attention of the reader to the many and varied factors which modify the response of the human to irritation. No claim is made for a complete coverage of these contributory influences, which modify the anticipated responses to any given situation and make the practice of any healing art an art, rather than a science and the application of the particular art truly "practice." Thus, with experience dawns recognition that in the care of human health the unexpected is likely to be the rule; that the textbooks describe the average, not the majority; and that the arts of diagnosis and prognosis are dependent, in large measure, upon the knowledge of functional neurology of the doctor and his skill in eliciting a thorough case history, including the habits, nutrition, eliminative status, toxic intake, etc., of his patient. These are modifying variables which make the practice of chiropractic and every form of healing a constant challenge and an intriguing pursuit.

As progress is made in the discussion of the tissue responses to the disturbing influence of the vertebral subluxation, the reader will be introduced to further variables and vagaries that change the response of the same tissues under peculiar circumstances and add complications to the well ordered practice of the doctor of chiropractic.

# CHAPTER IX

# Basic Architecture of the Nervous System

ONLY THE MOST primitive outline of the nervous system can be given in a single chapter of such a book as this and the reader must be referred to the classics of anatomy, as written by Gray, Cunningham, Piersol, Krieg and the multitude of other authorities. Yet for the discussion to follow to be complete and intelligible, it is necessary to touch upon the subject to provide a basis of common understanding between writer and reader.

The nervous system of the embryo commenced development at an early stage, first evidenced at the end of the second week of gestation, according to Curtis,[178] and developed from the ectodermal layer from which the integument, nails, hair and other important structures are derived. The relationship of the nervous system and the skin is of particular interest, since the skin continues throughout life to be a very important receptor organ for sensory perception, which keeps the central nervous system informed of changes in the environment. Hence, within the skin are those specialized end-organs stimulated by light touch, others by heat, still others by cold, different types of pressures and those for pain.

Nor is the skin the only structure to send information into the central nervous system. Every muscle, tendon, joint capsule, viscus and blood vessel, as well as the periosteum of bone and the perichondrium of cartilage supplies a continuous flow of afferent (sensory) information to the central nervous system. In addition, there are the organs of special sensation: the eyes, the ears, the nose, the tongue, which provide additional afferent impulses. In all there are five times as many fibres conducting impulses into the central nervous system as there are conducting from the central nervous system to the muscles, blood vessels, glands and organs supplied and controlled by this system, consisting of the brain and spinal cord.

As in the case of every organ and structure of the body, the nervous system is constructed of basic units, the cells, called neurones. The cell body, or cytone, differs little from cells of other tissues, having a nucleus, chromatin inclusions, etc. The distinguishing characteristic of a neurone is the greatly elongated processes that grow out from the cell body or cytone. The most primitive sensory neurone has a cytone that is bipolar in shape; that is, the cytone is spindle-shaped and from one pole a process of variable length grows outward toward the periphery and this is called the dendrite, conducting impulses toward the cell body; from the other pole of the cytone a process, which conducts away from the cell body, grows for a variable distance also. These neurones belong to the sensory division of the nervous system and the cytones have migrated away from the central nervous system to take up positions beyond the confines of the brain stem or spinal cord. Only a few examples of this embryonic type of afferent neurone remain in the adult, such as in the eye, the fibres responsible for the sense of smell, and from both divisions of the internal ear, serving both the orientation of the head in space and hearing.

The remainder of the afferent cytones of the human have assumed a unipolar appearance by the growth of the dendrite and axone towards each other until the appearance of a more or less round cytone with a common stem, which splits after a short distance into a dendrite and an axone, is the end result. This appearance and the term "split-axone" are deceiving, as dendrite and axone remain distinct in both structure and function. The cytones of these afferent fibres are grouped together into clusters to form ganglia, which have fibrous coverings and retain a distinct appearance. Such a ganglion is found in relation to every spinal nerve, close to the central nervous system (spinal cord) and upon a number of the sensory cranial nerves.

The dendrite and axone of a sensory nerve fibre may each measure several feet in length. An example of such length would be a nerve fibre that receives impulses from its end-organ in the joint capsule of the big toe, conducts these impulses to the cytone located in a ganglion within the vertebral canal in the lower lumbar region, from the cytone the axone passes into the spinal cord and assists in the formation of the Tractus Cuneatus to enter the skull prior to terminating by connection with a second order neurone in the Nucleus Cuneatus of the Medulla Oblongata, the continuation of the spinal cord within the cranial cavity.

A third type of cytone is found to be consistent for all efferent neurones, the Final Common Motor Pathway or Fibre. These are described as multipolar because there are a number of relatively short dendrites projecting from the cell, thereby permitting the cell body to be stimulated by impulses from a great many different sources, and a single long axone, which leaves the central nervous system, runs a variable course as an element of a nerve, reaches a somatic muscle, divides into fine filaments, each of which supplies a single muscle fibre. Each axone controls from fifty to one hundred and

fifty muscle fibres, (Guyton[179] has modified these numbers drastically in his latest edition to from three to two thousand muscle fibres),
and the entire complex, neurone and muscle fibres supplied, is
referred to as being a Motor Unit.

A fourth type, by far the most numerous, is the multipolar connector, internuncial, or intercalated neurone, which forms the bulk
of the central nervous system. These have numerous dendrites and a
single axone and the entire neurone is confined to the central
nervous system, with the exception of those belonging to the autonomic system. The latter send their axones out of the central nervous
system to make connections with the efferent, or effector, neurones
located in ganglia, or plexuses, relatively close to the organs to be
supplied. The majority of connector neurones permit the complexity
of activity and response of the central nervous system, which will
receive some consideration in the next chapter.

It should be noted that the cell body of each neurone is the
trophic centre for that unit, as confirmed by Minckler[180] and with
the electron microscope neurotubules of 200 to 300 Å diameters
have been demonstrated by Curtis, Jacobson and Marcus[181] with the
greater number found in the dendrites and axon hillock. Other investigators have hypothesized that these microtubules of varying size
provide conduction channels for protein molecules of differing sizes.
There has been some speculation as to whether this mechanism provides an explanation of the trophic influence of neurones upon the
tissues supplied.

## Sheaths of Fibres

The fibres outside of the central nervous system, whether dendrites or axones, and many of the fibres within the brain and spinal
cord, are insulated by a white, fatty material, called myelin and are
thus referred to as being myelinated fibres. It has been mentioned by
Guyton[182] that more than half of all afferent fibres of peripheral
nerves are of the type C (0.2 to 1.0 microns in diameter, conducting
at 0.2 to 2 meters per second, and poorly myelinated). This con-
serves space. Of course, all postganglionic autonomic fibres are of
this type. Where a great number of myelinated fibres are collected together within the central nervous system, the substance is white in
appearance and is called "white matter" to distinguish it from the
"gray matter," which is composed of cell bodies and unmyelinated
fibres. This nomenclature is used especially in discussion of the

central nervous system and modified slightly for description of the autonomic division of the nervous system.

The fibres outside of the central nervous system have a further sheath, called neurolemma, external to the myelin, which terminates at the surface of the spinal cord or brain stem. Until recent years it has been taught that the neurolemma was essential for regeneration of an injured axone or dendrite, and that there could be no regrowth of damaged fibres within the central nervous system, since these fibres are devoid of neurolemma. However, in recent years, investigators have been able to demonstrate regrowth of fibres within the confines of the central nervous system, following damage and Wallerian degeneration. Much of this work has been done in the University of Indiana.

The cells and fibres of the central nervous system are supported and bound together by additional cells of connective tissue, called neuroglia, which have many shapes and sizes, as well as names. Most of this connective tissue is derived from ectoderm, rather than mesoderm.

The brain and spinal cord are enveloped by a sheath of connective tissue, the Pia Mater. A potential space separates the Pia Mater from the second protective layer, the Arachnoid Mater. The Subarachnoid Space is a potential, honeycombed space, filled with cerebro-spinal fluid, which serves as a supporting and protective element and may serve as a source of nutrient to the delicate neural structures. Beyond the Arachnoid is a second space, the Subdural Space, filled with lymph, a fluid distinct from that of the cerebro-spinal fluid. The Dura Mater is the tough, fibrous, outer covering, which in the cranial cavity of the skull is fused with the periosteum to form the inner lining of the bones. Specialized folds of Dura Mater separate, support and protect various portions of the brain. In the vertebral canal the Dura Mater is separated from the walls of the spinal canal by the Extra-dural Space, filled with loose connective tissue, plexuses of veins and fat.

## The Medulla Spinalis

The spinal cord, with which we are primarily concerned in this consideration of the subluxation, extends from the level of the Foramen Magnum of the skull to the lower border of the body of the second lumbar vertebra, and is said to be composed of thirty-one segments, or neuromeres, to which is appended one pair of spinal nerves for each segment. Thus, there are thirty-one pairs of spinal nerves.

The periphery of the spinal cord is composed of white matter, innumerable fibres, each with its coating of myelin. These are arranged in named tracts or bundles and conduct nerve impulses either superiorly or inferiorly, some merely one or two segments, while others may traverse the entire length of the spinal cord and extend for some distance within the brain stem.

Those fibres, which are the axones of afferent or sensory neurones from peripheral structures, have unipolar cell bodies located in ganglia outside the central nervous system. Others are the axones of cell bodies located within the spinal cord segment and are a portion of one of the connector type neurones, with which the first order neurone has made synaptic connection in the segment of entrance and are now conducting the impulses to nuclei at higher levels. Still other fibres of the white matter may be axones of cell bodies located in higher brain centres, descending to influence efferent cells of the neuromeres. These fibres, without number and of different courses, origins, terminations and functions, are grouped together, according to a plan, into named bundles, tracts, or fasciculi and some will require further discussion in the course of these writings.

It should be noted that the afferent pathways occupy the periphery of the cord, the motor pathways from the higher centres are deeper, while the tracts which influence splanchnic function are even more deeply placed in closer proximity to the central gray matter of the cord. Lying adjacent to the gray matter on all four sides are the intersegmental tracts, or Fasciculi Proprii, which serve as the association fibres of varying length, linking segments in function, permitting the spinal cord to be truly a unit of structure and function. The thirty-one neuromeres, each with some degree of autonomy over those structures derived from the ectoderm, mesoderm and entoderm of the same embryological segment, are linked and integrated by the intersegmental pathways.

The central portion of the spinal cord is composed of gray matter in an H-shape, or butterfly-shape. As previously mentioned, gray matter is primarily an aggregation of cell bodies and unmyelinated fibres, hence the colour. This central mass of gray matter is divided into two posterior gray columns and two anterior gray columns, and the two symmetrical halves of the gray substance are joined by the gray commissure, in which may be seen the tiny neural canal, passing in a vertical direction and continuous above with the fourth ventricle, while ending inferiorly as the Terminal Ventricle of the Conus

Medullaris. The portion of each gray column, located in a neuromere, may be referred to as a horn. Thus, there is an anterior and a posterior horn in each half of each neuromere of the spinal cord.

The twelve thoracic segments or neuromeres and the first to the third or fourth lumbar segments, as well as the second and third, or third and fourth, sacral segments have, in addition to the anterior and posterior horns, lateral horns. Each of these portions of the central gray matter will now receive consideration as to their peculiarities of structure in this chapter and as to their specialized functions in the next chapter.

## The Anterior Gray Column

The anterior gray column is composed of multipolar cell bodies, which are all very similar in size and structure and all have numerous, relatively short dendrites, allowing for the reception of impulses from a number of sources. The axones of all of these cells leave the spinal cord, forming the thirty-one pairs of Anterior Nerve Roots, one pair for each neuromere.

By devious and variable routes the axones of each of these cells continue to the periphery to supply from 50 to 150 fibres of a somatic muscle. Each neurone and its associated somatic muscle fibres form a unit of function, a Motor Unit. All impulses that are destined to reach a particular group of muscle fibres do so by way of that efferent neurone only, which is, therefore, called the Final Common Motor Pathway, or Lower Motor Neurone. No matter the source of afferent impulses, there is only one motor neurone capable of conducting impulses to any given muscle fibre. Without integrity of this Final Common Motor Pathway the group of associated muscle fibres would lack the control of the central nervous system, undergo paralysis, loss of tone and degeneration would be their lot.

## Pain and Temperature

The Posterior Horn, or Column, is differentiated into a number of parts, each having cells of varying size and function. The tip of the horn is a crescent-shaped collection of cells of relatively small size and the whole has a jelly-like appearance, hence the name Substantia Gelatinosa of Rolando. This specialized group of cells receives the impulses of pain and temperature from the periphery by way of first order neurones, whose cells are unipolar in type and located in ganglia beyond the confines of the central nervous system. The axones of these cells enter the cord and ascend several segments prior to terminating in the Substantia Gelatinosa. This bundle of ascending fibres is called the Posterolateral Tract or Tract of Lissauer and is located between the tip of the posterior horn and the surface of the cord. The axones of the cells of the Substantia Gelatinosa then decussate in front of the Gray Commissure, forming the White Commissure, and turn upward as the Lateral Spinothalamic Tract, a fasciculus of the lateral white funiculus of the spinal cord. This tract continues throughout the remainder of the spinal cord, through the Medulla Oblongata, the Pons and the Mid-brain to reach the Thalamus where synaptic connection is made with the third order neurones. The latter conduct the impulses by way of their axones as a portion of the Internal Capsule and the Corona Radiata to reach the Postcentral Gyrus of the cerebral cortex, in which conscious awareness and interpretation of pain and temperature occur.

The above is the classical description of the pathway of a pain, but more recent investigations have demonstrated that this is the course for the delta type A fibres that conduct at the rate of three to twenty meters per second, resulting in the pricking type pain, synapse in the posterior nuclear portion of the thalamus. A second type of pain of a burning and aching sensation, conducted into the cord by type C fibres at 0.5 to 2.0 meters per second, synapse as above, turn upward and, as Guyton[183] describes this pathway, participate in the formation of the Spinoreticular Tract to terminate in the reticular areas of medulla, pons, and mesencephalon. The burning and aching pain fibres synapse in the intralaminar nuclei of the thalamus.

Melzack,[184] on the other hand, considers that pain may be due to the number of fibres stimulated and the rate of transmission, rather than the passage of signals over specific types of fibres.

## Light Touch

Deep to the above described area of the posterior gray column is another collection of cells of similar multipolar design, but slightly larger size, arranged in a somewhat sponge-like formation and named the Substantia Spongiosa. This group of cells receives impulses from the peripheral receptors of light touch, which have been conducted into the medulla spinalis by first order neurones, whose cell bodies also are to be found in the ganglion of the appropriate posterior nerve root. The axones of the cells of the Substantia Spongiosa decussate within the Gray Commissure and then take up their position as part of the Anterior Spinothalamic Tract in the anterior white column. The authorities are not in agreement as to the existence of the particular tract, but it has been thoroughly described by some, hence is included in this consideration.

Within the Medulla, the Anterior and Lateral Spinothalamic Tracts unite to form the Spinal Lemniscus, which, at a higher level, aids in the formation of the Medial Lemniscus, thereby losing identity but continuing to the Thalamus as described above. The third order neurones begin in the Thalamus and take a similar course to that previously mentioned. It should be emphasized that the axones of the thalamic cells reach the cortex without interruption, although the name of the fibre tracts through which they pass may be changed several times.

Another pathway for the sensation of light touch meets with greater unanimity of opinion among the neurologists. The first order neurones of light touch with neurones of proprioception from muscles, tendons, ligaments, joint capsules, etc., assist in the formation of each posterior nerve root and their unipolar cell bodies are part of each posterior nerve root ganglion. The axones of these neurones, upon entering the spinal cord, give off collaterals in the segment of entrance, as well as sending a division in an inferior direction as part of the Septomarginal System in the posterior white column. At different levels this Septomarginal Tract assumes different names, but the fibres and the function remain the same. These descending branches provide collaterals for each neuromere through which they pass and terminate at variable levels below their point of entrance.

The ascending divisions of the axones take part in the formation of the Tractus Gracilis or Tractus Cuneatus, depending upon the level of entrance. Those fibres, entering below the level of the mid-thoracic region, take part in the formation of the Tractus Gracilis, while those from mid-thoracic level superior take part in the structure of the Tractus Cuneatus, located lateral to the Gracilis. It is not until the Nuclei Gracilis and Cuneatus, on the posterior surface of the Medulla Oblongata, are reached that these first order neurones terminate.

The course of the second order neurones, whose cytones form the above mentioned nuclei, is complicated and must be considered in groups. Those, conducting the impulses of light touch and conscious proprioception, leave the nuclei as Internal Arcuate Fibres, decussate, forming the Great Sensory Decussation, turn upward as part of the Medial Lemniscus, above mentioned, reach the Thalamus to terminate by synaptic connection with the third order neurones, which continue the conduction of the impulses to the Postcentral Gyrus, as previously described.

## Proprioception

Other axones of cells in the Gracile and Cuneate Nuclei are called Anterior and Posterior External Arcuate Fibres. The Anterior External Arcuate Fibres, after leaving the nuclei, run forward in the lateral peripheral portion of the Medulla, decussate, continue posteriorly and superiorly on the opposite lateral surface to enter the Inferior Cerebellar Peduncle to reach the cortex of the cerebellum, while the Posterior External Arcuate Fibres take a more direct course, do not decussate, and help in the formation of the Inferior Cerebellar Peduncle of the same side to reach the cortex of the cerebellum.

Still more medial in the posterior gray column than the Substantia Spongiosum is another collection of multipolar cells of slightly less uniformity throughout the cord. In the thoracic segments, especially, these cells are aggregated into a well defined mass, called the Dorsal Nucleus, Thoracic Nucleus, Nucleus Dorsalis, etc., while in other regions the cytones are in scattered clumps and are then referred to as Clark's Vesicular Column.

First order neurones carry proprioceptive, or kinesthetic impulses from muscles, tendons, ligaments, joint capsules, etc., into the spinal cord by way of the posterior nerve roots and make synaptic connection with the dendrites of the cells, forming the above named nuclei. The axones of the second order turn upward as the Anterior and Posterior Spinocerebellar Tracts, which form the most peripheral tracts of the lateral white column. A few of the second order neurones have decussated and these enter into formation of the Anterior Spinocerebellar Tract. Neither of these tracts are concerned with conduction of impulses to consciousness, but, rather, the Posterior Tract enters into the formation of the Inferior Cerebellar Peduncle and the fibres terminate in the cortex of the cerebellum, while the Anterior Tract continues further superiorly to reach the lower border of the Mid-brain prior to turning posteriorly into the Superior Cerebellar Peduncle to enter the cerebellum and terminate in the cortex.

## Association

The remainder of the Posterior Gray Column is composed of scattered cells, referred to as the Reticular Formation. This collection of cells is for connector purposes, that is association of one area with another, either in segments above, below, the same side, or on the opposite side. The gray commissure is composed of cells of association also.

It must be emphasized that each first order neurone, upon entering the spinal cord, divides into an ascending and a descending branch from each of which collaterals branch at right angles to enter the gray matter to effect synaptic connection with the dendrites of one or more connector neurones. The axone of such an intercalated neurone may then travel forward into the Anterior Gray Horn to stimulate a motor, or efferent, neurone which then sends impulses out of the cord to cause contraction of the associated muscle cells of the Motor Unit. This forms the simplest Reflex Arc, which receives constant attention throughout the pages of this book.

The association fibre may have synapsed with cells of the Lateral Gray Horn to create activity in splanchnic structures rather than somatic muscle response, or a combination of responses may occur with equal facility. Each is considered a simple Reflex Arc.

Numerous association neurones in chain formations may become involved in the conduction of a nerve impulse to the opposite side of the cord or to segments superior or inferior to the point of entrance of the original axone into the spinal cord.

## Splanchnic Connections

The Lateral Gray Column, as found extending through the twelve thoracic segments and the first three or four lumbar neuromeres are peculiar in that these are connector neurones, whose axones leave the cord to aid in the formation of the anterior nerve root, to make synaptic connection with approximately five effector neurones, whose cell bodies are located in ganglia beyond the vertebral column, either in the Paravertebral Chain of ganglia or in Prevertebral Ganglia in relatively close proximity to the visceral structures to be supplied.

The cell bodies, which are concentrated in the ganglia, send their axones to blood vessels of the entire body, to some viscera, to the Erector Pili muscles of the skin and to the sweat glands of the skin as secretomotor fibres. The group of axones of the Lateral Gray Column are referred to as being Preganglionic Sympathetic Fibres and the entire collection as the spinal outflow of the Sympathetic Division of the Autonomic nervous system. The axones of the cells in autonomic ganglia are said to be Postganglionic Fibres. The Preganglionic Fibres are well myelinated and white in appearance, while the Postganglionic Fibres are poorly myelinated with a gray colour. Both forms boast neurilemma beyond the spinal cord.

The other division of the Autonomic nervous system, the Parasympathetic, is represented in the spinal cord by only those cytones grouped together to form the lateral horns of the second and third, or third and fourth, sacral segments. The axones of these cell bodies, which are also Connector Neurones and Preganglionic, myelinated fibres leave the spinal cord in the anterior nerve roots of the two sacral nerves and make synaptic connection with effector neurones, the Postganglionic, poorly myelinated fibres, which are very short and terminate in the viscera of the pelvis and lower abdomen.

The cranial outflow of preganglionic parasympathetic fibres is by way of five cranial nerves from the brain stem, III, VII, IX and X and the XI, with which we are not immediately concerned.

## Spinal Nerves

It has been previously mentioned that each segment of the medulla spinalis is distinguished by the attachment of one spinal nerve on each side. These nerves vary in size and in their fibre content. Harold Swanberg[185] reported in his book that there is a gradual increase in the supero-inferior diameter of the foramina from 8.5 mm. for the fourth cervical to 19 mm. for the second lumbar and a gradual decrease in size beyond this group. Swanberg[186] pointed out, after very careful measurements, that the space of the inter-vertebral foramina occupied by the nerve trunk varies from 1/12th to 1/3rd.

Each nerve trunk divides within the vertebral canal into an anterior and a posterior nerve root and each root is further subdivided into rootlets, or radicles, as it approaches the surface of the spinal cord. The rootlets of the anterior nerve are scattered over an area on the anterolateral aspect of each neuromere and are found to be composed of a great number of efferent fibres; the eight pairs of cervical roots are made up of somatic motor fibres only for the supply of voluntary muscle fibres; the twelve thoracic anterior nerve roots are composed of both somatic efferent or motor fibres and preganglionic sympathetic fibres, as are the first three or four lumbar nerves; the fourth and fifth lumbar nerves, the first sacral nerve, the fourth and fifth sacral and the coccygeal nerves have only somatic motor fibres in their composition; the second and third, or third and fourth, sacral nerves have, in addition to the somatic efferent fibres, preganglionic parasympathetic fibres; and the remaining sacral, whether it be the second or the fourth, is purely somatic efferent.

The posterior nerve root of each of the thirty-one pairs of spinal nerves are composed of the axones of the unipolar cells located in the Posterior Nerve Root Ganglia, which are located either in the intervertebral foramina or in the vertebral canal. Each posterior root is divided into a number of rootlets or radicles arranged in a vertical line as they pierce the surface of the cord through the floor of the posterolateral sulcus. Each root is considered by most authorities to be strictly afferent or sensory, returning impulses from receptor end-organs in the skin, muscles, tendons, joint capsules, ligaments, perio-steum, perichondrium, blood vessels and viscera.

The fibres of the posterior nerve roots vary in size in accordance with the type of impulses they must carry. The larger the diameter of the fibre, the quicker is the rate of conduction. The fibres of light touch are the largest and the fibres of pain and temperature are the smallest. It has been previously emphasized that each form of affer-ent impulse commands the path of specific fibres, which upon enter-ing the spinal cord or brain stem in the case of cranial nerves, are grouped together into separately named tracts, synapse with differ-ent groups of cells within the gray column and at differing levels. Furthermore, the second order neurones for each modality assist in the formation of distinct fibre tracts with their own peculiar termina-tion in higher brain centres.

As has been illustrated previously, some of the afferent impulses reach conscious awareness and many others do not, but, rather, create reflex responses before the conscious centres have had time to be cognizant of the stimulus, interpret the information, or react by sending the impulses along to motor centres which would stimulate the Final Common Motor fibres.

The afferent impulses arising in viscera are not readily appreciated as such by the cerebral cortex and it is most frequently necessary for the afferent fibres of the first order to make synaptic connection with the fibres of the second order whose function it is to conduct information from somatic structures. Upon arrival in the cerebral cortex, this information is interpreted as arising in a somatic struc-ture, rather than in the viscus. If this sensation be pain, it is called a Referred Pain. The doctor's constant awareness of this phenomenon provides him with diagnostic acumen and guards against mistaken direction of treatment.

Much of the proprioceptive or kinesthetic information derived from the articulations and muscles does not reach the level of consciousness, but is utilized for the postural and tonal adjustments of the human structure, against which the reflex and purposeful, voluntary, actions take place. Other proprioceptive information does have a direct pathway of conduction to the centres of awareness to provide information of the position of each and every part of the somatic body in space and in relation to the other segments. Further, this kinesthetic information is necessary for an appreciation of weight, size and shape of objects handled, etc.

It has been brought to the reader's attention previously that each afferent fibre, upon entering the spinal cord or brain stem, divides into an ascending and a descending branch from which collaterals are given off at right angles to the course of the fibre to enter the gray matter, where synaptic connections are made. Guyton[187] is more specific, stating that the C and delta type A fibres travel upward for 1 to 6 segments and the descending branches for from 1 to 4 segments prior to synapsing with cells of the posterior horn. Sherrington[188] has stated that the greater number of collaterals are given off in the segment entered by the afferent fibre and the spacing between collaterals becomes wider as the fibre passes further cephalad or caudad from its point of ingress. The collaterals may cause reflex action of the simplest form, involving only an efferent neurone. Or, many connector neurones may be disturbed in a pattern of intricate connections, involving higher brain centres and finally the Lower Motor Neurones or Final Common Motor Pathways.

It should be appreciated that reflex activity may be caused in the tissues and organs supplied by the sympathetic division of the autonomic nervous system or the parasympathetic division. These splanchnic structures may receive their impulses via either the spinal or cranial outflow. Furthermore, it is inconceivable to imagine a somatic reflex without a corresponding disturbance in splanchnic structures. Sherrington[189] stated that the idea of a simple two neurone reflex arc is an abstraction of convenience for understanding the function of the nervous system, but in reality the reflex response is likely to be "plurisegmental." That is, not only are more than two neurones involved in a simple reflex, but more than one segment of the spinal cord and more than one division of the nervous system would take part in integrated action or reaction.

## The Synapse

The association of the axone of one neurone with the dendrite of another occurs at a synapse, an anatomical structure of definite construction and specific function. The axone, or its collateral, breaks up into a tuft of thread-like fibrils to come into close relation, but not contact, with a similar end-brush of the dendrite of another neurone. The tiny space between these brush-like tufts may be decreased by a process of neurobiotaxis, or growth towards each other, as the synapse is utilized, thereby decreasing the resistance, making it easier for the next impulse to cross the gap to stimulate the second neurone. The synapse assures one-way conduction from axone to dendrite and the variable resistance offered by different synapses determines the pathway to be taken by an impulse. Most synapses are located in the gray matter of the central nervous system and in the ganglia beyond the confines of the neuraxis.

The description of a synapse supra has been modified drastically by electron microscopic studies which show that the axone fibril expand into a terminal bouton, containing vesicles and mitochondria, with a thickened membrane. These may be in very close relationship with a dendrite, a cell body or even the axone hillock or node of Ranvier of an axone. The latter two are hypothesized by Minckler[190] to be inhibitory in function, although this remains a question. Each second order neurone of the central nervous system may have synaptic connections which number into the thousands.

## Vascularity

No detailed consideration of the mechanism by which the subluxation disturbs the function of the nervous system could be undertaken without some attention being directed to the arterial supply and venous drainage of the central nervous system in general. Most of this consideration is to be devoted to the spinal cord.

As the two Vertebral Arteries, which have coursed through the foramina transversaria of the six superior cervical vertebrae, crossed the posterior arch of the atlas in the Sulcus Arteriae Vertebralis and entered the cranial cavity through the Foramen Magnum, begin approximating anterior to the Medulla, they give off a small branch. These two branches unite to form the Anterior Spinal Artery which descends in the Anterior Median Fissure for the entire length of the spinal cord. Each Vertebral Artery gives off a small Posterior Spinal Artery, which remains discrete and descends in close relation with the radicles of the Posterior Nerve Roots for the entire length of the cord. Thus, the cord has three arteries running vertically throughout its length, serving as a vertical anastamotic system between segments. In addition, a Spinal Artery enters through each of the intervertebral foramina in company with the thirty-one pairs of spinal nerve trunks.

As each artery enters the vertebral canal, it divides into an anterior and a posterior division to follow the course of the corresponding nerve roots. Each division divides, close to the surface of the medulla spinalis, into an anterior and a posterior branch to extend along the periphery of the cord, giving off tiny twigs that penetrate the white matter and break up into a capillary plexus for the supply of nutrition to the vertically travelling fibres of this white substance. The posterior branch of the posterior division joins or anastomoses with the Posterior Spinal Artery. A small vessel passes across the posterior surface of the cord to create an anastomosis between the two Posterior Spinal Arteries for each neuromere.

The anterior branch of the posterior division extends forward along the surface of the cord to anastomose with the posterior branch of the anterior division of the Spinal Artery, while the anterior branch of the anterior division continues to the anterior median line of anastomose with the Anterior Spinal Artery. Thus, a complete ring of arterial vessels has been formed for each segment, from which the periphery of the cord receives its arterial supply. The Anterior Spinal Artery provides at least one branch in each neuromere which pierces the floor of the Anterior Median Fissure to branch in a tree-like formation for the supply of most of the gray matter of that neuromere with only the periphery of gray matter receiving contributions from the numerous vessels of the white matter.

Since the above paragraphs were written, backed by such authorities as Cunningham,[191] Gray[192] and the latest edition of Gray[193] and others, the veracity of such an extended and intricate arterial supply to the spinal cord has been held up to question by Elliott[194] who provides evidence that there may be no more than four pairs of spinal arteries as tributaries of the three vertical spinal arteries. While such a contretemps may be forgiven with such august company as the classical anatomical authorities, it does dictate the necessity of modest alteration in the theoretical explanation of the mechanism by which the subluxation or fixation produces adverse neural responses. However, as advocated previously, chiropractic must stand four square with known facts.

Curtis, Jacobson and Marcus[195] in their text of 1972 describe these questionable arteries under the name Radicular Arteries and do agree with Elliott to the point of stating: "Most of the radicular arteries do not contribute a significant supply. The critical sources are the radicular arteries to segments C.6, T.10 and L.2. ... The actual border zones of circulation have been found to be segments T.4 and L.1."

Elliott has stated, "Most of these [radicular] arteries are insignificant and expend themselves on the roots without reaching the cord. ... Of a possible 30-odd on each side, only 5 to 8 connect with the spinal arteries, and since some pass only to the posterior artery, as few as 2 and seldom more than 4 feeders reach each longitudinal artery on each side. These may come in at any level and those on the two sides are not symmetrical.

"The actual state of affairs has ominous clinical consequences. Since wide gaps occur between the tributaries, the 'water-shed' between any two is a point of minimal blood supply; ... typically lower cervical levels or T.4 (Ziilch, 1954) are therefore peculiarly vulnerable to any circulatory deficiency; they are found, for example, to sucumb most easily to the oxygen-lack in pernicious anaemia. ... Interruption of any one radicular artery (or of the intercostal or other source of such artery) may cause softening and death of the nervous tissue supplied, because of inadequate anastomotic supply from above and below the effort will be like that of a cord transection, partial or complete."

The same author points out that in the lower thoracic or upper lumbar area a large radicular artery joins the anterior spinal artery as the arteria radicularis magnus. Elliott takes further issue with the classical description of the sulcal branches of the anterior spinal artery. His description is that these sulcal arteries pierce the floor of the anterior median sulcus and supply one side of the cord alternately for the most part and supply the anterior gray columns, central gray matter, and much of the white matter. The posterior spinal artery supplies the posterior gray column and part of the posterior funiculus. The superficial layer of the cord is supplied by the vasocorona, a network of small arteries from the three vertical spinal arteries.

As in other areas of the body, the terminal arterioles separate into the capillary plexus, through the walls of which oxygen and nutritive material are exchanged for carbon dioxide and other waste products of cellular metabolism. The capillaries then join to form tiny venules and these lead to the surface, forming veins in the Pia Mater.

The larger veins are located in the subarachnoid space and plexuses of veins in the extra-dural space, from which two or three thin-walled veins pass out of the vertebral canal via each of the intervertebral foramina to drain into a rich plexus of veins in proximity to the vertebral column. The veins, which traverse the intervertebral foramina, are peculiar in that they do not boast the usual valves and venous blood is permitted to pass in either direction. Increased pressure intra-thoracically or intra-abdominally causes the venous blood to be driven back through the veins of the intervertebral foramina of the region into the extra-dural plexus.

Elliott[196] varies in his description of the venous drainage of the cord from the classical texts. He states that 10 or 20 radicular veins conduct most of the venous blood from the extradural plexus through the intervertebral foramina to the external plexus and the levels of exit are variable. Again, a large venous trunk exists in the lower thoracic or upper lumbar area, the vena radicularis magna.

One observation is of particular interest to chiropractic physicians in the discussion of the extradural plexus: ". . . it is apt to form large varicosities like a 'tangle of worms,' which may extend two or three segments and press on nerve roots with symptoms of irritation or compression, or even compress the spinal cord itself."

The arterial supply and venous drainage of the intracranial structures is quite complicated and of little concern in the discussion of subluxation. Therefore, the reader is referred to the standard textbooks of anatomy to refresh his memory on any of the points that may not be clarified by the present volume.

CHAPTER X

# Significant Physiology of the Nervous System

CELLS OF EACH tissue of the body have their own specialized function; thus, muscle cells contract, gland cells secrete, red blood cells transport oxygen, and the white blood cells are phagocytic in action. Neurones, with their long processes, dendrites and axones, are peculiarly constructed for the very specialized function of conduction of the nerve impulse, an electro-biological phenomenon resembling electricity in many respects, yet differing from electricity in many other respects.

The axis cylinder and the dendrites correspond to wires for the conduction of electricity and the myelin as the insulation for same. Unlike the ordinary wire, the nerve fibre does not show equal insulation, or myelin, for its entire length, rather, it shows segmentation at frequent and equidistant intervals by a decrease, or lack, of myelin allowing the surface sheath of neurolemma to dip into close contact with the fibre. These constrictions are called the Nodes of Ranvier, where, according to I. Tasaki,[197] the fibre is found to be most readily stimulated by an electrical current. These nodes, or Constrictions of Ranvier, according to Maximow and Bloom[198] and Curtis,[199] occur from 50 to 1000 microns apart, the distance varying with the size and type of nerve fibre studied.

The quantity of myelin is not constant for all fibres but varies with the size and type also.

Postganglionic autonomic fibres, either sympathetic or parasympathetic, have a very thin layer or no myelin and, hence, a gray appearance. The preganglionic autonomic fibres are well supplied with myelin and difficult to distinguish from somatic fibres.

Feldenkrais,[200] in agreement with most authorities, has pointed out that the nerve cells, unlike most cells of the body, lose the ability to reproduce some considerable time before birth and that the increased bulk of the nervous system following birth is due to the increase in number of processes and their individual increase in diameter, as well as the addition of myelin, it might well be added.

Without myelination fibre tracts do not function within the central nervous system and such myelination for the greater percentage of these tracts takes place after birth. It is for this reason that the newborn and the infant are incapable of coordinated activity. As myelination progresses, the range and complexity of learned coordinated actions increase. An average nine-month-old child cannot be taught to do up buttons, no matter how persistent the teacher, because the nervous system is not myelinated to the degree necessary for such complicated and skilled activity.

While it was formerly held that myelin was fatty material produced by Schwann cells or neuroglia, the use of the electron microscope has altered this opinion. Crelin[201] now reports that oligodendroglial cells within the central nervous system and neurilemmal cells peripherally wrap around the fibre in a series of layers. The majority of the cytoplasm of these cells is lost and the cell membranes blend with layers of protein and lipid molecules alternating.

## Afferent Fibres

As W. E. LeGros Clark[202] has emphasized forcefully, the commencement of any sensory tract is not the first order neurones, but, rather, the specialized receptor end-organs, which are peculiar for each type of sensation. The receptors for the sensation of cold are thus different from those for heat, light, touch or pain. The nerve impulses aroused by adequate stimulation of each type of receptor are identical, although they may vary in their speed of transmission and their frequency. The resultant sensation is dependent upon the area of the cerebral cortex of termination. Thus, a sensation is dependent upon the specific receptors stimulated and the specific area of the brain into which the stimulus is conducted.

Clark[203] has pointed out also that a number of nerve fibres approach a specific sensory spot from different directions and that stimulation of that area causes impulses to reach the central nervous system by different fibres, resulting in a specific pattern of excitation in the central nervous system. This peculiarity of multiple supply of fibres to a limited area is related to the ability to localize accurately the source of stimulation upon the skin.

## Efferent Fibres

On the other side, it has been pointed out that each efferent fibre of the somatic system arrives at a muscle, where it divides into from 1 to over 100 fibrils, according to Minckler,[204] each of which makes contact with a single muscle cell and is the sole pathway of nerve impulses to that muscle cell, without which the cell would not only cease to function in an organized manner in keeping with the needs of the entire body and in accordance with the dictates of the central nervous system, but would undergo degeneration with a loss of its anatomical integrity. Guyton,[205] however, places the number of muscle fibres supplied by each nerve fibre at 3 to 2,000, as previously noted.

## Trophic Function

The nervous system is not only a controlling and integrating system, but has a trophic influence upon the tissues supplied. The October, 1958, issue of *Scientific American* carried an article entitled "The Regeneration of Body Parts by Marcus Singer,"[206] which states in part: ". . . the function of nerve which we know best is that of conduction. Nerve fibres carry messages from one nerve cell to the next, from the brain and spinal cord by way of nerves to every tissue of the body and back again. All our actions and thoughts depend upon this capacity of nerve cells. It seems proper that this system which is responsible for maintaining the wholeness of body function should also serve to repair the mutilated body. However, experiments on the salamander have shown that the nerve's role in regeneration is distinct from that in carrying messages. The growth function, for example, does not require the reflex circuits which are necessary to nerve conduction. Indeed, in the absence of all other innervation, sensory nerve ganglia implanted in regenerated tissue will enable it to continue growing.

"How nerve assists regeneration is poorly understood but most probably the nerve fibres give off substances which promote growth."

Marcus Singer further pointed out that the type of nerve fibres present was not important but the number is critical, or in his words: "A threshhold number of nerve fibres act in concert to induce the new growth — the individual fibre is ineffective."

In this same article, it was pointed out that J. M. Van Stone of Princeton University, L. W. Polezhayev of the U.S.S.R. and S. Meryl Rose of the University of Illinois had, among others, done various experiments to show the role of the nervous system in the regeneration of tissues. Singer makes this statement with which chiropractors would be in accord: "It is probably safe to assume that every organ has the power to regrow lying latent within it, needing only the appropriate 'useful dispositions' to bring it out."

As previously mentioned, microtubules have been found under electron microscopy to be a part of the neural fibres and that these vary in diameter. It has been hypothecated that these microtubules may conduct molecules of protein of variable size, which may play a part in the trophic function.

Chiropractors have been taught from the days of D. D. Palmer that the cells of the body have the knowledge, Innate Intelligence or homeostatic tendency, to know their own needs for growth, function, reproduction and repair; that the nervous system was, and is, supreme in coordinating and integrating unit function into organic function and into body function and action; that the nervous system is all-important in health and in disease; that those factors which interfere with normal neural activity result in disturbed organic, somatic and cellular function; that the disturbances of function are accompanied by the symptoms and tissue changes of disease.

Sachs[207] substantiates the above statement: ". . .every pathological condition is obviously associated with disturbances in the autonomic nervous system."

As this text progresses the reader will find more and more evidence of the truth of this statement and the interdependence of structure and function through the activity of the nervous system.

## Reflex Arcs

Progressing now from the single neurone and its peculiarities to the functional unit of the nervous system, the Reflex Arc is the next step in the understanding of the nervous system and its peculiar, complex and varied functions. As previously brought to mind, receptors in skin, tendons, ligaments, joint capsules, muscles, periosteum, blood vessel walls, internal organs, and the organs of special sensation such as the eye, ear, tongue, nose, etc., upon receipt of an adequate stimulus cause a nerve impulse to be initiated in an afferent neurone, which is charged with the responsibility of conducting the impulse into the central nervous system.

Most afferent neurones have unipolar cell bodies located in ganglia without the nervous system proper and in the instance of spinal nerves with which we are primarily concerned at this point, the ganglia are located on the posterior nerve root, occupying either part of the intervertebral foramen or the spinal canal, depending upon the level considered. The afferent fibre, as the axone of the unipolar cyton in a Posterior Nerve Root Ganglion, assists in the formation of a Posterior Nerve Root and one of the radicles of this root to enter the spinal cord through the floor of the Postero-lateral Sulcus of the cord.

According to Sir Charles Sherrington,[208] quoting Donaldson, there are three times as many of these afferent fibres entering the spinal cord as there are efferent fibres leaving the cord and considering the cranial nerves, the ratio of afferents to efferent fibres is 5 to 1.

Upon entering the cord, each afferent fibre divides into an ascending and descending branch, as well as giving of collaterals which immediately enter the gray matter of the segment of entrance to make synaptic connections with efferent neurones. In the words of Sir Charles Sherrington,[209] "Taken generally, for each afferent root there exists in immediate proximity to its own place of entrance in the cord (e.g., in its own segment) a reflex motor path of as low a threshhold and of as high potency as any open to it anywhere."

In other words, the collaterals given off from the afferent fibre enter the gray matter and either pass forward to make synaptic connection with the dendrites of the efferent, motor cytones of the anterior horn, or make synaptic connection with internuncial neurones which conduct the impulse forward to the motor cytones.

It must not be assumed that the writer is unmindful of the varied methods of synaptic connection and influence, such as terminal bouttons in potential contact with the cell body or even Nodes of Ranvier of an axone, but merely for the sake of simplicity and clarity the axone-dendrite connection is utilized.

Impulses are then carried out of the cord to the muscle cells, stimulating contraction. Thus, the most simple reflex arc is completed, but as Sherrington[210] has pointed out, "A simple reflex is probably a purely abstract conception because all parts of the nervous system are connected together and no part of it is probably ever capable of reaction without affecting and being affected by various other parts, and it is a system certainly never absolutely at rest."

However, to understand the workings of the nervous system it is essential to have the mechanism of the simple reflex arc clearly in mind that modifying influences of higher levels can then be appreciated. The reflex arc shows, according to Sherrington[211] and other neurologists, a slower speed of conduction than the length of the nerve pathway would justify and this time factor is greater for the weaker stimuli; the time of cessation of the motor reaction does not correspond exactly with the time of cessation of the stimulus to the receptor; the rhythms of end-effect and stimulus do not correspond exactly; the end-effect does not exactly correspond to the intensity of the stimulus; a single nerve impulse is resisted but a repetition of the stimulus overcomes the resistance — Temporal Summation; there is one-way conduction over a reflex arc, but conduction in both directions by a single nerve fibre; the reflex arc shows fatigue effects, while the nerve fibre is very resistant to fatigue; the resistance to the strength of stimulus necessary for conduction over a reflex arc varies greatly as compared to almost uniform resistance for the nerve fibre; the reflex arc shows a refractory period, inhibition, and shock to a much greater degree than the nerve fibre; the reflex arc is more dependent upon optimum blood and oxygen supply than is the fibre; drugs, anaesthetics and chemicals have a much greater influence upon the reflex arc than upon the fibre. All of the above variations between the reflex arc and the single fibre, or neurone, are considered to be the responsibility of the synapse, or synapses, associated with the reflex arc within the gray matter of the central nervous system.

## Strength of Stimulus

It has been clearly shown that the stronger the stimulus applied, the more the speed of the reflex arc corresponds to the speed of conduction of an ordinary nerve fibre of equal length. At first glance this might seem to obviate the application of the "All-or-none Law," but the strength of the nerve stimulus seems to be dependent more upon the frequency with which impulses follow one another along the nerve fibre and across the synapse than upon an increase in amplitude of a single impulse. The strength of the stimulus also determines to some degree the number of synapses crossed and, therefore, the number of efferent fibres activated and the degree of muscular contraction elicited.

To illustrate, a stimulus of a strength capable of activating a reflex arc is likely to stimulate an efferent pathway within the segment entered by the afferent fibre through the collateral given off within the segment, but, if the strength of the stimulus is increased, it may be capable of crossing the synapse formed by collaterals in the segment above or below, and if further increased, may well cross the more resistant synaptic junctions in segments more remote.

The synaptic connections made by the various collaterals have different degrees of resistance and this resistance also varies with the local conditions of the nervous system. An unexpected tap on the shoulder may cause a normal individual to turn his head and eyes to observe the source of such stimulus, but a highly irritable or nervous person may be startled, jump, throw up his arms, and even let out a screech. The normal person might do likewise, if he were walking through the dark, after seeing a horror movie, or the reaction might be even more severe and consciousness might be lost. This indicates the importance of the variability of irritation within the central nervous system, and the control of higher centres.

The subluxation will be shown to modify the local condition of the central nervous system and alter the response to stimulation and Chapter VIII has given some consideration to a few of the modifying factors.

At this point it must be brought clearly to mind that all afferents, somatic or visceral, make reflex connection with both efferent fibres of the somatic and autonomic divisions of the nervous system (Lockhart et al). Thus, an afferent fibre, either somatic or visceral, upon entering the gray matter will, through connector neurones, effect both lateral and anterior horn cells and somatic muscle will be stimulated, as well as visceral structures influenced. Albert Kuntz[212] makes this abundantly clear in his writings. In this way the subluxation has detrimental effects upon the functioning of visceral structures as well as upon muscles and other somatic tissues.

## Tonus

Afferent impulses are constantly entering the central nervous system from such sources as changes in temperature of the surrounding medium, the pressure of clothing upon the body, the degree of tension in muscles, the pull of muscles upon their tendons, the position of joints and from visceral structures within the cavities of the body. This constant stream of afferent impulses is transmitted to the efferent fibres of the somatic system to result in efferent impulses being transmitted to the muscles at the rate of 5 to 10 per second, according to Kreig.[213] Credit is given by Guyton[214] to the almost continuous discharge of neural impulses from the muscle spindles to cause excitation of the anterior motor neurones to result in muscle tone.

The more recent studies, utilizing surface and needle electrodes of the electromyograph, have cast serious doubt upon this explanation of tonus for Basmajian[215] states: "In no normal muscle at complete rest has there been any sign of neuromuscular activity, even with multiple electrodes."

The same authority in the area of electromyography states, "that the general tone of a muscle is determined both by the passive elasticity or turgor of muscular (and fibrous) tissues and by the active (though not continuous) contraction of muscle in response to the reaction of the nervous system to stimuli."

Such tone, or tonus, is that degree of contraction shown by normal resting muscle, which therefore has no slack to be taken up when action is indicated and which maintains the attachments in proper anatomical relationship. While such a muscle is said to be resting, it is nonetheless functioning by supporting the body, holding the articular surfaces of bones in contact and on guard for direction from the central nervous system to contract and produce movement.

Tonus is not a phenomenon exclusively confined to somatic muscle, but rather every normal organ, tissue and cell shows this watchful, waiting attitude. Any deviation from normal tone in a resting structure is abnormal and is referred to either as hypotonus or hypertonus.

Again Basmajian[216] emphasized, "If one keeps one's hands off a resting normal muscle, it shows no more neuromuscular activity than one with its nerve cut." This is not to suggest that the neural system is not largely responsible for muscle tone and its variation, as Basmajian has emphasized on the same page of his text, "To repeat, tone is a function of the nervous system controlling muscle but it also results from the natural elasticity of the muscular and fibrous tissue." He has been emphatic in assigning relative importance to the mechanisms responsible for tonus: "In the clinical appreciation of tone, the more important of the above two elements is the reactivity of the nervous system."

D. D. Palmer[217] considered "Tone" to be extremely important and stated: "Life is the expression of tone. In that sentence is the basic principle of chiropractic."

Those situations which modify the centripetal flow of neural impulses, disturb the centrifugal flow and, thereby, modify the tonus of somatic and/or visceral structures.

## Important Principles

By far the greater percentage of muscles are derived from the mesoderm of more than one embryonic segment and, thus, receive efferent nerve fibres from a corresponding number of spinal cord segments. These fibres have united outside of the spinal cord and the vertebral canal to form the motor portion of the nerve of supply to the muscle in question. It must be mentioned that there are afferents from, or to, a corresponding number of neuromeres and these assist the efferent fibres in the formation of the nerve of supply to the muscle. While it may be often referred to as the motor nerve of the muscle, it is, in fact, a mixed nerve with efferent, afferent fibres, as well as postganglionic sympathetic fibres for distribution to the blood vessels of the muscle and afferent fibres from the blood vessels, which may be thought of as being sympathetic afferents, but do not differ from the somatic afferents in appearance or location of unipolar cell bodies.

The electrical stimulation of the motor nerve has been shown to cause a greater contraction of the muscle than when the afferent limb of the reflex arc is stimulated, or when the fibres of a posterior nerve root are artificially stimulated. This Fractionation of the motor response to the normally elicited reflex, as mentioned by Krieg,[218] is due to the afferent fibres influencing a number of Motor Units in the segment of entrance, but these Motor Units may be for the supply of different muscles, therefore, a contraction could result in a small group of muscle fibres in several muscles and produce little appreciable effect, while stimulation of a motor nerve to a single muscle would cause a discharge of impulses into the majority of the muscle fibres of a single muscle and the resultant contraction would be obvious. In the words of Krieg,[219] "This principle is referred to as FRACTIONATION, implying that the strength of a reflexly induced contraction is only a fraction of the total possible contraction of the muscle."

The group of motor neurones, whose cell bodies may be located in the anterior horns of a number of spinal cord segments, supply a single muscle and is referred to as a Motor Pool. The Motor Pool seldom discharges all of its neurones at any moment and thus a muscle rarely contracts to its entire extent, but a percentage of the fibres contract, while the remainder rest and then the first group rests, while another group contracts.

A number of afferents, carrying impulses from different types of receptors, stimulate a portion of the Motor Pool, referred to as Convergence, to produce a stronger reflex response than when one type of receptor is stimulated alone. If the stimulus, arising from each type of receptor, is not sufficiently strong to elicit the reflex alone, the Summing of the several forms of afferent stimuli may be sufficient to result in a reflex motor discharge, Reinforcement. However, stimuli from several types of receptors may share common efferent pathways, thus, the end effect of stimulating both types of receptors may not be the total of contraction caused by adequate stimulation of each type individually, and this is referred to as Occlusion.

It should be noted also that an afferent stimulus may cause contraction of the flexor muscles on the same side, but result in contraction of the antagonistic muscles, the extensors, of the opposite side. An example might well be stepping on a tack, which would cause the foot to be withdrawn by flexing the knee and hip on the side of stimulation, thus throwing all of the body weight upon the opposite leg and hence, the extensors would be required to contract to support the extra load. Many examples could be provided to indicate that the single source of afferent impulses may result in opposite reflex reactions on the two sides of the body.

Several other important terms must be understood prior to considering the details of the effects to be expected by the interference to normal function by the subluxation. Inhibition is a poorly understood factor within the nervous system. Sherrington[220] propounded the idea of the existence within the various areas of the central nervous system, or within the Motor Pool, of conditions called Central Excitatory States and Central Inhibitory States.

He has shown that there are no inhibitory fibres to muscles to cause them to relax and that this phenomenon must, of necessity, be a central process and function and points out that it is not a peculiarity of either the afferent or efferent fibres, but, rather, an activity of either the synapse or the internuncial mechanism. He has quoted MacDougall's theory to explain the Central Excitatory and Central Inhibitory States.

With the advent of more precise micro-chemical investigation much has been learned about the method of stimulation, inhibition, and neural transmission. Guyton[221] mentions that the postsynaptic fibres may be inhibited by inhibitory transmitter substances produced by special type presynaptic fibres. In brief, it is hypothesized that this substance increases the permeability of the membrane of the neurone to potassium and chloride ions without altering the rate of sodium permeability. Several substances have been isolated as inhibitors, e.g., gamma aminobytyric acid, ammino acid glycine, but it is not settled that these are common to the human nervous system or are the only inhibitory substances.

With the development of fatigue, the resistance at the synapse between this collateral and the motor neurone is increased to the degree that the inhibitory and excitatory positions are reversed and the discharge of impulses now concentrates upon the efferent neurone to the flexor muscle. The flexor reflex arc now enjoys a

Central Excitatory State and the extensor reflex arc has a Central Inhibitory State prevailing.

Curtis, Jacobson and Marcus[222] indicate that inhibition is not clearly understood at this date but progress has been made with the discovery and investigation of the Renshaw cells, connector neurones in the anterior gray column, which are "activated by the firing of anterior horn cells." These cells then inhibit the action of other anterior horn cells for antagonistic muscles. The Renshaw cells are frequently inhibited (disinhibition) in their function.

It must be added that local conditions within the central nervous system, as discussed in Chapter VIII, may modify the degree of irritability without altering the predominance of this shifting excitatory-inhibitory state. In other words, altering the irritability does not abolish the mechanisms of excitation and inhibition, but, rather, accentuates or decreases the strength of the stimulus necessary to evoke the mechanism.

## Neuromere

Attention is next directed to the function of the individual neuromere of the medulla spinalis. It must be called to mind and kept clear at all times by doctors of chiropractic who aspire to be good diagnosticians and good locators of the vertebral subluxations, productive of the symptom complex, that all tissues derived from the ectoderm, mesoderm and entoderm of the embryological segment maintain afferent and efferent neural relation with the neuromere of the same segment. Thus, stimuli to any of the receptor end-organs of the segmental tissues create the greatest reflex response in somatic muscle fibres derived from the same myotome and blood vessels and visceral components formulated from the mesoderm and entoderm of that embryonic segment. Were the neuromere to be capable of function as a separate and distinct unit without the influence of higher brain centres, the volleys of afferent impulses from the receptors would stimulate the efferent neurones, resulting in hypertonicity of all muscle fibres supplied to the degree that spasticity would be the order.

It has been recorded previously that each afferent fibre, entering the cord, has the potential of influencing a number of segments, both superior and inferior to the point of ingress. Also, Sherrington[223] has been quoted as stating that all afferent fibres create a reflex response that is plurisegmental. This is essential, since the vast majority of muscles have been derived from portions of a number of myotomes and are, therefore, supplied with efferent fibres from more than one neuromere. Furthermore, the intersegmental tracts which bond a number of neuromeres into functional units and anterior horn cells, located in a number of neuromeres, but concerned with the control of a single muscle, into Motor Pools, have received brief consideration in prior pages.

Sherrington[224] has shown that the afferent limb of the reflex arc facilitates, by lowering the threshhold of response, the pathways within the central nervous system for other reflexes that are closely associated with the primary one and makes for the smooth integration of one reflex with the next necessary for a continued action. Also, as a reflex contraction takes place in a muscle, the receptor end-organs of that muscle, its tendons and the articulations moved are stimulated to return afferent stimuli to the neuromeres which serves to reinforce the reflex. The muscle continues to respond to efferent impulses for a short time after the original afferent stimulus has ceased to be applied, the After-discharge. The presynaptic fibres, by stimulating the efferent neurones of the Motor Pool, cause a potential that persists at least 15 milliseconds; or, parallel connector neurones may be activated and discharge at slightly varying times into the efferent neurones; or, collaterals from the efferent neurones may stimulate a variable number of connector neurones which have synaptic relation with the same efferent neurones and, therefore, re-stimulate by Reverberation. The details are to be found in Guyton's[225] text. At the same time, it is pointed out by Guyton[226] that the antagonistic muscles are inhibited to permit smooth and effective action of the agonists. As the latter shorten, there is a decrease in the signals from the muscle spindles, but an increase in activity of those in the antagonist, due to the stretching, especially if the movement is sudden. The antagonists may then change to prime movers (agonists) and the part moved may be restored to its resting position.

## Proprioceptive Influence

The proprioceptive afferent supply is constant and maintains the tonus of the musculature. These are of low intensity and do not suffer fatigue readily, but are interfered with by other forms of reflex activity of higher intensity, but of short duration. The latter soon suffer fatigue and the resting posture is resumed.

Sir Charles Sherrington[227] is the authority for the information that the proprioceptive arcs of the more headward segments have a reflex influence over larger fields of somatic musculature than do those of lower neuromeres. To illustrate this point, it has been clearly described by Krieg[228] how the afferent impulses from the receptors in the muscles and ligaments of the neck have an important influence upon the tonus of not only the cervical muscles themselves, but also the muscles of the four limbs. Turning the neck toward the right, for example, increases the tone of the muscles of the right limbs and decreases the tonus of the left limbs. Anterior flexion of the neck causes an increase of tone of the flexors of the arms and the extensors of the legs, while posterior nodding results in a directly opposite distribution of tonus.

The proprioceptive information from the structures of the neck tend to cause reflexes that bring the neck into proper alignment with the head (Neck Righting Reflexes) and then the segments of the trunk are brought into alignment by the segmental stretch reflexes. Higher levels of influence may also play an important part in these reflexes, since it is difficult, if not impossible, to separate the levels of the central nervous system into functional units, except in an arbitrary manner for descriptive purposes.

Matzke and Foltz[229] describe the important influence of the vestibular system via fibres in the medial longitudinal bundle which synapse with internuncial neurones to reach the anterior horn cells of the cervical region, especially.

Summing up the basic somatic function of the spinal cord prior to a glance at the higher forms of control and modification, Krieg[230] is utilized as the authority who clearly points out that protection, muscle tonus, basic reflexes for standing and walking, and the capacity to funnel stimuli from a variety of sources into definite motor channels of response are important basic functions of the cord, as is the propensity to delay or prolong the response to sensory stimulation. Guyton[231] writes that muscle spasm that was formerly explained as being due to metabolites, has been found to involve spinal cord reflexes. Ischemia, severe cold, excessive exercise sends afferent impulses into the cord, resulting in muscle contraction by reflex action, which further stimulates afferent receptors and increases the reflex activity until a spasm is the result.

## Higher Levels of Influence

The afferent fibres of the vestibular division of the eighth cranial nerve from the semicircular canals are intimately associated with the proprioceptive system and through connector neurones, whose cell bodies form Deiter's Nucleus (Lateral Vestibular Nucleus) and the axones of these cells descending through the entire length of the anterior white column of the cord as the Vestibulospinal Tract, or Bulbospinal Tract, influence the motor cells of the homolateral side and modify the tonus of the entire musculature.

The Reticular Formation of the brain stem adds a controlling influence to the basic reflex activity of the spinal cord. This is a series of clumps of cells scattered throughout the medulla, pons and mid-brain. It serves to coordinate the somatic activity with the visceral needs and those of the organism as a whole at any one moment. It may form new reflex responses or modify older spinal forms.

The complexity of this Reticular system may be best illustrated by the information provided by Curtis, Jacobson and Marcus[232] that each cell receives impulses from at least 1,000 neurones and connects with 10,000 neurones. Afferent pathways of the spinal cord, cranial nerves, higher brain centres of both somatic and visceral import feed information to this system for integration and appropriate motor response.

That portion of the Reticular Formation occupying the lower medulla is concerned with the reflexes of coughing, swallowing, vomiting and respiration, each of which require the cooperative effort of many somatic muscles.

It should be appreciated that the axones of the cells of one of the reticular nuclei, such as the centre for vomiting, would descend into the spinal cord to effect stimulation of anterior horn cells at a number of levels to provide widespread somatic muscle contraction either in concert or in smooth sequence. The vomiting reflex is most frequently elicited by afferent impulses from the stomach via the Vagus nerve to the Nucleus of the Tractus Solitarius, from which connector neurones stimulate the cells of the centre in question, causing a discharge of impulses into the Motor Pool for the diaphragm in cervical segments three to five, especially cervical four; the Motor Pool for the abdominal muscles in thoracic segments five to lumbar segment two; and the pelvic floor in sacral segments four and five. In addition, autonomic centres are also activated to produce the reverse peristalsis of the stomach, the relaxation of the cardiac sphincter and the salivation which occur, as the somatic muscles suddenly contract to greatly increase the intra-abdominal pressure, propelling the stomach content up the oesophagus.

The axones of the middle reticular nuclei in the pons and the inferior reticular nuclei in the medulla pass down in the Medial Longitudinal Fasciculus to enter the spinal cord as the Medial Reticulospinal Tract and are believed to cause somatic response to visceral afferent stimuli.

The Lateral Reticulospinal Tract is derived from the nuclei in the pons, whose axones, unlike those above mentioned, decussate and descend into the lateral white column of the spinal cord.

The fibres of the Anterior Reticulospinal Tract are crossed axones from cells in the tegmentum of the mid-brain and are thought to be short neurones in a chain formation.

All of these tracts are closely associated with the intersegmental tracts of the spinal cord and with the Extrapyramidal System. This system has yet to be understood completely, due to the complexity and difficulties of experimentation. Hence, differences of opinion exist between neurologists of the present.

## Posture

It has been proven that the Extensor Thrust which develops as a result of contact of the feet with a firm surface, producing stimulation of the proprioceptive endings and a massive Stretch Reflex response, is a function of the spinal cord to form the most basic background for posture. To this is added increased tonus of the flexors to create rigidity of the limbs, Limb Supporting Reaction, and a degree of trunk fixation by the Reticular Nuclei of the medulla to produce Reflex Standing.

The Stretch Reflex of the cord resists passive movement of a joint, but under the influence of the Reticular Nuclei of the medulla the limb is permitted to be moved and then tone of the muscles maintains the new position which is useful for posture and is a modification of the Stretch Reflex. Part of the Inferior Reticular Substance of the medulla acts as the bulbar suppressor centre to inhibit all somatic muscle tone upon stimulation, but must be influenced by higher centres or spasticity results, which appears to be a contradiction. One such area of higher control has been found in a narrow area of the cerebral cortex immediately anterior to the motor cortex of the anterior lobe, the precentral gyrus.

The Shifting Reaction is also under the control of the Inferior Reticular Substance. Thus, with one foot touching the floor and the other held in a flexed position, any shifting of the body weight toward the flexed leg side causes an immediate increase in the tone of the extensor muscles of the flexed leg to prevent falling.

The Reticular Formation in the region of the vestibular nuclei in the medulla and inferior pons seems to integrate proprioceptive stimuli from the cord levels with the stimuli from the semicircular canal system to cause the condition known as Decerebrate Rigidity which resists gravity. All of these influences over the cord are concerned with Static Reflexes, keeping the body in one position. The Righting Reflexes which are necessary to restore normal posture, after it has been disturbed, are under the control of areas still higher in the neuraxis.

The Righting Reflexes are an integration of afferent impulses from the proprioceptors of the cervical articulations and muscles, from the eyes and from the labyrinths of the internal ears, which have reached the Red Nucleus of the mid-brain by way of the Medial Longitudinal Bundle. The impulses are then discharged down the Rubrospinal Tract which decussates and descends to the motor cells of the cervical segments to modify the muscle tone and position of the head in space. The afferent information from the neck muscles effects a reflex by way of reticular nuclei in the mid-brain which cause contraction of lower spinal muscles to produce the Neck Righting Reflex, and the stretch reflexes initiated by the afferents in the muscles and joints of these lower segments result in contraction of the lower segmental muscle in progression until the entire trunk is brought into alignment.

Body on Head Righting Reflexes are mediated through the mesencephalic reticular nuclei without the influence of the semicircular canals and is due to contact of one side of the body and head when the animal is lying on its side. The head is first righted and then neck and body follow.

There are also Body on Body Righting Reflexes by which afferents from the trunk segments are integrated in the mid-brain reticular formation to right the body and bring the feet into contact with the ground.

Visual Righting Reflexes in man are more potent than the labyrinthine reflexes. The extra-ocular muscles cause the eyes to focus straight ahead, then the afferents from the extrinsic muscles of the eyes cause the necessary action of the muscles of the neck to move the head into such facing that the ocular muscles are in balanced equilibrium. The afferent impulses from the muscles of the neck cause the lower segments to be brought into alignment and the stretch reflex from segment to segment completes the adjustment of the entire body to the position assumed by the eyes. The cerebral cortex and Red Nucleus are essential for the control of these reflexes.

The Superior and Middle Reticular Nuclei have the ability to augment the stretch reflex.

The Cerebellum adds a controlling influence over many of these basic reflexes. The anterior lobe regulates the tone of postural muscles and stimulation of this area causes a loss of tone of the extensor muscles without an increase in the flexor tone and its destruction results in spasticity of the extensors.

The middle lobe of the cerebellum has been described by Krieg[233] as responsible for strengthening muscular contractions, particularly of the limbs; strengthening the stretch reflexes; normalizing the timing of voluntary actions.

The posterior lobe, when destroyed, is seen to have influenced the reflexes necessary for the erect posture, for the body sways and the feet are planted wide apart; and, if one side is damaged, the head turns to the side of the lesion and the victim staggers to the opposite side.

In the erect posture Basmajian[234] has demonstrated that the Iliopsoas is the only muscle that is constantly active and he suggests that it functions as a "vital ligament to prevent hyperextension of the hip joint." However, with the subject placed with one foot on each of two scales it will be readily observed that the completely static, quiescent posture cannot be retained for many moments. The same authority considers that slight activity of the intrinsic muscles of the back and of the thighs is sufficient to adjust the weight distribution around the gravity line and retain balance.

## Volitional Movements

Upon this background of reflex activity of the spinal cord and its modifications by higher levels into purposeful posture and basic movements so far described in a most limited manner without attempting to exhaust the many areas of influence, the voluntary, fine movements take place, due to the stream of impulses from the precentral gyrus by way of the Pyramidal Tracts, the greater proportion of which decussate to the opposite side. These tracts contain axones from two types of cells in intimate anatomical relationship in the cortex of the cerebrum. If the true pyramid cortex is destroyed or its fibres interrupted, a flaccid condition of the supplied muscles results. However, if damage occurs to the cells or axones of the cells, slightly further anterior in the precentral gyrus, spasticity is the order.

The pyramidal system has greatest concern for the movements of skill and finesse, such as are performed by the fingers and to a lesser degree the forearms, toes, feet and some of the muscles of facial expression, as well as those of the larynx and tongue for speech.

One final point must be made relative to the neuromere. Each afferent volley that creates a somatic muscle response also creates an alteration of visceral function through the corresponding sympathetic fibres, if present in that segment, or by coursing to the appropriate neuromere of controlling influence. As Sachs[235] has stated: "Every response of the organism to a situation in the external environment is associated with a disturbance in the internal environment."

Kuntz[236] has clearly stated the proposition that visceral and somatic afferents have reflex relationship with both visceral and somatic efferent fibres.

The influence of the autonomic cells of the medulla spinalis will receive consideration and discussion as the neural mechanics of the subluxation as a disturbing factor to the harmonious function of the body unfold in later chapters.

With this naive introduction to the functioning of the central nervous system attention is now directed to the intricacies of the intervertebral foramen and its environs.

# CHAPTER XI

# The Intervertebral Foramina and Environs

A DISCOURSE SUCH as this would be in no way complete were a discussion of the intervertebral foramina, their content, associated and related structures neglected. Again, no claim to an exhaustive coverage of the subject can be made, but, rather, a review of significant features and those aspects essential to an understanding of the subluxation, as envisioned by the writer, must receive consideration.

Some interesting information is to be derived from the investigations of Harold Swanberg.[237] Careful measurements were made of an adult male vertebral column 75 cm. in length, presumably from occipital condyles to the tip of the coccyx. The measurements made of the vertical diameter of each intervertebral foramen from the third cervical to the fifth lumbar inclusive, omitting the clefts for the first and second cervical nerves and the foramina for the sacral and coccygeal nerves, provide a total of 29.65 cms., or approximately 40% of the overall length with an average of 12.9 mm. of vertical height for each foramen. Assuming that the remaining eight openings were consistent with the average findings, there would be an additional 10.32 cms. for a total of 39.97 cms. and this would be about 53.3% of the total length of the vertebral column.

D. D. Palmer[238] was not unmindful of these interesting facts and stated in part: "The spinal column of an adult measures about 2 feet 2 inches. The intervertebral discs occupy about 1/4 of the space, or about 6 inches all told. The average thickness of all the intervertebral cartilages is about 1/4 of an inch. They increase in thickness from an 1/8th of an inch in the cervical, to 1/4 inch in the lumbar region."

Swanberg[239] measured the thickness of the intervertebral fibrocartilaginous discs at their posterior and anterior borders and his figures indicate that the posterior borders account for a total length of 9.25 cms., or 13.3% of the spine's length, while the anterior borders of the discs give a total of 15.15 cms., or 20% of the length. Also, the average disc composes approximately 31.2% of the anterior wall of an intervertebral foramen.

Gray's *Anatomy*[240] mentions that the discs account for approximately 1/4 of the length of the vertebral column.

Swanberg[241] calculated that the spinal nerve trunks occupy from 1/12th to 1/3rd of the space in an intervertebral foramen and the largest nerve trunks measure 7 mms. in vertical dimension. He pointed out that the thoracic region offers the greatest protection to the nerves and has the least range of motion between vertebrae and the cervical nerves have the least protection, yet this region enjoys the greatest range of movement. It is suggestive and significant that the thoracic nerve trunks contain preganglionic sympathetic nerve fibres for visceral control, thus, are deserving of greater protection than those concerned with somatic supply only.

## General Considerations

A brief review of the boundaries of a typical intervertebral foramen must receive first consideration prior to reviewing the exceptions and regional peculiarities.

From the posterolateral angle of each vertebral body a pedicle projects posteriorly and somewhat laterally. Each pedicle forms the floor of the superior vertebral notch and the roof of the inferior vertebral notch. The body of the vertebra forms the anterior boundary of each notch and the root of the superior articular process forms the posterior boundary of the superior notch, while the root of the inferior articular process limits the inferior notch posteriorly.

When two contiguous vertebrae are articulated, the notches form the majority of the boundaries of an intervertebral foramen. To complete the foraminal walls, it is necessary to mention the posterior border of the intervertebral fibrocartilaginous disc which accounts for approximately one-third of the anterior boundary of the average intervertebral foramen. The posterior wall of the intervertebral foramen is composed of the superior articular process and just the root of the inferior articular process of the vertebra above, since this inferior projection extends posterior to the superior articular process.

In some areas at least, the thin, loose articular capsules are associated intimately with the content of the intervertebral foramina as portions of the posterior boundaries.

To this general description, the exceptions are more frequent than the rule, as will be noted in the following specific descriptions.

## Content of the Intervertebral Foramina

It is necessary to first generalize prior to particularizing. Of course, the largest and most important structure passing through every intervertebral foramen is the nerve trunk, that short section in which the fibres of anterior and posterior nerve roots commingle before dividing into anterior and posterior primary rami, each of which is composed of afferent and efferent fibres. It has been estimated that the afferent fibres outnumber the efferents by three to one in the nerve trunk.

Swanberg[242] has indicated that the nerve trunk lies about 1/80th of an inch from the superior pedicle of the foramen and, therefore, occupies the superior portion of the foramen, especially in those instances in which the nerve takes up a mere 1/12th of the foramen and at most 1/3rd of the space.

In the majority of instances, the posterior nerve root ganglion also occupies a portion of the intervertebral foramen. However, these ganglia for the lower lumbar, sacral and coccygeal nerves are most frequently found within the vertebral canal.

Another nerve of import to this consideration and to the function of the organism is the recurrent spinal nerve, or meningeal nerve, that passes back into the vertebral canal by way of the intervertebral foramen. Although this is a mixed nerve, having afferent and efferent fibres as components, the efferent fibres are postganglionic sympathetic fibres from cytones in the associated paravertebral sympathetic ganglion for distribution to the blood vessels of the vertebrae, nerve roots, meninges and spinal cord. The afferents have receptor endings in the articular capsule, the intervertebral disc, posterior longitudinal ligament, meninges and blood vessels. There are no axones of anterior horn cells in the recurrent spinal nerves, as there are no striated muscle fibres to be supplied within the vertebral canal.

The meningeal nerves were well known to and appreciated by D. D. Palmer,[243] who wrote: "At its exit, the spinal nerve divides into two branches, the anterior and posterior somatic branches. Just before it divides, it gives off a small branch which returns inward. The anterior of the two divisions is joined by a branch from the sympathetic cord called ramus communicans. This latter gives to the recurrent branch a filament from the sympathetic. These two form one nerve which, returning through the intervertebral foramen, supplies innervation to the fibrous membrane which forms the outermost covering of the brain and spinal cord. It, also, sends branches to the vertebrae and vertebral ligaments."

Furthermore, he stated on the same page of his textbook: "If the innervation of the recurrent nerve is interfered with by pressure, it becomes irritated, molecular action is increased, there is greater vibration, and the heat becomes more intense, causing pathological conditions varying from headache to that of brain fever; or spinal

150

irritation, deviating from neurasthenia to vertebral caries."

A spinal artery enters through each intervertebral foramen for distribution as previously described. The source of each spinal artery varies according to the region, but the distribution and function remain as revealed by the modern authorities quoted.

The venous blood accumulated in the plexus of veins in the extra-dural space of the vertebral canal finds escape via several thin-walled, valveless veins that pass through the intervertebral foramen to join the vertebral venous plexus externally located.

Although the spinal cord of the adult terminates about the level of the superior border of the second lumbar vertebra, it should be re-iterated that a spinal artery, with vena commitantes, accompany every spinal nerve through the corresponding intervertebral foramen. Thus, there are thirty-one pairs of recurrent spinal nerves to supply the thirty-one segments of the spinal cord and thirty-one pairs of spinal arteries. The anastomoses with the anterior and two posterior spinal arteries which run vertically the full length of the cord receive postganglionic sympathetic fibres via each recurrent spinal nerve, also.

The nerve trunk is ensheathed in a sleeve of dura mater which has enveloped both of the roots and the posterior nerve root ganglion. The arachnoid mater and pia mater envelope the anterior and posterior nerve roots separately and intimately. The dural sheath of the nerve trunk appears to lose its identity within the intervertebral foramen by becoming continuous with the fine, loose, areolar tissue that forms a reticulum in the remaining space of the intervertebral foramen, giving support within its meshes to soft fat.

A variable number of minute lymphatic channels are found to leave each intervertebral foramen and are continuous with the sub-dural space of the sheath of the nerve trunk, offering additional means of return of the protective layer of lymph to general circulation.

Some authors, although none of the authorities of anatomy known to this writer, have described a thickening or accumulation of the connective tissue to form suspensory ligaments for the nerve trunk. Be this as it may, the contention to be formulated in future pages does not rest upon the presence or absence of such ligaments.

## Escape of the First Cervical Nerve

Now that the generalization has received brief consideration, attention is directed to each area of the vertebral column and the outstanding variations from the typical intervertebral foramen, commencing superiorly and progressing down in an orderly fashion.

As D. D. Palmer[244] forcefully brought to the attention of his students and readers a number of times in his textbook, "The first pair of cervical nerves emerge above and the second below the atlas in grooves, where there is an abundance of room and no vertebral notches to slide together; they cannot be occluded. The first and second pair of cervical nerves cannot be pressed or squeezed between the occiput and atlas or in the cleft between the atlas and axis, and yet there are many diseases resulting from their displacement."

As D. D. has emphasized, the first cervical nerve leaves the vertebral canal not by a true intervertebral foramen, but through the sulcus arteriae vertebralis in the posterior arch of the atlas immediately posterior to the lateral mass, in company with the vertebral artery which arose as a branch of the subclavian artery and travelled superiorly through the foramina transversaria of the upper six cervical vertebrae. Upon leaving the foramen in the transverse process of the atlas, this comparatively large artery takes a tortuous course around the lateral mass of the atlas, through the sulcus, into the vertebral canal, to turn superior through the foramen magnum, piercing the dura and arachnoid maters, to join its fellow at the lower border of the pons in the formation of the basilar artery of the circle of Willis. It is from the vertebral artery that the cervical spinal arteries are derived for the supply of meninges, spinal cord, vertebrae, etc. It is from the vertebral arteries also that the posterior spinal arteries and the branches which unite to form the single anterior spinal artery are derived to extend downward the entire length of the spinal cord.

It is of interest to note that the first cervical nerve escapes from the vertebral canal posterior to the articular process, or lateral mass, rather than anterior as is the usual in previously described foramina. The lateral mass overhangs the anterior portion of the sulcus and gives attachment to the free border of the posterior atlanto-occipital membrane which completes the margin of the opening. In a percentage of cases the free border of this membrane becomes ossified to complete a fixed foramen. The posterior atlanto-occipital membrane corresponds to the ligamentum flavum between laminae of the lower vertebrae and is attached to the superior border of the posterior arch of the atlas inferiorly and to the posterior margin of the foramen magnum superiorly. The margin of the foramen magnum is above the opening under discussion, but the mechanism of movement is such that the occiput cannot close this foramen, as contact would occur between the posterior arch of the atlas and the occiput before posterior nodding of the occiput becomes excessive. Thus, the vertebral artery and first cervical nerve are protected from osseous encroachment.

The first cervical nerve lies under the vertebral artery, separating the artery from the floor of the sulcus. Upon division of the nerve trunk, the anterior primary ramus proceeds anteriorly along the lateral surface of the lateral mass, medial to the vertebral artery, to pass in close relation to the medial margin of the rectus capitis lateralis which it supplies. It continues through the space between this muscle and the rectus capitis anterior, to which a twig of supply is given, as well as a fine branch to the longus capitis muscle, then turns inferiorly over the anterior margin of the transverse process of the atlas in intimate relation with the posterior wall of the internal jugular vein. The posterior primary ramus, the larger of the two, escapes from under the artery into the suboccipital triangle to divide into a number of branches for the supply of the suboccipal muscles and there may be a small cutaneous branch for the occipital region.

The anterior division is joined by a gray ramus communicans from the superior cervical sympathetic ganglion before joining the anterior ramus of the second cervical nerve to forfeit its identity. Some of these postganglionic sympathetic fibres travel centralward in the anterior division until the junction with the posterior primary ramus is reached and then turn out in the latter for distribution to the postvertebral structures.

## Second Cervical Nerve

Again there is an atypical situation and some detail is necessary to appreciate the peculiarity of the avenue of egress of the second cervical nerve.

There is no true intervertebral foramen for this nerve, nor is the arrangement similar in detail to that above described for the first nerve. The superior articular facet for articulation with the atlas is supported on the posterolateral portion of the body and the anterior portion of the strong pedicle, thereby being part of the anterior boundary of the slit-like aperture for the escape of the second nerve from the vertebral canal. The inferior articular process of the atlas and the loose articular capsule complete the anterior boundary, while the lamina of the axis forms the floor; the superior margin is formed by the posterior arch of the atlas; and the anterior free border of the posterior atlanto-axial membrane comprises the posterior limitation of the opening.

The posterior nodding of the head and dorsi-flexion of the cervicals would be most inclined to close the passageway, but such possibility is forestalled by the locking of the posterior arch of the atlas and the laminae of the axis prior to any serious reduction in size of the aperture.

The posterior primary ramus of this nerve is considerably larger than the anterior ramus and upon crossing the lamina passes under the inferior margin of the obliquus capitis inferior muscle to divide into medial and lateral branches which lie, for the most part, on the external surface of this muscle. The medial branch is called the greater occipital nerve and is predominantly sensory to the posterior scalp as far as the vertex, while the lateral branch supplies muscular branches to the splenius, longissimus capitis and semispinalis capitis.

The anterior primary ramus passes between the transverse processes of the atlas and axis, between the vertebral artery and the posterior intertransverse muscle which extends from the superior border of the transverse process of the axis to the inferior border of the transverse process of the atlas. The ramus then turns anterior, lateral to the vertebral artery, to pass between the longus capitis and levator scapulae to divide into ascending and descending branches to form loops with the first and third anterior primary rami, thereby losing individuality.

It should be mentioned that the anterior division receives a gray ramus communicans, as does every spinal nerve, from the superior cervical sympathetic ganglion. Furthermore, some of the postganglionic fibres, upon uniting with the anterior ramus, extend toward the nerve trunk to turn out in the posterior primary ramus and the recurrent spinal nerve. This is also true of all spinal nerves.

## Typical Cervical Intervertebral Foramina

The superior and inferior vertebral notches of the remaining vertebrae of the cervical region are of almost equal depth and, in accordance with the measurements provided by Swanberg,[245] create intervertebral foramina of an average vertical dimension of 9.75 mm. The posterior borders of the intervertebral discs account, on the average, for 2.83 mm. of the diameter. It may be computed that the body of the superior vertebra contributes 3.46 mm. to the anterior wall of the foramen, the disc 2.93 mm., and the body of the inferior verte-

154

bra an additional 3.46 mm. for a total of 9.75 mm.

The superior and inferior boundaries of the foramina are the pedicles of contiguous vertebrae and the posterior boundary is formed by the articular pillar, composed of the inferior articular process of the segment above and the superior articular process of the one below. The loose articular capsule unites these processes and acts as the actual posterior limitation of the intervertebral foramen. Hence, it is conceivable that injury to the articulation could result in an excess of serous fluid in the joint cavity, distending the capsular ligament to encroach upon the content of the intervertebral foramen.

It should be noted that the articular processes form the posterior limit of each intervertebral foramen from that for the third cervical nerve to the last true intervertebral foramen for the fifth lumbar nerve. Further, the content of each has been previously described.

The spinal nerves occupy the grooves on the superior surface of the transverse process of the vertebra below, which is formed by the true transverse segment posteriorly and the rudimentary costal process anteriorly and floored by the costotransverse bar which also forms the lateral boundary of the foramen transversarium for the vertebral artery. The spinal nerve divides into its anterior and posterior primary rami as it passes posterior to the vertebral artery.

The posterior primary ramus turns back in intimate relation with the lateral surface of the superior articular process and medial to the posterior intratransverse muscle, thus, does not extend sufficiently far laterally to reach the extremity of the transverse process. This ramus divides into a medial and a lateral branch for supply of the post-vertebral muscles and the skin, although the sixth, seventh and eighth cervical nerves may have no cutaneous branches.

The anterior ramus continues laterally beyond the limits of the transverse and is between the anterior and posterior intertransverse muscles, then emerges between scalenus anterior and scalenus medius. Each anterior ramus is joined by a gray ramus from the appropriate paravertebral sympathetic ganglion and a short distance beyond loses its identity by participating in either the cervical plexus for the first four or the brachial plexus for the lower four rami.

Prior to leaving this consideration of the cervical nerves, it should be emphasized that each cervical nerve trunk is composed of somatic efferent and afferent fibres only, and that each ramus has, in addition to these somatic fibres, postganglionic sympathetic fibres received from a gray ramus communicans extending from the paravertebral sympathetic chain.

## Thoracic Intervertebral Foramina

The thoracic intervertebral foramina, according to Swanberg,[246] show a gradual increase in vertical measurement from the first to the twelfth, ranging from 10 to 16 mm. with an average of 12.8 mm. The average thickness of the posterior borders of the fibrocartilaginous discs seems to be 2.96 mm.

The superior vertebral notches are almost imperceptible, except for the first thoracic, while the inferior notches are deep. The anterior wall of the intervertebral foramen is formed by the posterolateral surface of the body of the vertebra above and the fibrocartilaginous disc. In all but the tenth, eleventh and twelfth thoracic intervertebral foramina, the head of a rib and its capsular ligament assist in formation of the anterior boundary of the foramen.

The majority of the posterior wall of the foramen is formed by the superior articular process of the vertebra below and only the root of the inferior articular process, as it fuses with the pedicle of the vertebra above, contributes to the most superior portion of this wall. Due to the facing of the articular facets in this area of the column, the superior portion only of the articular capsule is in relation to the content of the intervertebral foramen and could be considered a portion of the wall. The exception to the latter statement may well be the joint capsule for the articulation between twelfth thoracic and first lumbar articular processes, since the inferior process of the twelfth is transitional in character and does not face as frankly laterally as those of true lumbar vertebrae; thus, the superior and medial borders of the joint capsule are related to the content of the foramen.

The posterior primary ramus of each thoracic nerve travels posteriorly in close relation to the joint capsule of the articulation to divide into a medial and lateral branch for the supply of the postvertebral musculature and the posterior cutaneous portion of the trunk.

The anterior primary ramus of each of the first eleven thoracic nerves extend laterally, lying anterior to the intertransverse ligament and muscles in those areas where the latter are present, to become the intercostal nerve for supply of the muscles of the thorax and abdominal wall. The twelfth thoracic nerve lies between the twelfth thoracic vertebra and the first lumbar vertebra and is called the subcostal nerve as it passes laterally below the twelfth rib.

It must be reiterated that each anterior primary ramus receives a gray ramus communicans from the appropriate sympathetic ganglion and the postganglionic sympathetic fibres make their way through both the anterior and posterior primary rami and all of their branches for distribution to blood vessels of the somatic muscle, bone and skin, as well as to the sudoriferous glands and erectores pili muscles of the skin.

Each anterior primary ramus of the thoracic nerves give off a white ramus communicans, composed of the axones of the lateral horn cells, which are preganglionic sympathetic fibres to synapse within the paravertebral or prevertebral ganglia with the postganglionic neurones. Afferent fibres from visceral structures contribute to the formation of the white ramus communicans, nerve trunk and posterior nerve root of each of the thoracic segments in contradistinction to the somatic efferent and afferent fibres only found in the nerve trunks and roots of the cervical nerves.

The spinal arteries, which enter each intervertebral foramen, are derived from several sources and must be considered in separate groups. Those for the first two thoracic foramina are branches of the posterior intercostal divisions of the superior intercostal artery, itself a branch of the costocervical trunk of the subclavian artery.

Here it may be well to mention that the spinal artery accompanying the eighth cervical nerve through the intervertebral foramen has been derived from the deep cervical artery, the other division of the costocervical trunk.

From the third thoracic down, the spinal arteries are twigs from the posterior branches of the posterior intercostal arteries, derived from the descending aorta. That for the twelfth thoracic foramen is derived from the posterior ramus of the subcostal artery which is the last branch from the descending thoracic aorta.

## Foramina for the Lumbar Nerves

The superior vertebral notch of each lumbar vertebra is distinct but shallow in comparison to the depth of the inferior notch. The foramina have an average vertical measurement of about 16.9 mm. with the posterior border of the disc accounting for approximately 8 mm. of this dimension, according to the research of Swanberg.[247] Only the superior rim of the inferior lumbar vertebral body aids in the formation of the anterior wall of the intervertebral foramen.

The posterior limitation of the foramen is formed in largest measure by the inferior articular process of the superior vertebra with the superior articular process of the vertebra below contributing to a lesser degree. The articular capsule of the average individual may

157

come into relationship with the content of the foramen at the superomedial aspect of the articulation, since the wide set superior
articular processes have curved facets which face primarily medially
and posteriorly and the inferior facets of the vertebra in juxtaposi-
tion are more closely set to fit between the above mentioned. Such
arrangement and facing carries the capsule away from the content of
the intervertebral foramen to a considerable degree.

The lumbar nerve trunks increase in size from the first to the fifth.
The fifth and first sacral nerves have been found to be the largest of
the entire thirty-one pairs and upon measurement by Swanberg,[248]
found to be 7 mm. in diameter.

The posterior primary ramus of each lumbar nerve spirals posteriorly between the inferior articular process and the medial free border
of the medial intertransverse muscle to divide into medial and lateral
branches for the supply of the postvertebral muscles and skin of the
back.

The anterior primary rami of the first and second, perhaps the
third and even the fourth, are found to give off white rami communicantes for connection with the paravertebral and prevertebral
ganglia, as above discussed. Of course, every anterior ramus of a
spinal nerve receives a gray ramus communicans from the paravertebral ganglion associated with it.

The anterior primary divisions travel lateralward and inferiorly,
either posterior to the psoas major muscle or between the fasciculi of
muscle fibres within the structure of the muscle. These divisions soon
lose identity as they join in the formation of the lumbosacral plexus.

The spinal artery for each lumbar intervertebral foramen is a contribution from the posterior branch of the lumbar artery, four pairs
derived in series with the posterior intercostal arteries from the posterior aspect of the descending abdominal aorta. The fifth lumbar
artery is a branch of the iliolumbar artery, derived from the posterior
trunk of the internal iliac artery.

### Sacral Foramina

The intervertebral foramina for the sacral nerves have become
complicated by the fusion of the segments into a single wedge-shaped
bone, the sacrum. The true foramina remain for the nerve trunks
much as has been described in the more cephalic region, although the
boundaries have become ossified to form openings of fixed and permanent size. The pedicles continue to form roof and floor; the

anterior wall is formed by the bodies and ossified intervertebral disc; the posterior limit is the column formed by the fused articular processes. Thus, a fixed, smooth-walled foramen exists for the trunk of each of the superior four pairs of sacral spinal nerves.

The complications arise as the anterior and posterior primary rami seek to escape to the corresponding surfaces of the sacrum via four pairs of anterior sacral foramina and four pairs of posterior sacral foramina. To appreciate the formation of these sixteen openings it becomes imperative that a review of the sacral fusion be undertaken.

In the development of the sacrum there were five sacral vertebrae, each having the elements of a typical moveable vertebra. As growth progressed, the discs ossify to form a continuous column of bone with the bodies; the costal elements forming the boundaries between anterior foramina, greatly enlarge and ossify, forming the lateral mass of the sacrum and the lateral boundary of each foramen. Through each of these foramina passes the anterior primary ramus of one sacral nerve and the accompanying structures, such as the meningeal nerve and the spinal artery and veins.

The posterior surface reveals the fusion of the spinous processes and interspinous ligaments to form the median sacral crest; the fusion of laminae; the obliteration of the articular processes, creating an articular crest marked by four tubercles, which bound the posterior sacral foramina medially; the fusion of the elements of the transverse processes and intertransverse structures creates the lateral sacral crest, marked by four tubercles, which bound the posterior sacral foramina laterally, while the transverse processes separate the foramina.

The laminae of the fifth sacral segment fail to form, leaving the terminal end of the sacral canal open as the sacral hiatus. The inferior articular processes are known as the sacral cornua and are united to the coccygeal cornua by the intercornual ligament on each side. This completes the posterior border of the slit-like aperture that corresponds to an intervertebral foramen for the escape of the small fifth sacral nerve trunk from the canal. Upon division, the anterior ramus grooves the lateral margin of the rudimentary fifth sacral body, passing through a foramen whose lateral boundary is the lateral sacrococcygeal ligament, from the rudimentary transverse process of the first coccygeal segment to the lateral angle of the sacrum. The posterior ramus descends posterior to the rudimentary coccygeal transverse process.

The coccygeal nerve escapes from the sacral hiatus below the

coccygeal cornu and divides into a small cutaneous posterior ramus
and an anterior ramus which continues around the lateral margin of
the first coccygeal segment.

Each sacral and the coccygeal anterior primary ramus receives a
gray ramus communicans from the paravertebral ganglionic chain of
the sympathetic system and these postganglionic sympathetic fibres
of the gray ramus are distributed through the branches of both the
anterior and posterior rami, as is true for all spinal nerves.

The anterior rami of the second and third, or third and fourth,
sacral nerves give off a bundle of fibres, which correspond to a white
ramus communicans, but these two pairs do not pass to the sympathetic ganglia, but enter the pelvis as preganglionic parasympathetic
visceral branches and are the sacral outflow of the parasympathetic
system. It must be appreciated that from the third lumbar nerve to
the coccygeal nerve there is no further sympathetic outflow, or white
rami communicantes, and no other spinal nerves than the two sacrals,
above mentioned, contribute fibres to the parasympathetic division
of the autonomic system.

The spinal arteries for the sacral foramina are branches of the
lateral sacral artery from the posterior trunk of the internal iliac,
which extends inferiorly on the anterior surface of the sacrum just
lateral to the anterior foramina. Each spinal artery, of unusually large
size in comparison to those previously discussed, enters through the
anterior foramen, supplies twigs to the content of the true intervertebral foramen and vertebral canal and then proceeds out through the
posterior foramen to supply the muscles and skin of the area over the
dorsum of the sacrum. These arteries, in fact, correspond more
closely to the posterior ramus of the posterior intercostal arteries and
only the twig given off within the sacrum to enter the true intervertebral foramen should be deserving of the title, "spinal artery."

The latter twig is long, since it must follow the course of the
greatly elongated nerve roots to reach the corresponding segments of
the spinal cord to form the usual anastomosis and supply the neuromere.

### Meningeal Nerves

As a conclusion to the chapter of general background review pre-
paratory to the consideration of the mechanisms by which the subluxation and vertebral distortion alter the function of the nervous
system, it is fitting that the nerve supply to the structures associated

with the vertebral foramen and the intervertebral foramen should receive consideration in a little more detail.

Gerald Burke[249] utilized the term Nervus Sinu Vertebralis that has been called by others Recurrent Spinal or Meningeal Nerve, states: "The existence of this immensely important nerve has apparently escaped recognition by the profession at large. It is not specifically described in any textbook, even those on anatomy and surgical anatomy." How unfortunate that Dr. Burke did not have access to pages 38 or 326 of D. D. Palmer's text of 1910, for this nerve is described. This author's original *Gray's Anatomy*, 23rd edition, 1936, makes mention of this series of nerves. While the good orthopaedist was extremely critical of chiropractic physicians in his text, he would have found that nearly any member of this profession could have informed him relative to these meningeal nerves.

As *Gray's Anatomy*[250] has mentioned, every spinal nerve trunk provides a meningeal branch, or recurrent spinal nerve, prior to dividing into anterior and posterior primary rami. Each meningeal nerve is composed of afferent fibres and postganglionic sympathetic fibres. The latter have been derived from cell bodies in a paravertebral sympathetic ganglion associated with the spinal nerve by a gray ramus communicans. Upon entering the anterior ramus, some of the unmyelinated fibres follow the course of the anterior ramus and its various branches, other fibres turn back into the trunk, then into the meningeal nerve and others into the posterior primary ramus. Those sympathetic fibres, distributed via the meningeal nerve, are vasomotor for the control of the vessels to the adjacent vertebral segments, the various branches and the neuromere itself.

The afferent fibres of the meningeal nerve are distributed to the blood vessels, the periosteum of the vertebra in the region of the intervertebral foramen, the disc, the posterior longitudinal ligament, the ligamentum flavum, the capsular ligaments, the meninges covering the neuromere, the nerve roots, posterior nerve root ganglion and the spinal nerve trunk.

The muscles, tendons, fascia and skin derived from the same embryonic segment retain connection, both efferent and afferent, with the neuromere of the same segment. It must be emphasized that the skin and muscles may, in the course of development, have migrated a considerable distance and, in the adult, may not lie in close association with the intervertebral foramen and origin of their spinal nerve, a factor which complicates both spinal analysis and diagnosis.

Those muscles which have retained their segmental characteristics, such as the rotatores, the intertransversarii, the interspinales, the intercostales, etc., are supplied by a single neuromere. On the other hand, sheets of muscle, such as the externus obliquus abdominis, are dependent upon many neuromeres for fibres of both afferent and efferent supply. Despite the plurisegmental supply, it must be appreciated that the afferent impulses returning to each segment have a modifying influence upon the function of each individual neuromere. Disturbances to the structures supplied by the recurrent spinal nerve may thus be reflected in the other somatic structures supplied by the same neuromere and these disturbances may add further to the alteration in nerve supply to visceral structures dependent upon the same neuromere.

It has been observed by experimental neurologists that afferent impulses have a more profound influence within the neuromere the closer the receptor end-organ is located to the neuraxis. Furthermore, Sherrington[251] and others have pointed out that noxious afferent impulses tend to dominate reflex pathways. Hence, injury to the vertebral column creates a bombardment of the spinal cord with noxious, or nociceptive, afferent impulses from a source in intimate relation with the neuraxis and supplied by the recurrent spinal nerve. There is little wonder that the disturbances resulting are so profound and far reaching. The doctor of chiropractic is justified in his concern for spinal structure and function, as the following pages seek to establish.

# CHAPTER XII

# General Effects of the Subluxation

THE MECHANISM BY which the vertebral subluxation disturbs the neural function is one of considerable complication and requires consideration under a number of headings for clarification of description, although each is an integral part of the whole and difficult to separate from the other ingredients of the phenomenon. Nor is it possible to always describe each portion of the mechanism in chronological order, nor assign a degree of importance to each, other than in a most arbitrary manner. The reader may wish to re-arrange the order of importance of each phase of the mechanism and this should be possible without any loss of value to the entire consideration. It is doubtful that any one phase can be discarded without a loss of much that is important to a complete understanding of the manifold disturbances that may transpire in consequence of a spinal subluxation. Furthermore, not all of the possibilities have received the degree of enlargement to which they are entitled. There is little doubt that future research may reveal facts of inestimable value in the completion of the explanation of the mechanism by which the subluxation disturbs function.

The writer would emphasize that each phase of the mechanism is but a portion of a complicated, interrelated, interacting, interdependent biological response of the body to a structural disrelation brought about by stresses, either of the external or internal environment, or by a combination of many.

Furthermore, the end results of the disturbance to the neural function varies in general with the area of the subluxation within the vertebral column, the state of irritability of the nervous system and the condition of the tissues supplied at the time of the subluxation. The state of the chemistry at the effector end-organs plays an important role in the response of the various tissues to the neural disturbances attendant upon subluxation. Each of these factors must receive consideration in proper sequence.

As has been apparent, the writer has little sympathy with the view that ordinary subluxation of a vertebral segment creates direct pressure or transmitted pressure through the content of an intervertebral foramen upon the nerve trunk sufficient to interfere with its function, or that a subluxation always decreases neural conduction. Rather, the teachings of D. D. Palmer[252] are favoured, "The larger share of diseases are the result of too much vital force; consequently, energy is not hindered, kept back, prevented, obstructed, or shut off, but accelerated, hastened, quickened, urged, hurried, the volume and force is augmented."

On occasion, direct pressure upon a spinal nerve trunk does occur, but this is not an instance of the chiropractic subluxation. Rather, this is an example of serious local pathology or trauma. Fracture-dislocations, luxations of cervical vertebrae, pathological destruction of the vertebral body with collapse and displacement of segments, true herniation of the nucleus pulposus of the intervertebral discs, exostoses, etc., are a few examples of problems that may create direct nerve trunk pressure or impingement. The reader is referred to good, standard orthopaedic texts for the symptomatology of such conditions. Conviction should dawn that any similarity between the symptom pictures of direct nerve pressure from pathology and trauma and the chiropractic subluxation is purely and simply coincidental, if not accidental.

Since there is complete agreement with the thought expressed by D. D. Palmer,[253] "When we consider that the spinal cord is freely moveable within the spinal canal and that the spinal nerves are afforded ample space for their emergence from the intervertebral foramina, we will see that normal movements do not compress either the spinal cord or spinal nerves," a brief look at the subluxation through the eyes of the author might be the first logical step in the consideration of the adverse influences of the subluxation.

## The Subluxation

The disrelation of a vertebral segment in association with the contiguous vertebra, or vertebrae, is not visualized as a partial dislocation, as the term implies, but, rather, as a disturbance of normal function of a vertebral segment, which would be better expressed by the term "Fixation," which is a less pretentious, shorter, but more limited, term than Dr. Pinkenburg's[254] "vertebral articular kinetic aberration." Thus, the vertebra in question is within its normal range of motion with its facets continuing to articulate with those of the vertebrae above and below. Such a Fixation does not alter the size of the associated intervertebral foramina materially, yet the disrelation, or disturbed kinetic function, does have profound significance for the neuromere and nerve trunk.

The subluxation, or fixation, may be demonstrated by x-ray

visualization of the involved area by carefully measuring and comparing adjacent vertebrae. While the full spine, standing A-P x-ray plate has been utilized extensively by chiropractors since Dr. Warren L. Sausser, a New York State chiropractor, made the first such exposure in 1932, the subluxation, or fixation, may be detected by the "orthodox," so-called diagnostic film taken of a local area primarily to reveal the details of osseous structure and determine the presence or absence of pathology. Many ingenious methods have been developed for the utilization of the Roentgen rays for the detection of the fixation by some of the best minds in the field of chiropractic radiology. No matter the technique of radiology employed, the true subluxations are revealed to the skilled chiropractor, as the abnormal facing of the subluxated vertebra remains a constant finding at rest, or at any point in the range of motion. In other words, the subluxated vertebra takes part in the motion of the area but its facing is always at variance with the normal for the position assumed.

While the sophistication of diagnostic radiological interest has led to a de-emphasis and depreciation of the full-spine roentgenogram by all too many chiropractors, no other x-ray study is charged with a similar volume of analytical information to assist the doctor of chiropractic in determining the fundamental structural problem underlying the patient's symptom complex.

Better A-P techniques and more extensive use of the lateral full-spine exposures are indicated, if this profession seeks to extend its reputation as the specialists of human structure and remain in the vanguard of those interested in the spine. This is not to deprecate diagnostic radiology in the hands of the chiropractic profession, but, rather, to emphasize that one must not be forfeited for the other. Both are essential. However, the specialists in human architecture will find the richest practical rewards in a deeper study of the spinograph.

The research conducted in the field of cineradiography of the spine by Dr. Illi of Switzerland and the late Dr. Earl Rich of the Lincoln Chiropractic College, as well as the addition of this sophisticated equipment to the research departments of the National and Northwestern Colleges, promises to reveal new and extensive information relative to the spine in motion that will be of assistance to every chiropractor and of rich benefit to the millions of patients dependent upon chiropractic for a health service.

The educated fingers of the doctor of chiropractic are capable of detecting the slight alteration of facing of the offending vertebra and the failure of the segment to move normally through its full range of motion.

The trained eye often detects the area of limited motion. Devices, such as the plumb line and its many elaborate modifications, have been developed to assist the chiropractor to visually locate spinal problems and subluxations or fixations. One of the best of these instruments has been developed by Dr. Lyman C. Johnston, Research Director of the Canadian Memorial Chiropractic College, and named the Panoramic Plumb-line Posturometer. The Posturometer has special interest for those chiropractors interested in total body contour and posture and materially aids in the determination of basic distortion and compensation, as well as assisting in the localization of the subluxations or fixations.

Furthermore, muscle tension, particularly of the deeply seated segmental muscles, are detectable on palpation and serve as important signposts to those exploring the spine for subluxations by digital means.

At times, the altered temperature of the overlying, or associated, dermatome may be elicited by the sensitive finger tips, but more consistently by the wide variety of thermographs which have been invented to measure, compare and record the temperatures of the two sides of the vertebral column.

Chronicity of vertebral fixation results in alterations in texture of the skin, subcutaneous tissues and associated muscles. The skin of the corresponding dermatome has been found to vary from a thin, glossy texture to a thickened, roughened, discoloured patch, resembling a calus formation. Such alterations of the skin have been described by Pottenger[255] and osteopathic researchers who reported their findings in a book, *The Pathogenesis of Disease Following Vertebral Lesion*, edited by Louisa Burns, Chandler and Rice.[256] The thickened form of cutaneous reaction to the fixation may be observed with the unaided eye and the more subtle colour changes, due to vascular alteration, may be detected by such instruments as the Visual Nerve Tracer, invented by Dr. Geo. W. Adelman of Brockton, Massachusetts.

Infra-red photographs have been utilized also to determine the sites of subluxations as indicated by vascular changes in the dermatome.

The subcutaneous tissues are disturbed in texture by the alteration of nerve supply and demonstrate to the palpating fingers a variety of textures, ranging all the way from a "slimy" feeling of "skin-slip" to a granular disposition.

The musculature demonstrates to the exploring fingers departures from the normal resiliency of contracted muscles through a wide range of apparent fibrotic change to the cord-like, stringy band of the chronic contracture.

Instrumentation of a different principle can detect the subluxation by the change in electrical conductivity that occurs in the corresponding dermatome in response to altered activity of the sudoriferous glands as a concomitance of vertebral fixation and altered nerve supply.

The most convincing evidence for the patient, however, is the acute, subjective tenderness experienced when the probing finger reaches the site of fixation. In many instances the patient is not aware of a "sore spot" in the particular region of the spine and his pain and other symptoms may be far removed from the offending vertebral segment.

Motion study techniques have been devised that range from the most simple to the most ingenious and elaborate to make abundantly clear that the subluxation is in reality a limitation of the normal range of vertebral movement. It is anticipated that the cineradiographic research sponsored by the American Chiropractic Association will bring forth rich rewards of knowledge relative to the spine in motion.

There can be little remaining doubt in the mind of a patient that subluxations do occur when he has experienced the deft thrust of the skilled doctor of chiropractic, felt the segment move, heard the sound produced by the changing tension of the holding elements, experienced a new freedom of motion in the region and often a marked relief of pain almost immediately. It becomes difficult to "sell" such a person upon the idea that subluxations or fixations exist only in the fevered imagination of the chiropractor and that any beneficial response or alleviation of symptoms occurred by way of suggestive therapeutics. This is the conviction that organized allopathic medicine has diligently attempted to foster in the minds of the public for a great many years with an ever decreasing degree of success.

Another type of individual that cannot be made to believe that subluxations do not exist in the vertebral column is the one who, in desperation, has sought the services of a doctor of chiropractic for an ailing pet — dog, cat, or even a horse on occasion. The adjusting of animal spines has proven efficacious in many instances to the surprise of veterinarians and even the chiropractors themselves.

Both the osteopathic and chiropractic professions have done animal experimentation to determine the effects of producing and correcting spinal disrelations. The most exhaustive report of any of the research projects is to be found in the previously mentioned book, *The Pathogenesis of Visceral Disease Following Vertebral Lesions*, edited by Burns, Chandler and Rice[257] of the American Osteopathic Association.

## Disturbance of the Neurological Bed

The production of a fixation by any of the stresses previously discussed disturb the receptor endings in the joint capsules, ligaments, intervertebral disc, muscles, tendons, etc. Such disrelation causes a flow of afferent impulses into the neuromere, which is no longer bilaterally equal as would normally be the case with the area at rest. The excess stimulation which is persistent alters the function within the neuromere and those above and below for a variable distance. Such afferent impulses succeed in making synaptic connection with the motor pool of neurones in the anterior gray horns through either collaterals or internuncial neurones. Muscular contraction results, or is perpetuated.

The most noticeable muscular contraction is to be found in the segmental muscles, such as the Rotatores and the deepest layer of the Multifidus. This is not to suggest that the muscle fibres derived from the self-same segment, but whose identity has been lost in the welter of complicated divisions and unions of the mesoderm of the same myotome, do not experience an increase in tonicity. Rather, due to the intermingling and intricacy of fibre arrangement, those fibres supplied by the same neuromere may experience a degree of hypertonicity without being readily detected by palpation. However, with the addition of the time factor, there may be a demonstrable change in texture of the long postvertebral muscles as fibrosis develops.

The musculature supplied by the anterior primary ramus of the nerve trunk associated with this neuromere does not escape alteration in tonus either. However, this is not readily demonstrated by the usual methods of examination.

Lest there be confusion created by the above, it must be made abundantly clear that not every fibril supplied by every efferent neurone whose cytone is located in the anterior gray horn of the involved neuromere experiences an increase in neural stimulus. This is far from the fact that is being utilized. Those muscles, whose action is antagonistic to the prime movers, are inhibited by a decrease in tonus of the constituent myofibrils by a decrease in nerve impulses passing outward from the appropriate motor pool. Furthermore, the antagonists of the opposite side of the vertebral column and trunk generally would experience a degree of inhibition. For a simple example: if the Rotatores of the right side of the column were stimulated to contract, the Rotatores of the left side would be inhibited. As previously mentioned, this phenomenon is one of changed irritability of the motor pools within the central nervous system and not a peripheral experience.

As has been brought to the attention of the reader, the mechanism of inhibition is poorly understood by the neurological research workers, although it is discussed in a most knowing manner. The best explanation seems to this writer to be that of Sherrington,[258] who has pointed out unequivocally that there are no inhibitory fibres to somatic muscle leaving the central nervous system, and that inhibition is thus a central function. Furthermore, the connector neurones for each motor neurone provide collaterals for the efferent neurone of antagonistic predisposition. When the one becomes the prime activator, a reduction of synaptic resistance occurs at the collateral from its antagonist and the neural charge is drained from the antagonist to reinforce the stimulation of the prime mover, thereby simultaneously decreasing, or inhibiting the neural activity of the antagonist.

Curtis, Jacobson and Marcus[259] have mentioned that the afferent fibres from the stretch receptors of a prime mover through collaterals and internuncial neurones inhibit the antagonistic muscle. Further, that the activity of the efferent neurones of control of the prime mover also stimulate the Renshaw neurones of the anterior gray horn with an inhibitory effect upon the neurones of the antagonist. As the efferent neurones of the prime mover depolarize, the cell membranes of the efferent neurones of the antagonist becomes hyperpolarized and resistant to stimulation (inhibition). The chemical mediator of this change in resistance is unknown, but the chloride conductance is known to increase.

Further, there may be inhibition of efferent cells without a change in resting membrane polarity and this seems to take place at the synapse between axone and dendrite.

Guyton[260] has devoted a number of sections to the discussion of central inhibition and points out that an afferent fibre entering the spinal cord may give off a collateral which stimulates an inhibitory fibre which secretes inhibitory substance at its synaptic connection with the fibres that are the final common motor pathway for control of the antagonist to the prime mover (agonist) under consideration.

Many factors modify the determinant of selection of the particular motor pool to be stimulated by the centripetal stimuli from the receptor nerve endings above mentioned. It cannot be foreseen and prognosticated for any patient or individual the muscles that will become hypertonicized by the abnormal quantity of afferent impulses aroused by a fixation or subluxation. However, there are those that are most frequently involved and are to be expected to show the greatest amount of tonal disturbance.

The anterior horn cells are not the only cytones affected. The afferent impulses will also involve the lateral horn cells for the control of the vascular bed of the musculature experiencing hyperactivity. It has been demonstrated by Best and Taylor[261] that active muscle requires 20 to 30 times the amount of oxygen demanded by resting muscle and the source of oxygen is dependent upon increased arterial blood supply.

Krogh has been quoted by Pottenger[262] as having demonstrated that in guinea pig muscle there are 85 active capillaries in each square millimeter of resting muscle and 2,500 capillaries active in the same quantity of muscle during contraction.

To provide such an increase in arterial flow the vascular bed of the musculature must undergo dilation. Again, such activity is dependent upon a decrease in neural supply to the tunica media of the arteries and arterioles, strongly suggestive of a central inhibitory state of the preganglionic sympathetic group of cells in the lateral gray horn.

It has been postulated by Guyton[263] that a portion of the hypothalamus may be stimulated, especially by the cerebral motor cortex, with the impulses relayed in the sub-collicular area which, in turn, activates special preganglionic sympathetic cell bodies of the lateral horn of the cord. These neurones then stimulate postganglionic sympathetic fibres to the vessels of muscle and perhaps by the secretion of acetylcholine result in vasodilation. It is not clear as to whether cord reflex influences could have a similar response.

Furthermore, the vascularity of the corresponding dermatome is greatly decreased, as may be detected by the thermocouple and other heat measuring instruments, as well as by photographic techniques mentioned.

This phenomenon has been investigated by Dr. Matsunaga[264] who discovered for himself a decrease in skin temperature of the embryologically associated paravertebral dermatomes in all cases of pleurisy, 91% of heart disease, 80% of upper G-I disorders, and 78% of pulmonary tuberculosis. While his findings give no indication of vertebral kinetic aberration, nor the serial occurrence of these phenomena, they merely indicated the interrelationship of somatic and visceral tissues, emphasizing that dysfunction of one type of tissue is likely to be accompanied by reflective dysfunction in the other.

Associated with this vascular activity, the sudoriferous glands are activated by stimulation of other preganglionic sympathetic neurones of the lateral gray horn, which, in turn, activate the postganglionic fibres distributed through the posterior primary ramus of the nerve trunk at the level of subluxation or fixation. This activity of the sudoriferous glands may be detected by sensitive instruments capable of measuring the resistance of the skin to minor electrical currents. The activity of these glands alters the electrolytes present on the surface of the skin and hence its conductivity.

It should be appreciated from the above that, like the somatic neural supply, there is a central inhibitory state of some sympathetic preganglionic cytones and a central excitatory state of others. This same situation must be extended to include the supply by these autonomic neurones of visceral structures within the cavities of the body, which will be done later.

Noxious afferent impulses may arise from any of the holding elements injured by the stress, or trauma, which was the causative factor in producing the fixation. Such impulses take precedent over the proprioceptive impulses and result in the necessary muscle contraction to produce the "splinting" action required to fix the injured articulation, thereby preventing further motion that might well aggravate the injured tissues (Hilton's Law[265] ).

If the injury has been caused by sufficient mechanical force to strain, or sprain, the articulation and its holding elements, these noxious afferent impulses may result in a plurisegmental response with extensive postvertebral muscle spasm and pronounced vertebral distortion, although the traumatized segment may continue to demonstrate the greatest degree of distortion and more asymmetry of motion than the other segments involved. From a practical point of view, treatment and adjustive procedures directed to the area generally may be to little avail unless the primary segment of involvement is corrected, either inadvertently or by design. The well qualified, efficient doctor of chiropractic will have determined the prime offender and directed his care of the region to the specific involved vertebra.

Tissue damage in the vertebral column follows the same laws of response as any of the other tissues and histamine-like chemical substance is liberated, called necrosin, or bradykinin by some authorities such as Guyton.[266] Bradykinin is considered by Guyton[267] to be, at least, one of the chemicals released by traumatized cells, which may directly stimulate the receptors of pain. This chemical causes a greatly increased permeability of the capillaries, permitting extravasation of the blood plasma into the tissue spaces with much protein and fibrinogen escaping also. The interaction of necrosin and fibrinogen tends to cause a coagulation and a "brawny edema" around the damaged cells. This swelling produces pressure upon the receptor nerve endings in the area to perpetuate the flow of centripetal noxious impulses into the spinal cord.

It must be appreciated also that tissue injury calls forth a local vasodilation, due to the response of the minute vessels to the chemical products released from the damaged tissues and a more pronounced vasodilation of the larger arterioles through the alteration of neural supply to the vascular bed. It has been postulated by Guyton[268] that a portion of the hypothalamus may be stimulated, especially by the cerebral motor cortex, with the impulses relayed in the subcollicular area which, in turn, activates special preganglionic sympathetic cell bodies of the lateral horn of the cord. These neurones then stimulate postganglionic sympathetic fibres to the vessels of muscle and by the secretion of acetylcholine result in vasodilation. It is not clear as to whether cord reflex influences could have a similar response. Sherrington[269] mentioned that the exteroceptors, interoceptors and proprioceptors influence very readily the vascular musculature and that the kinaesthetic receptor fibres particularly influence the vascular bed of the somatic musculature.

Such a response is recollective of another central inhibitory state involving cells of the lateral gray column of the spinal cord. It would appear that there are two mechanisms involved; one, an active response to necrosin and the other, a passive dilatation of vessels resultant from a decrease of neural impulses reaching the tunica media of larger arterioles and arteries. That there is, in fact, a dependence upon the nervous system for much of the vascular response to tissue injury is demonstrated by the practitioners of Yoga who are able to hold live coals in their hands, push needles through their flesh, and do other remarkable feats without their tissues demonstrating the usual inflammatory responses. These phenomena of control appear to be dependent upon the ability of the individual to influence his nervous system and prevent the usual, normal response to noxious impulses.

The edema, above mentioned, may involve the tissues of the intervertebral foramen, thereby exerting an abnormal degree of pressure upon the trunk nerve. However, it is problematical as to whether such edema ever exerts sufficient pressure to damage the nerve trunk, and thereby decrease its ability to conduct. If such were the case, muscles supplied by the fibres of that nerve trunk would demonstrate paralysis to the degree that they are dependent upon the fibres of that particular trunk for efferent supply and those tissues, skin, muscles, ligaments, blood vessels and viscera, supplied by that trunk would be lacking in sensation, or evince a degree of anaesthesia consistent with their dependence upon the nerve trunk for centripetal fibres. These factors are rarely demonstrable in association with an ordinary subluxation.

It is more consistent with fact to postulate that the edema of the intervertebral content stimulates the receptor end-organs of the epineurium of the nerve trunk, sending further noxious afferent impulses back into the cord via fibres of the recurrent spinal nerve, through the nerve trunk and the posterior nerve root. Again, these tend to summate with those impulses above discussed to result in "splinting" of the articulation by postvertebral muscle contraction and the vascular changes thus far discussed.

Nor are the responses confined to the local area of the medulla spinalis into which the afferent fibres make their entrance. Both kinaesthetic and nociceptive impulses spread cephalad to involve higher neural centres. The noxious impulses may be transmitted by their connection with cells of the Substantia Gelatinosa of Rolando at the apex of the posterior gray horn. The pathway to the post-central gyrus of the cerebral cortex has been briefly described in a previous chapter. In this area of cortex appreciation, localization and interpretation occur. Many side effects might well be discussed, such as the influence the cells of the thalamus may have upon centres in the diencephalon, which have a generalized, or specific, regulatory influence upon the autonomic components of the nervous system, depending upon which group of cells may be activated. Suffice it to draw attention to the possibilities of complicated responses at higher levels as a result of centripetal impulses aroused by a vertebral fixation.

The kinaesthetic or proprioceptive impulses may be conducted into the cord by fibres which turn cephalad upon entrance into the cord to form part of either the Fasciculus Gracilis or Fasciculus Cuneatus, give off collaterals, especially in the segment of entrance, and travel headward in the posterior white column. The pathway followed by these impulses also received previous consideration.

In all of the diverse influences from the disturbances of the neural bed of the tissues upset by the fixation could be found adequate explanation for the vast majority of adverse responses of the human to vertebral fixation, but this would be to ignore other factors that would seem to be of very real significance and modifying predisposition.

Later chapters dealing with the fixations of each region of the vertebral column will emphasize the visceral disturbances possible and the mechanisms by which such functional and tissue changes engendered by the vertebral distortion come to pass.

## Arterial Disturbances

While the vascular disturbances of the somatic tissues at the site of fixation have received some consideration above, attention must now be directed to the vessels of the nerve trunk, roots and radicles, as well as the neuromere specifically.

It should be recalled that a previous chapter devoted attention to the origin and distribution of the spinal arteries, one of which enters through each intervertebral foramen. The contained nerve trunk, posterior nerve root ganglion and nerve roots are supplied by this artery which then continues on to supply the radicles.

The possibility of disturbance of the autonomic nerve supply to these vessels by the overactivation of the centripetal nerve fibres, due to the irritating influence of the fixation or subluxation, is very real. The afferent impulses entering the spinal cord may have either an excitatory or an inhibitory influence upon the efferent neurones of both the anterior and lateral gray horns within the segment of entrance and may involve neuromeres both superior and inferior to the point of entrance. Furthermore, the same afferent impulses have both an excitatory and an inhibitory effect at the same time. Such a disturbing influence is further modified by the local conditions existent within the neuromere at the time.

Should the subluxation stimulate centripetal fibres and cause them to discharge into the preganglionic sympathetic neurones concerned with the vasomotor control of the spinal artery of the fixated segment, an increased supply of nerve impulses to the smooth muscle fibres of the tunica media would result in vasoconstriction and a decrease in arterial supply to the neural structures. Decreasing the arterial blood supply to the nerve trunk and, especially, to the gray matter of the cord segment reduces the quantity of both oxygen and nutritive material transported to these important structures with a subsequent alteration from normal of their function.

While the cytone is the primary source of nutrition for the neurone, due to the length of its fibres, other sources of supply are necessary for adequate function. The authorities appear in agreement with Gray[270] that a Node of Ranvier occurs about every 1 or 2 mm. along the course of the nerve fibre and each of these constrictions acts as an additional region for metabolic intake. Through the capillary plexuses in close association with the fibres, an interchange of oxygen, nutrition and the metabolites of neural activity takes place. Thus, the interchange between blood and axoplasm may be accomplished with the minimum of resistance at these areas where the myelin sheath is all but absent and the neurilemma comes into intimate relation with the axis cylinder.

The passage of the nerve impulse is dependent upon the extracellular fluid, as well as upon the neurone itself, and any changes of the electrolytes of the intercellular fluid would alter the conductivity of neural signals. This homeostasis of the intercellular fluid is dependent upon free and normal interchange of fluids within and without the capillary plexuses. Any disturbance to the circulatory bed can only have detrimental influences upon the ability of the fibres of the nerve trunk to conduct in conformity with the needs of the tissues supplied and the demands of environmental changes.

It is suggested that the detrimental effects of the fixation or chiropractic subluxation and the osteopathic vertebral lesion is due in substance to the alterations in the milieu and nutrition of the fibres of the nerve trunk, rather than to any excess of pressure, per se, upon the trunk as a direct concomitance of the edematous condition described by the osteopathic researchers, as reported in the textbook *The Pathogenesis of Visceral Disease Following the Vertebral Lesion*, by Burns, et al.[271]

The dense capillary plexus within the nerve has been described in detail by Wyke,[272] who indicates that such a plexus extends longitudinally, fed by arterioles from arteries of supply to neighbouring muscles. The nutrient, oxygen and metabolite exchange takes place at the Nodes of Ranvier. Alterations of either quantity or quality of blood supplied will result in aberrations of neural function.

Sherrington[273] pointed out that the blood supply, narcosis, fatigue and other factors have a very real influence upon the functioning of the nerve fibres and the nervous system as a whole. The same authority, Sherrington,[274] brought to the attention of his readers the fact that the nerve trunk conduction is disturbed in its ability to conduct but slowly by a decrease in blood supply, but reflexes suffer very quickly from anoxia.

As has been quoted previously, Best and Taylor,[275] as well as other experimental physiologists, have demonstrated that direct nerve pressure does not shut off the passage of the nerve impulse along the nerve fibre. Therefore, attention should be directed to the neuromere itself for a better understanding of the functional disturbances that may arise from the fixation of vertebral segments.

The alteration of arterial supply to the neuromere may be readily influenced by the postganglionic sympathetic fibres carried by the meningeal nerve for distribution to the anastamotic network of arteries that pierce the periphery of the cord to form a rich capillary plexus in relation to the fibres of the white matter and the cells and fibres of the gray matter. Disturbance to circulation within the neuromere, due to vasoconstriction or vasodilatation, must alter the conductivity of neural impulses, reflexes and the general state of neural activity. The disturbances of circulatory integrity to the neuromere has the potential of creating a multitude of complex responses far in excess of those following altered conductivity of a nerve trunk.

It must be emphasized that, although modifications by modern authorities relative to the arterial supply of neuromeres have been discussed, the alteration of the calibre of the lumen of those arterioles which do supply the cord segment is likely to have a greater disturbing influence than previously assumed due to the paucicity of vessels but a dependence of the neural cells upon adequate blood supply.

Wyke[276] has emphasized that neurones neither store glucose, nor adequately convert other substances for their metabolism, thus are dependent upon adequate blood supply for both glucose and oxygen, plus the co-enzyme, thiamine. The quantity of calcium ions in the extra-cellular fluid is critical to the function of the neurones, also. A low concentration of calcium ions decreases the sodium ion influx and decreases the action potential.

It has been stated by Curtis, Jacobson and Marcus[277] that brain cells must receive a continuous supply of oxygen and glucose lest damage occur. Since the cells of the gray matter of the spinal cord are similar in nature and function, it follows that they must have an optimum supply continuously or suffer unfavourable consequences.

Sherrington[278] discussed briefly the adverse influence upon the reflexes of asphyxia. This is, of course, a disturbance within the segment of the spinal cord, due to insufficient oxygen reaching the neural structures via the arterial supply. One of the causes of such asphyxia could be the result of vasoconstrictive sympathetic nerve impulses transmitted from the lateral horn cells over preganglionic sympathetic fibres, through the anterior nerve root, the nerve trunk, into the anterior primary ramus, to leave via the white ramus communicans to reach a paravertebral sympathetic ganglion, in which synaptic connection is made with the postganglionic fibres. These rejoin the anterior primary ramus by way of a gray ramus to reenter the spinal canal by way of the intervertebral foramen, to distribute these fibres to the smooth muscle fibres of the walls of the spinal artery and its various branches.

It should be recalled that the gray matter of each neuromere is dependent in large measure for its arterial blood supply upon a branch or arteriole from the anterior spinal artery which extends vertically downward in the anterior median fissure.

A tiny branch of the anterior spinal artery pierces the floor of the fissure and branches in a tree-like formation to supply the majority of the gray matter of the neuromere. The periphery of the gray matter, especially the posterior horn, derives arterial blood from those arterioles that have pierced the periphery of the cord to supply principally the white tracts.

The afferent impulses that have entered the segment may stimulate the lateral horn cells and send out vasoconstrictor impulses to result in constriction of the spinal artery and its branches, decreasing the supply of arterial blood to the neuromere, which, in turn, disturbs the reflex activity within that segment.

This is not to suggest that there is ever a frank ischemia of the neuromere as a concomitant of the vertebral fixation for, as has been demonstrated in previous pages, the vertical and circular anastomoses preclude such a possibility, but as Krieg[279] has stressed, the very sensitive nature of the neural elements to changes in their environment, that is the intercellular fluid, which, in turn, is dependent upon the vascular system for its homeostatic state, makes it unnecessary to have a wide variation of the tissue fluids to disturb the functioning of the cytones.

The more modern writings of Boyd[280] are in complete agreement with Krieg, as evinced by the statement: "It is the delicate balance of electrolytes and water that serves to maintain the constancy of the internal environment, the importance of which Bernard was the first to emphasize." There is no question that this internal environment or extracellular fluid is dependent upon adequate circulation for its stability of homeostasis.

Cobb[281] has shown that nerve cells may alter their rate of discharge with the variations in available oxygen within the tissue fluids and that an oxygen debt may develop with increased activity of the cells which exceeds the supply of oxygen, despite an increased blood flow. He has thoroughly described the stages of structural distortion of the cytones as a response to anoxemia and other irritants. Swelling appears first, chromatolysis and later disappearance of the chromidial substance, swelling of nucleus and the dark staining property of the nucleolus. If the process continues, the cells shrink and become pyknotic and dark with many spike-like processes. Function alters to the point of complete cessation, a situation most unlikely as a result of a vertebral fixation. However, an aberration of function is to be anticipated, due to the minor alteration in the arterial supply.

Furthermore, Cobb[282] has mentioned that cerebral cells degenerate after 3 minutes and 10 seconds of complete anoxia, but those of the medulla spinalis may withstand 15 minutes of complete lack of oxygen and still recover. Curtis et al[283] state that brain damage occurs after 4 to 5 minutes of anoxia and 10 to 15 minutes of lack of glucose.

Magoun and Rhines[284] report the findings of Harreveld, Marmont and Harreveld, who have found that asphyxia and anoxia have a very selective detrimental influence upon the neurones of the spinal cord. It has been shown by these researchers that internuncial or intercalated neurones suffer destruction from anoxia, while the anterior horn cells and the fibres entering via the posterior nerve roots remain intact and functional. As a result of this form of disturbance, the reflexes become hyperactive, having been freed from some of the inhibitory influence of the internuncial system of neurones.

It is of interest to note that Cobb[285] has reported that there are about 200 to 300 mm. of capillaries active for each cubic millimeter of white matter and 600 to 1000 mm. for each cubic millimeter of gray matter, thereby providing for the greatest oxygen and nutritional supply to the most active portions of the nervous system. Disturbance to the supply of arterial blood would interfere most conspicuously with the functioning of the gray matter.

Freeman[286] has observed and others have confirmed his observation that the nervous system utilizes glucose for its metabolism and any disturbance of the quantity available upsets the normal functional integrity of the neurones. An increase in quantity available in the tissue fluid increases the threshhold of response and exercises an inhibitory influence, while the reverse situation, a decrease in available glucose, raises the excitability of the neurones for a period of time and results in an erratic function. This latter observation has been stressed particularly by Abrahamson.[287] The transport of glucose to the cells is, of course, dependent upon the adequacy of arterial supply consistent with the functional needs of the moment.

Stanley Cobb[288] mentions that acetylcholine can only be formed at the neural terminals and the next neurone can only respond to acetylcholine when adequate glucose is available for the functional integrity of the neurones. Since the mechanism by which the stimulus is transmitted from one axone to the dendrite of the next neurone at the synaptic junction is through the medium of acetylcholine release by the axone's terminal endings, it may be appreciated how essential adequate nutrition via optimum arterial blood distribution must be.

From these references to the necessity for competent oxygen and nutritional supply by means of the arterial and capillary bed of the neuromere, it is hoped that the reader may appreciate the complexity of possible responses of the neural structures to the simple vertebral fixation or subluxation. The afferent bombardment, caused by the fixation, disturbs the vasomotor control by the lateral horn cells of somatic, neural and also visceral structures supplied from the same neuromere. The latter disturbances will receive consideration as attention is directed to each area of the spinal cord.


## Venous Derangement

While it is true that the venous division of the vascular system is also under the direct controlling influence of the sympathetic nervous system, more attention will be devoted to the mechanical domination over the venous return from the associated neuromere created by the fixation of a vertebral segment. Cobb[289] has demonstrated that arteries, veins and even capillaries of the central nervous system have myelinated and postganglionic sympathetic nerve fibres accompanying them.

It must be appreciated that the distal ends of the capillary plexuses are continuous with the venules and that any failure of free venous drainage would create a back pressure into the capillary bed and a resultant passive hyperemia or congestion. Each artery has one or two, usually two, venae commintantes leaving the neuromere to take part in the formation of a rich plexus. A further network of veins from the meninges in the formation of the venous plexus in the extradural space of the vertebral canal can be demonstrated. The latter plexus of the extradural space is drained by several thin-walled veins which exit through each intervertebral foramen. These veins lack the customary valves, thereby permitting the blood to flow in either direction with equal facility.

There are several possibilities and probabilities by which the vertebral fixation may impede the venous flow from the extradural plexus. Free movement is important throughout the body for the propulsion of venous blood along its course back toward the heart. There seems little reason, or evidence, to doubt that movement of the spinal column aids in the promotion of venous flow through these intervertebral veins.

A vertebral fixation eliminates the alterations of intervertebral pressure, as normal movements play upon the area. It can be appreciated that the majority of movements change the thickness of the intervertebral fibrocartilaginous disc which forms an integral portion of the anterior wall of the intervertebral foramen. Dorsiflexion of the spine narrows the posterior border of the discs involved. Lateral flexion narrows the discs on the concave side and increases the thickness on the convex side. Anterior flexion also increases the posterior thickness and narrows the anterior borders. Such a play of alternating pressure and relative negative pressure acts as a pumping mechanism to propel the venous blood on its way beyond the point where valves within the veins make return impossible.

A second factor is added by the fixation to disturb the free egress of venous blood from the extradural plexus through the veins of the involved intervertebral foramen. As the osteopathic researchers, Burns et al,[290] demonstrated, the vertebral fixation results in an edematous condition within the tissues of the intervertebral foramen. Such pressure may be sufficient to inhibit the free flow of venous blood through the thin-walled veins without being sufficient to create a pressure upon the nerve trunk of such magnitude as would be necessary to disrupt the conductivity of the fibres of this structure.

The lack of pumping and the impeding pressure within the intervertebral foramen decreases the flow of venous blood, creating an increase in pressure within the extradural plexus with resultant increase in hydrostatic pressure within the veins of the neuromere. A passive venous congestion results. Such a minor degree of stagnation may result in a minor anoxia of the neural tissues.

Cobb[291] has quoted Barcroft as describing three types of anoxemia, the anaemic, anoxic and the stagnant. Due to the minor degree of back pressure exerted by the venous stagnation, the arterioles and proximal ends of the capillary plexuses are unable to supply the optimum of arterial blood with its oxygen and nutrition. Hence, the neural tissues may be disturbed in function much as described under the previous heading.

The failure of the capillaries and venules to remove the carbon dioxide and other metabolites may accentuate the problem. Cobb[292] has pointed out that asphyxia causes an increased permeability and dilatation of the minute vessels with the formation of edema, extravasation of errythrocytes to form a red infarction.

It must be obvious that the fixation of a single vertebral segment is unlikely to create sufficient back pressure to result in a red infarction. However, it is more common for the acute subluxation or fixation to be accompanied by a limitation of motion of a number of segments above and below. This is particularly true when the fixation occurs as a result of mechanical trauma to the area and injury to the holding elements with the application of the principle expressed as Hilton's Law.[293] That is, the noxious impulses entering the neuromere stimulate the motor neurones to cause the musculature to contract in a "splinting" action to put at rest the injured segment, but as Sherrington,[294] in particular, has emphasized, the efferent response to a centripetal stimulus is plurisegmental. Therefore, the postvertebral muscles over an area of the spine are likely to engage in this "splinting" activity and a number of segments experience a degree of fixation which decreases with distance from the primary source of nociceptive stimuli.

Such limitation of motion of an area of the spine accentuates the venous embarrassment and thereby contributes to a more pronounced degree of venous stagnation above described. The neuromere of primary involvement suffers the greatest ill-effects with those adjacent experiencing a progressively lesser degree of stagnation with distance from the site of primary fixation. Thus, the disturbance created by a single acute fixation is rarely simple and the possible aberrations are almost legion.

It is not the intention of the writer to leave the impression that the usual subluxation or fixation produces a gross venous stagnation, but, rather, that the mild passive congestion, as a resultant to vertebral fixation, contributes to the alteration of the environmental fluids, thereby disturbing the normal functioning of the cells and fibres of the neuromere, or neuromeres, involved and contributes to the disturbances created by faulty arterial supply, as a result of abnormal sympathetic innervation of the vessel musculature, which, in turn, has been the response to afferent impulses arising in the holding elements of the subluxated vertebra.

## Fatigue

Such a dissertation on the vertebral fixation, or chiropractic subluxation, would be in no way complete were consideration not given to the detrimental influence of fatigue as it relates to the neural mechanisms.

The bombardment of the neuromere by proprioceptive and nociceptive impulses has fatiguing influences which are not uniformly consistent for all the neurones affected within the segment. Sherrington[295] has made mention of this fact.

Krieg[296] has brought clearly to his readers' attention that the proprioceptive fibres and the motor fibres stimulated by them appear to be almost indefatiguable, while connector neurones and other elements of the nervous system, inclusive of the sympathetic neurones, show the ill-effects of fatigue in a relatively short period of time.

This is consistent with needs of the body's economy(Guyton[297]). The somatic musculature must maintain a degree of tone at all times and the basic tonal mechanism involves the afferent receptors in muscles and tendons, their centripetal nerve fibres and the efferent limb of the reflex arc. Upon this fundamental mechanism for the maintenance of a degree of muscle contraction all other modifying influences, both local and from higher levels, of the organized nervous system, play in a ceaseless modification of muscle tone in response to the changes of external and internal environment.

It is not surprising then that the postvertebral muscle contraction, once established by the causative stress, is capable of perpetuating its own contractile state long after the original source of irritation has passed away. The other neural elements are not so fortunate and do undergo alterations of cellular integrity as a result of fatigue, thereby modifying their functional capacity.

The first result of constant stimulation of nerve cells has been described by Kuntz[298] as being an enlargement of the cell body and a displacement of the chromaffin granules, which are essential to nerve impulse propagation, to the periphery of the cell after 15 minutes of stimulation. As the stimulus continues, the nucleus swells and the Nissl granules begin to disintegrate, or as Freeman[299] states, chromatolysis begins. The nucleus becomes eccentric and then the cell and nucleus begin to shrink in size with loss of its conductivity. Continuation of the fatiguing process may result in irreparable damage to the neurone and loss of function.

Pottenger[300] indicates that the first functional change, due to fatigue, is lessening of synaptic resistance and a more erratic response. As the fatigue process is accentuated, there is an increasing loss of ability of the nerve impulse to be transmitted across the synapse and a decline in the transmission of neural signals to the effector organs. Inasmuch as the neural supply to the tissues not only modify their functional capacity, but also have a trophic influence upon them, it is obvious that neural fatigue will result first in increased function of the tissues, followed by declining function as the stimuli decrease and finally, disturbance of integrity as the trophic influence of the nerve fibre is lost.

It is to be noted that these changes are almost a repetition of those of anoxia.

Fatigue of neurones is not confined to the spinal cord segments, but may involve the postganglionic sympathetic system. Thus, the afferent impulses entering the cord from the site of fixation may continue to activate the preganglionic sympathetic neurones of the lateral gray horn, sending out impulses to the cells in the appropriate paravertebral ganglion, which are concerned with the supply of a portion of the vascular bed and/or a viscus. Kuntz[301] has quoted researchers who have demonstrated that the postganglionic cell bodies respond to fatigue in a manner similar, if not identical, to that of the cells of the central nervous system. Thus, it may be that in some instances the disturbance in function is of a central nature, while in others it is more peripheral, involving the ganglionic cells.

Sherrington[302] has stated that fatigue is demonstrable for the pathways of sensory conduction to higher brain centres for conscious interpretation, thereby decreasing the conscious awareness of any form of afferent stimulation, including pain.

The neurological authorities appear to be in agreement that the phenomenon of fatigue involves the synpatic junction and is closely allied to the production of acetylcholine at the terminal endings of the axones. Furthermore, the production of acetylcholine is dependent upon adequate amounts of chromidial substance within the cell body. In the early stages of stimulation, the cell body increases in size, the Nissl granules are prominently displayed and the synaptic junction functions in a normal manner, due to the optimum production of acetylcholine at the synapse. In the early stage of fatigue, the chromaffin granules migrate to the periphery of the cell body, and as Pottenger[303] has established, the synapse permits an "easier transmission" of the neural signals. As chromatolysis progresses, there is a decline in the production of acetylcholine at the synapse and a raising of the threshhold resistance of the synapse. The final stage of fatigue, is, of course, the almost total absence of Nissl granules, the failure of production of acetylcholine at the synapse, and a cessation of neural impulse transmission across the synapse. Those effector organs at the terminal end of the efferent fibres are first overstimulated, gradually deprived of adequate stimuli, and then suffer from lack of neural signals and their trophic influence. Degenerative changes may then appear within the cells deprived of this trophic control.

It must be appreciated that the Nissl granules are considered to be stored nutrition for the metabolic function of the neurone and these are dependent upon adequate nutritional replenishment through the blood-vascular channels.

The electron microscope has aided in determining that the Nissl bodies are densely packed endoplasmic reticula studded by ribosomes which are spherical particles about 180 Å in diameter with protein synthesis occurring on their surfaces. Each is composed of approximately 50% RNA and 50% protein bound by magnesium ions, according to Minckler.[304] The same author shows an illustration of the normal and injured neural cell body and states: "If a neurone's supply of RNA and succinic dehydrogenase is depleted through function, high concentrations are found in the surrounding glia."

Nutrition supplied by the arterial blood stream below the level of requirement for the activity experienced by the neurones would soon contribute to the evils of fatigue, or predispose the neurones to fatigue. Other current authors agree with the older authorities and have added details of understanding of the biochemistry. Curtis et al[305] have stated: "This response is similar to the response of a nerve cell when there is insufficient blood supply, which produces an ischemic neurone."

Perhaps from these suggestions, as to the mechanisms by which the fixation of a vertebral segment may disturb the function of the components of the associated neuromere and, in turn, those tissues both somatic and splanchnic, supplied, it may be appreciated that the process is far from a simple mechanical pressure upon the nerve trunk.

The consideration has been far from exhaustive, the details of histologic structure and chemistry as discussed by Curtis et al[306] are beyond the competence of this author and would add nothing to the present discussion. Other factors will appear as each region of the spine is considered. As the researchers in the field of neurology continue to establish additional facts relative to the functioning of this amazingly complicated system, the necessity for further modification in the theory of chiropractic will make itself obvious and remain an ever present challenge to the active minds of students, practitioners, educators and researchers within the profession of chiropractic. Unless the challenge of continuous progress is accepted by each generation of doctors of chiropractic, the profession will not long remain in the vanguard of the healing arts.

CHAPTER XIII

# Detrimental Effects of the Cervical Subluxation

THE PREVIOUS CHAPTER has been devoted to the general mechanisms by which the vertebral fixation may disturb a nerve trunk and the associated neuromere. In this chapter and several hereafter, further detailed consideration must be given to the more specific detrimental effects of the vertebral kinetic aberration in relation to altered function in splanchnic and somatic tissues. Some additional disruption of neural function, due to the peculiarities of the local vertebral areas and cyto-architecture of the medulla spinalis, deserves consideration.

The upper cervical area is one of those regions, by virtue of its peculiar anatomical construction and the intimate association with the brain stem, that is deserving of extensive special discussion. Thus, the greater part of this chapter will refer to the upper cervical segments.

From the time of D. D. Palmer,[307] doctors of chiropractic have been cognizant of the unusual osseous formation of the atlas and axis and the virtual impossibility of subluxations to create pressure upon the first or second cervical nerve trunks. The profusion of symptoms and functional changes as a resultant of distortion of these two spinal segments has been amply demonstrated by the clinical response to the adjusting of these vertebrae. It is doubtful that any school of chiropractic thought, each with its individualized technique of vertebral correction, has neglected this extremely potent area, while several have featured this portion almost to the exclusion of the remainder of the vertebral column.

What appears on the surface to be a paradox, unfolds in an orderly and reasonable fashion when attention is directed toward the more subtle disturbances created by the segmental fixation. Certainly, direct nerve pressure cannot explain the multiplicity of responses, nor does the idea of cord pressure fulfill the requirements when studied from an anatomical and physiological viewpoint.

There can be no denial that cervical fixation disturbs splanchnic function and such inconsistency of facts dictates the wisdom of seeking a sound explanation of these inconsistencies in the field of physiological neurology.

186

## Peculiarities of the Cervical Cord

The gray matter of the cervical segments of the spinal cord is not composed of any group of cytones concerned with the efferent supply of visceral structures, including the vascular channels. In other words, there are just somatic efferent cytones and the cells of connector neurones, some of which receive impulses from the fibres of posterior nerve radicles.

Gray[308] has shown that the anterior gray column of the cervical cord, especially in the cervical enlargement, is large and broad, while the posterior column is long and narrow and there are no lateral gray horns composed of preganglionic sympathetic cell bodies in any of the segments.

The afferent fibres of the posterior nerve root, especially of pain and temperature, upon entrance into the cord turn upward for several segments prior to making synaptic connection with the Golgi Type I cells of the Substantia Gelatinosa of Rolando. This necessitates the fibres of, at least, the upper three posterior nerve roots entering the medulla oblongata before synapsing. In this structure, the Substantia Gelatinosa has been named the Nucleus of the Spinal Tract of the Trigeminal Nerve.

It is of interest to note that the Spinal Tract of the Trigeminal Nerve descends on the lateral surface of the Nucleus and some of the fibres continue on downward beyond the confines of the medulla as part of the Posterolateral Tract, or Tract of Lissauer, of the upper cervical region. Gray[309] specifies that these pain and temperature fibres synapse, "as far down as the second cervical segment."

Minckler,[310] on the other hand, states: "Of the branches of cranial nerve V, the ophthalmic pain and temperature fibres descend farthest in the descending root (to cervical segments); the maxillary fibres descend an intermediate distance, and the descending mandibular fibres extend the shortest distance (to the lower third of the medulla)." However, no indication of the number of cervical neuromeres involved is provided, but the indications are that both ophthalmic and maxillary fibres end in the cervical cord.

Krieg[311] states that this tract ends in the second cervical neuromere. Still other authorities submit evidence to show that some of these first order afferent neurones of the Trigeminal Nerve may descend as low as the fifth cervical segment. However, for future use in this discussion, it will be accepted that the second cervical neuromere is the lowest extension of these fibres.

Another peculiarity of the anatomy of the cervical region is the group of cell bodies in the lateral portion of the anterior gray column of the first five neuromeres, according to Gray,[312] whose axones are directed through the lateral white column to emerge on the lateral surface of the cord as the radicles, or rootlets, of the Spinal Accessory (XI Cranial) Nerve. While this root enters the cranium through the foramen magnum, is joined by fibres from the vagal nuclei and escapes again via the jugular foramen, these cervical fibres supply the sternocleidomastoideus and trapezius muscles. The cranial root is composed of vagal fibres, which run a short distance with the somatic fibres of the Accessory before returning to the Vagus for distribution.

Another collection of motor cytones that modify and enlarge the anterior gray column is that found in the fourth and fifth neuromeres for the motor supply of the diaphragm by way of the Phrenic Nerve.

Further contributions to the cervical enlargement, which includes segments from the third cervical to the second thoracic, according to Gray's[313] description, are made by additional efferent cells of the anterior gray column concerned with the motor supply of the muscles of the upper extremities.

A number of Golgi type I neurones of the gray matter contribute to the formation of the Sulcomarginal Fasciculus which, in turn, is continuous with the Medial Longitudinal Bundle of the medulla, as described by Gray.[314] The descending fibres of the Medial Longitudinal Bundle or Fasciculus extend downward into the region of the cervical cord to especially influence the neurones of control over the muscles that move the head, as described by Krieg,[315] in response to visual and vestibular reflexes.

The Tectospinal Tract is especially prominent in the cervical portion of the cord and loses its identity beyond this region. The cells of this tract are located in the superior corpus quadrigeminum of the opposite side and subserve visual reflexes, which are primarily concerned with movements of the head and neck and, on occasion, the protective movements of the arm.

The Olivospinal Tract is another bundle of fibres to be found exclusively in the cervical cord, with doubtful origin in the medulla near the inferior olivary nucleus and function unknown to Gray.[316]

These are some of the oddities of the cervical region of the medulla spinalis. Several others will be mentioned as this discourse unfolds. It demonstrates the customary tracts found in the other regions of the cord, but not above discussed specifically. Most of these

188

tracts are larger in the cervical segments because, if motor tracts, few fibres have had the opportunity to synapse in the gray matter and if sensory, they are the consolidation of fibres contributed at each neuromere below to increase in number from below upward.

With this sketchy review of the outstanding peculiarities of the region of the cord, attention is directed to the disturbances created by fixation of cervical segments.

## Somatic Symptom Complexes

In addition to the local pain, tenderness and muscle spasm attendant upon the acute subluxation, especially those resulting from mechanical force that traumatizes the holding elements, the subluxation of one or more of the upper five segments is particularly prone to the production of an acute torticollis or spasm of a portion of the trapezius muscle.

Utilizing the noxious impulses from the holding elements, as an example, it may be seen that the unusual bombardment of such impulses entering the cord by way of the pain fibres of the meningeal nerve, nerve trunk, posterior nerve root and the radicles, turn upward in the Tract of Lissauer for several segments prior to synapsing with the second order neurones of the star-shaped variety in the Substantia Gelatinosa. Collaterals of these first order neurones may make direct synaptic connection with the anterior horn cells, or through one or more internuncial neurones of the Golgi Type II form, stimulate the motor neurones, causing the postvertebral muscle contraction called "splinting," to fix the injured articulation and thereby prevent further injury or irritation. If the stimulus is sufficiently strong, or the irritability of the neurones is increased, a "spill-over" may take place to involve many additional efferent neurones.

The longus capitis and longus colli muscles on the anterior surface of the cervical column may become contracted, as well as one or more of the scalenus anterior, medius or posterior muscles. All of these muscles lateral flex the cervical column to the side of contraction, but the scaleni rotate the head toward the opposite side, while the longi rotate the head to the same side. The scaleni, being the stronger, would be responsible for the direction of head rotation.

The spread of impulses might well involve the motor pool of the Spinal Accessory nerve and thereby create muscle hypertension, or even spasm, of the sternocleidomastoideus and/or the trapezius. The former flexes the cervical spine to the same side and rotates the head to the opposite side, while the trapezius also rotates the head to the opposite side.

Utilizing Pflueger's fourth law,[317] which states that, if reflex excitement extends to other motor nerves than normally utilized, the direction of the spread is from below upward, it can be appreciated that a subluxation of any cervical vertebra could result in the acute muscle spasm of torticollis.

Although pain has been utilized as the type of afferent stimulus in this example, the following may serve to demonstrate the mechanism by which a subluxation, whose afferent impulses remain below the level of conscious awareness, may lay the groundwork for the production of an acute torticollis in response to an additional minor stimulating experience which, of itself, would be incapable of triggering such a violent response.

The proprioceptive impulses arising in the holding elements of a fixated segment of the spine may bombard the motor pools, whose cells have been made more irritable by the vascular and nutritional disturbances produced by the fixation, as discussed in the previous chapter. Together these may have created a central excitatory state, but insufficient in degree to produce the acute muscle spasm of torticollis. This individual now sits in a draught, chilling the skin of his neck. The afferent impulses aroused by this new stimulus now enter the spinal cord by way of special afferent fibres of the posterior nerve root to summate with the proprioceptive impulses from the area of fixation to activate beyond normal response the motor pools that have been made more irritable by the vascular and nutritional aberrations produced by the subluxation. A stream of efferent impulses results in the sudden, severe muscle spasm of acute torticollis. Now is added an additional stream of afferent impulses, some of which reach the postcentral gyrus to be experienced as severe pain, while yet others add to the bombardment of the efferent neurones to perpetuate and increase the muscle spasm.

Such a condition responds to the careful, gentle, skillful ministrations of the chiropractor, or may run its course as fatigue develops and the spasm gradually subsides. At times, accidental correction of the cervical subluxation occurs and the person has no further problem. In other instances, one severe bout of spasm and pain has hardly been forgotten before another exacerbation strikes. Still other unfortunates experience a cessation of the pain and acute muscle spasm, but retain difficulty in straightening their necks and carrying their heads in the proper facing. Allowing such a condition to continue, results in contractures of the muscles and great difficulty, or impossibility, in obtaining a complete correction.

## Complications

It would be negligent to discuss the problem of torticollis without acknowledging that the doctor of chiropractic periodically encounters a case of this nature which responds well to his ministrations for the relief of the acute problem, but has recurrences despite every attempt to normalize the subluxated vertebrae. If the practitioner, in his original examination, has overlooked investigation of those structures supplied by the Trigeminal Nerve, he now does so with the expectation of finding a source of irritation that continues to reproduce the cervical fixation and contributes to the central excitatory state of the motoneurones, making the insignificant additional forms of irritation sufficient to "trigger" another acute attack of torticollis. This may be an example of Facillitation.

Such sources of Trigeminal irritation may be ocular, nasal, dental or from the paranasal sinuses. Thus, the patient may require another branch of the healing arts to receive complete correction of his problem, since it is not within the purview of the chiropractic physician to prescribe corrective lenses, extract teeth, etc.

To utilize a practical example that the mechanism may be better appreciated, let it be assumed that the patient has an apical dental abscess, an impacted tooth, or postextraction infection, etc. Such irritation stimulates nociceptive fibres of either the maxillary or mandibular divisions of the Fifth Cranial Nerve. Upon entering the pons by way of the sensory root, these fibres turn inferiorly as components of the Spinal Tract of the Trigeminal Nerve to synapse with the second order neurones, whose cell bodies form the Nucleus of the Spinal Tract, previously discussed. While the primary function of these second order neurones is to relay the impulses to the thalamus, there is every clinical evidence to indicate that some connector fibres descend to stimulate the motor fibres in the upper cervical segments, especially those of the postvertebral muscles concerned with dorsiflexion of the head and neck. Such reflex movement is demonstrated by the withdrawal of the head from sources of potential danger, as seen when a foreign particle enters the conjunctival sac of the eye and the head is immediately jerked back in dorsiflexion. The dentist's drill causes a like attempt to withdraw the head reflexly.

Unilateral irritation of the fibres results in a flow of noxious impulses that may demonstrate Pflueger's first law,[318] "If stimulation of a sensory nerve be followed by a unilateral reflex movement, the latter always occurs on the side to which the sensory nerve belongs." As a result, contraction occurs in the postvertebral muscles on the same side as the source of dental irritation with fixation, or subluxation, of the associated vertebra or vertebrae. Now the complications above discussed may be repeated.

It may be comprehended that the adjusting of the cervical spine is followed by repeated muscle contraction and fixation until the primary source of irritation is discovered by the chiropractor and removed by the dental surgeon. The patient should return to the chiropractor following any dental work to have cervical adjustings until the alveolar irritation has subsided and the vertebral and muscular functions have been normalized. In fact, all oral surgical cases could benefit from the postoperative care of a doctor of chiropractic, because such alveolar trauma is more than likely to produce cervical fixations, which may not undergo spontaneous correction and remain as sources of further discomfort and more serious problems.

What has been said above for the dental irritants applies to those other structures, whose irritation stimulates the nociceptive fibres of the Trigeminus. The oculist, optometrist, nasal surgeon, etc., may be an essential ally of the doctor of chiropractic and the latter could serve admirably to benefit the patients of these specialists, following their professional services. These practitioners would be amazed at the improvement and speed of recovery of their patients were the chiropractor utilized for the correction of the subluxations experienced by such patients. While chiropractic may not be a panacea, chiropractic could play a useful and supportive role for every other branch of healing, as there is a need for the correction of vertebral fixations in every case of sickness or injury. When this realization dawns upon the other professions and cooperation is the rule, rather than the exception, patients will experience a marked improvement in their health service.

## Spasms of the Hyoid Muscles

Another very unpleasant complex experienced by some patients with an atlas, axis or third cervical fixation is the unilateral spasm of muscles attached to the hyoid bone. Most of these muscles are supplied by fibres of the first, second and/or third cervical nerves via the Ansa Hypoglossi. This sudden contraction may occur as the person

192

yawns, dorsiflexes his neck or stretches.

There is a sudden discomfort, inability to swallow or speak, but very little true pain. The individual is startled and usually grasps his throat, which, in most instances, is sufficient to release the spasm and permit free motion of the hyoid. This is an alarming experience and more nuisance value than serious, but the recurrences are likely to prompt the sufferer to seek professional help. The chiropractor is capable of explaining the problem and making the necessary osseous corrections that alleviate this misery. Many of these patients have been reassured and told it is "just nerves" by practitioners of other schools of thought, a platitude of little comfort when the patient fears strangulation at any moment.

The mechanisms for such a symptom phenomenon have received consideration previously. It should also be recognized that the Trigeminal irritations, as discussed, may be underlying causative factors, as every upper cervical fixation must be considered to be a response to Trigeminal irritation until investigation has eliminated such a possibility.

The presence of an upper cervical subluxation seems to be essential for this phenomenon to manifest itself and cervical correction relieves the problem. It would seem that the noxious impulses, travelling down the Spinal Tract of the Trigeminal to synapse in the Nucleus of the Spinal Tract, are conducted by these second order neurones or their collaterals to the motor pool of control over the Hyoid muscles. These impulses create a Central Excitatory State and predispose the efferent neurones to stimulation by the centripetal impulses from the locus of cervical subluxation.

## The Diaphragm

The Diaphragm is the most important single somatic muscle. Paralysis of the Diaphragm results in the cessation of life itself, as respiration is embarrassed to the degree that life cannot be sustained.

The Diaphragm, as has been previously mentioned, acts as an accessory heart in propelling the venous blood from the lower extremities, pelvic and abdominal cavities back through the Inferior Vena Cava to the right atrium of the heart.

The nerve supply to such an important structure is of considerable concern to the chiropractor. Hence, marked attention is devoted to the third, fourth, fifth and sixth cervical vertebrae, because between these segments emerge the fibres of the third, fourth, fifth cervical nerves destined to form the Phrenic Nerve for motor supply to the Diaphragm.

The fourth cervical spinal segment is usually the apex of the cervical lordosis and often the apex of a scoliosis with considerable rotation. These stressors contribute afferent impulses to the associated neuromeres. If frank subluxation, or fixation, occurs in addition, the Diaphragm may be stimulated to the point of acute unilateral spasm, which may be as painful as the acute torticollis and productive of greater anxiety on the part of the patient.

Most frequently these acute spasms occur without warning with a sudden paralyzing stab of pain, as though a knife had been driven through from the xiphoid process to about the eighth thoracic vertebra. Respiration is arrested for a short interval and then becomes shallow and hurried. The afflicted individual experiences great anxiety and may note pain in the base of his neck, his shoulder and even down his arm. Should this occur on the left side, even the physician may consider the possibilities of a coronary thrombosis. However, the blood pressure is more frequently elevated than lowered and cardiograms are negative.

If the referred pain is to the right shoulder, the doctor may first think in terms of cholelithiasis or other biliary problem. Some cases have considerable referred pain into the abdominal region, since afferent fibres return to the lower six thoracic neuromeres from the Diaphragm. Such symptoms have led to all manner of diagnostic abdominal explorations.

The writer was called to one patient, who experienced pain down both thighs and had flexion of both hips, due to associated contraction of the Psoas Major muscles. The most difficult phase of care was, as so frequently is true in this condition, convincing the patient that the "Grim Reaper" was not standing at her bedside.

The chronic Diaphragm contraction is much less dramatic and almost universal in occurrence. The universality of this problem is probably a result of the chronic bombardment of these associated neuromeres by afferent impulses aroused by the mechanical stresses above mentioned and the response of the Diaphragm to the emotional state of fear, worry and anxiety.

The disturbances of structural integrity and the causative influence of afferent impulses from the Diaphragm in the production of cervical subluxations have received consideration in a previous chapter.

Another frequent disquieting experience is the bout of "hic-cups," which in the relatively rare patient becomes so protracted and severe as to endanger life. While many forms of irritation may contribute to the production of this peculiar response, the subluxation is one of major importance and it is doubtful that any severe attack of this malady develops without the presence of a fixation of one or more of the associated vertebrae. The knowledgeable doctor of chiropractic would seek to determine the presence of a structural problem in the mid-cervical region first, but would not be unmindful of the lower six thoracic segments to which the afferent fibres of the Diaphragm return. Thus, a lower thoracic subluxation may contribute impulses to those connector neurones which subserve the Diaphragmatic control by ascending the spinal cord to synapse with the efferent neurones of the motor pool in the third, fourth and fifth cervical neuromeres.

Chiropractic adjusting of subluxated vertebral segments has brought to an end hiccups, after all other methods have been to no avail. There are those instances, however, when chiropractic techniques fail miserably, for as Kuntz[319] has enumerated, aortic aneurism, pulmonary carcinoma, peritonitis, carcinoma of stomach, liver, kidney or adrenal gland may be the causative factor. All of these result in the abnormal reflex through irritation of the fibres of the Phrenic Nerve and are unlikely to respond to conservative methods of any kind.

## The Upper Extremity

The arm and shoulder girdle are supplied with afferent and efferent fibres from the fifth to the eighth cervical anterior primary rami and that of the first thoracic, with a few sensory fibres from the second thoracic. As is, no doubt, known to the reader of this book, those rami take part in the formation of the Brachial Plexus, in which a rearrangement and regrouping of fibres occur to provide named nerves composed of fibres of more than one neuromere.

Fixation of any of the above mentioned vertebrae may disturb the normal functioning of the arm in accordance with the mechanisms discussed in Chapter XII. Only one peculiar condition affecting the arm will receive brief consideration here — the Scalene Syndrome.

As John Favill[320] has outlined, the Scalenus Anterior, Medius and Posterior are supplied by fibres of the fourth, fifth, sixth and seventh and eighth cervical nerves, thus may be disturbed by subluxations of the corresponding vertebrae. Due to the passage of the Brachial

Plexus between the Scalenus Anterior and Medius, according to Gray's[321] description, contraction of these two muscles, resulting from the excess stimulation produced by the cervical fixation, might well bring mechanical pressure to bear upon this plexus to produce many of the symptoms of this syndrome.

The passage of the subclavian artery between these same muscles may be responsible for some of the vascular phenomena associated with the complex, as the mechanical pressure interferes with the normal arterial supply.

In most instances, patients exhibiting this painful syndrome demonstrate marked postural faults, which permit the thorax to droop and flatten, thereby narrowing the space between the Scalenus Anticus and Scalenus Medius. The added contraction with increase in thickness of these muscles then becomes sufficient to exert pressure. The doctor of chiropractic may then be faced with a problem of postural and local subluxation correction.

The faulty posture also decreases the space between the attachment of the Scalenus Anticus and the first rib, permitting pressure upon the artery, as well as adding to the mechanical strain upon the vertebral segments which serve as transitions or apices of curves. This latter stress further adds to the bombardment of neuromeres by nociceptive impulses and contributes to the contraction of muscles and the aggravation of the problem.

## Compensatory Influences

Chiropractors have long been cognizant of the descending compensatory efforts of the spine in response to upper cervical subluxations and the mechanisms by which this is explained presents an interesting challenge to the chiropractic profession. The compensatory distortions, as a concomitance of basic distortion, have been thoroughly described by such chiropractic authorities as Willard Carver,[322] H.G. Beatty,[323] Hugh B. Logan,[324] and touched upon in an earlier chapter. A description of the neurology responsible for the ascending compensation is unknown to this writer.

Maintenance of the head in proper relation to the environment is of fundamental importance, especially to visual experience. It is of little surprise, therefore, that every effort is made by a number of neurological mechanisms to assure this correction of position in relation to the horizon. These function together in a harmony of cooperation, but must be separated for purposes of description.

Krieg[325] has described the effects of proprioceptive impulses from the ligamentous structures of the upper cervical segments which are concerned with establishing the proper relationship of the head to the body. Presuming then that a fixation of the atlanto-occipital complex exists in which the occiput is shifted to the left, it can be appreciated that, due to the shape of the condyles and superior articular facets of the atlas, the entire head is tipped right with the right ear lower than the left. Such a distortion could exert a degree of tension upon the ligamentous structures on the left, resulting in an excess of proprioceptive impulses bombarding the left side of the cord with the result that an increase in contraction occurs in the lateral flexor muscles of the cervical column, thereby establishing a right scoliosis. Such a scoliosis may be exaggerated beyond the needs of leveling the head and this condition then stimulates afferent fibres of the right to stimulate lateral flexor muscles and thereby create a left scoliosis of the upper thoracic region of a lesser degree to establish a balanced compensation and permit the eyes to regain the horizontal disposition.

Another contributing system of afferent fibres are those that ascend from the spinal cord to the reticular formation of the brain stem. These are concerned with a higher level of reflex integration or are the proprioceptive fibres of the superior cervical nerves, as established by Krieg.[326] From the reticular substance the impulses are conducted inferiorly by fibres of the Reticulospinal Tract and Medial Longitudinal Fasciculus to modify the activity of the effector neurones and contribute to the balancing of the head in proper relation to the horizon.

Curtis et al[327] has confirmed this Reticulospinal Tract as taking origin from the Nucleus Reticularis Gigantocellularis in the lower medulla. These authors have established that this system has an important control of posture and stabilizing the visceral function.

Having the head tipped, as suggested for the above mentioned fixation, would also involve stimulation of afferent vestibular fibres distributed to the maculae of the labyrinthine system of the low side and a corresponding decrease of stimulation on the opposite side. These impulses are then transmitted by the vestibular nerve to the nuclei in the brain stem and the Lateral Vestibular Nucleus in particular. The axones of this group of cell bodies descend as the Vestibulospinal Tract to stimulate the efferent neurones in an attempt to re-establish the normal relationship of the head in space and thereby contribute to the production of the scolioses.

Gray[328] has pointed out that vestibular impulses travel from the Superior and Lateral Vestibular Nuclei in fibres which aid in the formation of the Vestibulospinal Tract of the ipsilateral side to effect an influence upon the motor cells of the antagonistic muscles.

The vestibular system has an even greater influence upon the tonus of the muscles of the eyes and has a more far reaching modifying control over the postural muscles than the present discussion warrants considering.

The afferent impulses aroused by the fixation of the head in a tipped position, as per this example, may be transmitted over second order neurones from the posterior gray horn, to decussate, take part in the formation of the Spinotectal Tract, to reach the Superior Corpus Quadrigeminum, the reflex centre for integration of the eye movements. From this reflex centre the impulses travel via the Tectobulbar Tract to the nuclei of the cranial nerves of control of the ocular muscles.

Minckler[329] gives credit to the Spinotectal Tract for carrying sensations from the skin to the nuclei for eye muscle control.

Reversing the process, it may be established that were the head to be tipped and visual images appreciated on a slant, it would be disturbing to the afflicted person. Thus, the visual fibres of the Optic Nerve enter the Superior Colliculus via the superior brachium, synapse, and new fibres leave as part of the Tectobulbar or Tectospinal Tracts to decussate. Krieg[330] has discussed the fibres of the Tectobulbar Tract that enter the upper cervical segments of the cord to influence the motor cells, including those of the Spinal Accessory Nerve. The Tectospinal Tract not only makes connection with the efferent neurones of the cervical region but probably descends for the entire length of the cord. By this system, further influence may be exerted to establish a leveling influence upon the head by establishing such spinal compensations as may be necessary by the primary distortion.

It must be apparent that any distortion, fixation or subluxation that the cervical column may experience has the potential of creating disturbances such as have been described. Space and the patience of the reader do not permit detailed discussion of each.

As Sherrington[331] has established, the proprioceptive system of the more cephalic segments has a controlling influence upon "vast fields of the skeletal musculature," while the others deal with "limited regions of the musculature." From this presentation there should be little speculation as to the reason for the emphasis placed upon cervical techniques by almost every school of chiropractic thought.

## Visceral Symptom Complexes

Having covered some of the somatic problems created by cervical fixation, it is fitting that an investigation of the means by which these disrelations disturb visceral function should be undertaken. Such problems are common and not the exception, as might be expected in view of the lack of splanchnic efferent neurones arising from the cervical neuromeres. There is a wealth of information relative to the influence of the visceral afferent fibres upon the functioning of the somatic efferent neurones, but a paucity of references relative to the visceral disturbances initiated by somatic afferent impulses. It is, therefore, necessary to synthesize the facts as revealed by general physiology of the nervous system to acquire the required authoritative backing for the explanation of visceral malfunction in response to cervical fixation.

However, it has been shown that fibres of the Spinal Tract of the Trigeminus descend at least to the second cervical neuromere before synapsing in the Substantia Gelatinosa. Krieg[332] notes that fibres of the Tractus Solitarius, which are the first order neurones from pharynx, larynx, bronchi, lungs, stomach, carotid sinus and arch of the aorta, descend into the cord for several neuromeres.

Rasmussen[333] has brought forth the information that the afferent fibres of the lung and pleura, either by way of the Vagus or spinal nerves, have "special connections with the upper four or five cervical segments."

Krieg,[334] in his description of the Tractus Cuneatus, discusses the superior course of the sensory fibres of the posterior nerve roots of the upper cervical nerves, turning upward with this tract and making synaptic connection in the Nucleus Cuneatus. As a result, some of the neurones of this Nucleus are connector in type to travel "to the primary motor cells of the cranial nerve nuclei."

Another fact that bears repeating is that every afferent fibre, upon entering the medulla spinalis, divides into ascending and descending branches, as well as giving collaterals to the gray matter of the neuromere of entrance. The ascending divisions of the upper cervical nerves have no other recourse than to enter the medulla oblongata to synapse with the gray matter of that structure.

Recalling the disturbing influences of the fixation discussed in Chapter XII, it may be reasoned that these unusual neural extensions into the medulla will experience similar alterations in their functional capacity, as do the neural elements common to the cord. That is to say that the subluxation of an upper cervical vertebral segment disturbs the arterial supply to and the venous drainage from the corresponding nerve trunk, nerve roots and neuromeres. Such disturbance of vascularity and nutritional status involves the upper neuromeres and the more distal portion of the medulla oblongata, thereby altering the irritability of the components. Superimposed upon these deleterious influences there is the addition of unbalanced proprioceptive impulses and noxious neural signals from the involved somatic structures. There can be little reason to doubt the likelihood that the controlling neural pools for visceral structures, located in the gray matter of the medulla, are caused to react in a manner productive of functional aberrations in the visceral structures supplied.

The upper cervical fixation commonly bombards the neuromeres with noxious impulses that travel up in the Tract of Lissauer, into the lower part of the Spinal Tract of the Trigeminus, to terminate in the Nucleus of the Spinal Tract. Frequently a "spill-over" takes place into the second order neurones of the Trigeminal system, which ordinarily carry information from intracranial structures, such as the meninges and blood vessels, supplied by the V Cranial Nerve. When these impulses have passed through the thalamus and reach the postcentral gyrus, the unfortunate experiences headache. Other factors may contribute to the production of headache, such as vascular disturbances and tension of the musculature attached to the skull, etc., but the phenomenon of "spill-over" appears to be one important factor.

Clinically, it is well known that upper cervical fixations frequently produce nausea and vomiting with or without headache. The second order neurones from the portion of the Nucleus of the Tractus Solitarius, which Krieg[335] has described as the vomiting centre, are distributed to the motor neurones essential for the activation of the somatic muscles necessary for greatly increasing the intra-abdominal pressure and to the autonomic motor neurones essential for the reverse gastric peristalsis, salivation, etc.

In view of the descent of fibres of the Tractus Solitarius into the cervical segments and the ascent of cervical afferent fibres into the medulla, it is not surprising that the afferent impulses from a fixation may spread to over-stimulate irritable neurones of the Nucleus of the

Tractus Solitarius to produce the phenomenon of vomiting.

The intimate relation of the cells of the Nucleus of the Spinal Tract of the Trigeminal Nerve with the fibres conducting noxious impulses into the cord by way of the posterior nerve roots of upper cervical nerves and the intimate connection that exists between this nucleus and the Dorsal Nucleus of the Vagus facilitates the disturbance of Vagal function. Through such neural connections and the alterations of irritability created by the fixations, the possibilities of visceral symptoms become very real and probable. Coupled with the clinical evidence there can be little doubt of the pernicious influence of the cervical subluxation upon visceral control by the Vagus.

Detailed discussion of the possible pathways to the other cranial nerve motor nuclei, which may be disturbed by suboccipital fixation, should not be necessary. The same principles apply and the clinical evidence is available to substantiate the contention that cervical subluxations do, in fact, result in inimical functions of the organs and structures supplied.

It might be well to briefly consider the apparent selectivity of effect of these noxious impulses from the cervical fixation in a nucleus, such as the Dorsal Nucleus of the Vagus, which is concerned with the supply of numerous organs. Certainly, few patients are to be found who exhibit disturbances of every structure supplied by this nucleus in response to a cervical subluxation, but any one or more splanchnic effectors may demonstrate functional alteration.

The condition of irritability, or degree of Central Excitatory or Inhibitory State, of the different motor pools composing the total nucleus will, in a large measure, determine the response. The history of the group of neurones may have canalized certain pathways, making access more readily available to "spill-over." Thus, a patient who has previously had bouts of bronchitis, is prone to demonstrate symptoms in this system in response to the fixation, while another may experience gastro-intestinal problems, due to his previous disturbances.

Another factor of import is the presence, or absence, of fixations lower in the spine that may be influencing the sympathetic supply to the same viscus. To illustrate, the symptoms from excess vagal stimulation may be exaggerated in the event that the sympathetic supply has been decreased as a result of a chronic thoracic fixation, or the symptoms would be less severe were the sympathetic signals reaching the viscus normal or in excess.

The local chemical balance of the effector organs plays an important determining role as to the response of any organ to alterations in its nerve supply. This has been demonstrated by Pottenger.[336] In his discussion of the permeability of neural membranes, Guyton[337] has shown that calcium in the intercellular fluid is responsible for the stability of the membrane. A decrease permits greater irritability and an increase of calcium has an inhibitory consequence.

Wyke[338] has reported that a high concentration of calcium ions in the tissue fluid decreases the influx of sodium ions into the neurone and the magnitude of the action potential.

## Ganglionic Disturbances

Before leaving the cervical area of the spine, another possible form of neural disturbance is deserving of consideration. The sympathetic ganglia of the cervical region lie in such intimate relation to the vertebrae and to the anterior cervical muscles, Longus Colli, Longus Capitis and Rectus Capitis Anterior Major, that the trauma productive of the cervical fixation may have had direct injurious effects upon one or more of these muscles. Another possibility is that the vertebral fixation produces reflex contraction and thickening of the muscle, thereby bringing pressure to bear upon the ganglion in question.

Oppenheimer,[339] writing in the *Journal of Surgery, Gynecology and Obstetrics*, discussed in great detail neural disturbances from spinal pathology or trauma under the heading: "The Swollen Atrophic Hand." In this condition, he mentioned finding narrowing of one or more of the intervertebral foramina from the fourth cervical superiorly, an unexpected finding, since the cervical nerves five to eight and the first thoracic are concerned with the innervation of the upper extremity through the Brachial Plexus. The explanation of such a symptom picture requires investigation beyond the nerve trunk as it passes through an intervertebral foramen and attention is directed to the sympathetic ganglionic chain for adequate understanding of the problem.

As Albert Kuntz[340] points out that the Superior Cervical Sympathetic Ganglion sends postganglionic sympathetic fibres inferiorly in the interganglionic ramus for distribution via gray rami communicantes of cervical nerves lower than the first four, to which it normally and consistently supplies such fibres for distribution to the blood vessels, sudoriferous glands and the Erector Pili muscles. Thus, the fibres descending from their cell bodies in the Superior Cervical Ganglion may travel with other postganglionic fibres from the Middle

202

Cervical Ganglion to the fifth and sixth cervical nerves and extend into the arm and hand to have a pronounced effect upon the vessels and trophic function of the muscles and bone structure. Disturbance of neural supply to such vessels may have a marked influence upon the trophic activity, leading to the swelling, demineralization of bone, thinning and glossing of the skin, etc., so thoroughly described by Oppenheimer.

Other fibres of the same ganglion may continue their descent to escape in the seventh and eighth gray rami communicantes to be distributed in the corresponding nerves. Such is the complexity of the nervous system.

The explanation of such symptoms would appear to require either direct involvement of the Superior Cervical Sympathetic Ganglion by the upper cervical fixation or a central disturbance. The latter will receive consideration first. The afferent impulses from the holding elements of the subluxated upper cervical segments enter the cord by way of the posterior nerve roots of the associated nerves to synapse with connector neurones which descend the cord to attain the levels of the lateral gray horns in the upper thoracic segments, which are in reflex relation. It may even be that some of the descending branches of the afferent fibres entering the cervical neuromeres may travel down into the upper thoracic segments, since it is necessary for the sympathetic cells to be continually apprised of the needs of the tissues over which they have control and those whose vascular bed they modify. This source of impulses alters the discharge of the preganglionic sympathetic neurones, whose axones leave in the anterior nerve roots of the upper thoracic neuromeres, then through the white rami communicantes to reach the ganglionated chain, turn up through the various ganglia and interganglionic rami to reach the Superior Cervical Sympathetic Ganglion, in which synaptic connection is effected with the postganglionic fibres above discussed. In this circuitous manner the disturbance of the integrity of structure in the upper cervical segments may result in the tissue changes in the hand.

Due to the location of the Superior Cervical Sympathetic Ganglion, it is possible that D. D. Palmer[341] was correct when he said: "An atlas displaced to the right or left may cause tension on one or both of the sympathetic chains of ganglia which pass in front of the transverse processes."

Furthermore, Mennell[342] discusses in his textbook the possibilities of slight disrelation of the transverse processes of upper cervical vertebrae in instances of fixation. He suggests that, due to the thinness of the anterior vertebral muscles, the cervical sympathetic chain may be stretched and irritated and credits this disturbance of structure with being the cause of some migraine-like headaches.

The anterior cervical muscles, above mentioned, may have sustained injury from the mechanical force that produced the subluxation of vertebral segments. Local swelling or a haematoma may appreciably increase the thickness of the muscle involved. The reflex contraction of the same muscles in response to the fixation would, in itself, create the increase in thickness to bring continuing pressure against the ganglion.

These mechanical pressures may have a direct influence upon the functional capacity of the cells within the ganglion or may have a more complicated course of disturbing influence. The covering of the ganglion is supplied with afferent fibres which may be stimulated by the mechanical irritation of pressure, sending impulses back into the cord and thereby disrupting the normal efferent outflow through reflex activity.

The symptoms that may develop from derangement of the centrifugal impulses passing outward over the postganglionic sympathetic fibres of the Superior Cervical Sympathetic Ganglion are almost legion. It may be that the pupil of one eye is noticeably dilated, the eye is more prominent and the palpebral aperture is widened. One symptom may be present without the others or these may all be exaggerated in the complex called exophthalmos. The sympathetic fibres from this ganglion innervate the Dilator Pupillae muscle to produce the dilation of the pupil; Muller's muscle in the floor of the orbital fossa and the thin sheet of smooth muscle in the fascial sheath of the eyeball responsible for the prominence of the eyeball. The involuntary muscle fibres in the superior and inferior palpebrae are activated by other fibres from this ganglion and are responsible for the wider palpebral aperture.

The reverse symptom picture, Horner's Syndrome, of constricted pupil, sunken eyeball, narrowed palpebral aperture, would be suggestive that the trauma resulted in a degree of disturbance to the ganglion sufficient to interfere with the outflow necessary to maintain normal tonus in the above mentioned smooth muscle fibres, or for some reason the parasympathetic fibres have been overactivated.

The afflicted individual may not have any of these symptoms, but may have severe Trifacial neuralgia, tic douloureux, as a result of ischemia of the Gasserian ganglion of the Trigeminal Nerve, due to the overactivity of the postganglionic sympathetic neurones of the

Superior Cervical Sympathetic Ganglion which supply the vessels and result in vasoconstriction.

These are but examples of the symptom complexes that may arise in the head from disturbance to the Superior Cervical Sympathetic Ganglion. Headaches, tinnitus aurium, Meniere's syndrome, etc., may be others, but space dictates that more distant areas receive consideration.

Some fibres from this ganglion help to form the pharyngeal plexus and oesophageal plexus with a few fibres to the larynx. More important are the Superior Cardiac Nerve and the fibres for distribution through the Phrenic Nerve. The Superior Cardiac Nerve on the left helps to form the superficial cardiac plexus and the one on the right the deep cardiac plexus. Increasing the activity of these sympathetic fibres increases the rate of cardiac contraction, modifies conductivity within the heart muscle and its contractile power. The larger branches of the coronary arteries are supplied with vasoconstrictor fibres. Overactivity of sympathetic supply may result in increased heart rate, or tachycardia, and/or constriction of the coronary arteries to give rise to attacks of angina pectoris as the arterial supply falls below the work-load requirements.

Overactivity of supply to the respiratory tract may cause susceptibility to infection, due to the lower resistance of the mucosa when a relative ischemia from vasoconstriction prevails, as has been discussed by Kuntz.[343]

The reverse of many of these symptoms may be worked out by an application of neurological knowledge and should require no further discussion in these pages.

Fortunately, the Middle and Inferior Cervical Sympathetic Ganglia are not so prolific in their distribution of fibres. It must be appreciated that the Middle Cervical Ganglion lies anterior to the transverse process of the sixth cervical vertebra and supplies gray rami communicantes to the fifth and sixth cervical nerves. The Inferior Cervical Sympathetic Ganglion lies anterior to the transverse process of the seventh cervical vertebra and contributes gray rami communicantes to the seventh and eighth cervical nerves. It is to be recalled that both of these ganglia are in close proximity to the Longus Colli muscle and the great vessels of the neck. Injury sustained by this muscle may result in swelling, or even a haematoma, at the site of trauma, thereby bringing pressure to bear upon the ganglion closely associated therewith.

Both of these ganglia contribute postganglionic sympathetic fibres, by way of the gray rami to those nerves which form the Brachial Plexus, namely the fifth to eighth cervicals and, by way of the named nerves formed by this plexus, follow down into the arm, forearm, hand and supply the vessels of muscle, bone, connective tissue and skin. In the skin fibres are distributed also to the sudoriferous glands and the Erector Pili muscles.

The Middle Cervical Ganglion contributes fibres of a postganglionic nature by way of the Middle Cardiac Nerve to the deep cardiac plexus, through which they pass to influence the heart's activity, as previously mentioned. Fibres from this same ganglion accompany the Inferior Thyroid Artery and while it seems that there is little research data to indicate that the cells of the thyroid gland are under direct neural control of either the sympathetic or parasympathetic division of the autonomic nervous system, there is evidence that the quantity of blood flowing through the thyroid has a marked influence upon its secretory activity. This is to be expected, since glandular tissue cannot long function efficiently without the constant supply of the "raw materials" by the blood stream with which to synthesize the complex secretions.

It cannot be denied that the chief controlling factor of the thyroid is the anterior hypophyseal thyrotropic hormone. However, irritation that overactivates the vasoconstrictor fibres of the vascular bed of the thyroid could result in a marked reduction in thyroid function, hypothyroidism.

Curtis, et al,[344] has mentioned that in addition to the common symptoms of hoarseness, general muscle weakness and pain, as well as delay in the relaxation phase of the deep tendon reflexes may be observed in hypothyroidism.

Severe disruption of the ganglion or the influence of fatigue factors, previously discussed, could result in marked vasodilation within the thyroid with hyperthyroid symptoms of perspiration, exophthamos, dilated pupils, tachycardia and decreased gastric secretion.

The same authors have added to the symptoms of hyperthyroidism psychomotor hyperactivity, also myopathies and even periodic paralysis.

It is possible to show that the function of the hypophysis cerebri is influenced primarily through the hypothalamico-hypophyseal tract with the cell bodies in nuclei of the hypothalamus, and to a lesser degree by postganglionic sympathetic fibres whose cytones are located in the cervical sympathetic ganglia and whose axones control the calibre of the vessels of the hypophysis. By circumnavigation, it may be shown that the ganglia of the cervical region may influence the function of the thyroid gland as they disturb the vascular bed of the pituitary gland, modify its secretion and alter the response of the thyroid and other endocrine glands as a direct result.

The Inferior Cervical Ganglion contributes the Inferior Cardiac Nerve to the deep cardiac plexus for the innervation of the heart. Fibres form a plexus on the Vertebral Artery and others on the Common Carotid, then the Internal Carotid Artery, by which the majority of the vascular supply of the brain is controlled. Here it may be pointed out that many peculiar symptoms may arise from disturbance of neural control of the vessels within the cranium, e.g., headaches, symptoms simulating mild strokes, or cerebrovascular accidents, which, in reality, are due to the cortical ischemia produced by a vasospasm of an artery of supply. Much space could be utilized to expand upon these phenomena.

Other fibres from this ganglion assist in the formation of plexuses on the Subclavian and Internal Maxillary Arteries, which subserve vasomotor control of these arteries and their branches. It would be well to appreciate the distribution of the branches of the Internal Maxillary Artery and be prepared to justify recurrent colds, since the ischemia that may be produced in the respiratory mucous membrane lowers resistance to the filterable virus and the secondary infection of the other micro-organisms. (Kuntz)[345]

Still other fibres become integral parts of the Phrenic Nerve for distribution to the mediastinal and central diaphragmatic pleura, as well as the Diaphragm itself. Again, these fibres are primarily vasomotor in nature and the symptoms caused their altered functions are not likely to be obvious.

This coverage of the topic of cervical fixation has not been exhaustive, but the other regions of the vertebral column must receive attention before the patience and perseverance of the reader have been drained.

# CHAPTER XIV

# Responses of the Thoracic Neuromeres

WHILE THE CERVICAL region of the spinal cord offers many peculiarities of structure and function with complications that make description most involved, the thoracic neuromeres are much more straightforward and present less complication of discussion. These segments with the first two, three or four lumbar neuromeres are, nonetheless, of infinite importance to the physiology of the entire structure. There is no tissue that is not dependent upon the neural outflow from one or more of these segments for its function in both health and disease, since these are the segments responsible for the vasomotor control of the vessels throughout the entire body. In addition to the modification of vascular supply, these neuromeres have other somatic and splanchnic modifying influences, deserving of detailed consideration.

It was this region of the spine that produced the gratifying improvement in the hearing of Harvey Lillard, which led to the establishment of an entirely new and distinct branch of the healing art — the chiropractic profession.

D. D. Palmer[346] described the birth of chiropractic in these words: "On September 18, 1895, Harvey Lillard called upon me. He was so deaf for seventeen years that he could not hear the noises on the street. Mr. Lillard informed me that he was in a cramped position and felt something give in his back. I replaced the displaced fourth dorsal vertebra by one move, which restored his hearing fully."

It was recognized very early in the history of chiropractic by D. D. Palmer,[347] that one of the most frequent locations of the vertebral fixation was the twelfth thoracic and he has made mention a number of times in his textbook of its importance. In his own words is to be found this statement: "I have found the last dorsal to be the one most frequently displaced, as it is not as well braced as are other vertebrae; the third cervical subluxated oftener than any other cervical; the atlas comes a close second and the fourth next in frequency."

Attention must first be directed to the anatomical peculiarities of the thoracic and first two or three lumbar neuromeres, if a clear mental picture is to be acquired of the disturbing influences of the vertebral subluxation. The student of chiropractic also must learn to appreciate the thoracic and lumbar segments, which are intimately concerned with splanchnic function and are, in turn, frequently the site of visceromotor reflexes, pointing an accusing finger to the functionally disturbed viscus for the chiropractor to use as a guide in his diagnostic and analytical investigation. Such muscular contractions were called by Willard Carver,[348] "Motor Reaction," and he had worked out an elaborate system of explanation as to the structural and visceral problems associated with Motor Reaction. A study of Carver's work is commended to every chiropractor, especially his descriptions of Motor Reaction, basic distortion and compensation. For the doctor desirous of conserving time, the essence of Carver's investigations are to hand in the text, *Anatomical Adjustive Technic* by Homer G. Beatty, D.C.[349]

## Anatomical Peculiarities

Gray[350] has described the thoracic portion of the spinal cord as being small and almost circular on cross section. The anterior and posterior columns of gray matter are very slender and nearly uniform in width. The distinguishing feature in cross section is, of course, the lateral gray column in each symmetrical half of the cord.

The lateral gray column is composed of the cell bodies of the preganglionic sympathetic neurones. Each cell is relatively small and multipolar in type to allow for a multiplicity of connections with afferent fibres from the structures supplied, the collaterals of afferent fibres of somatic structures, connector neurones of the local level, as well as connectors from numerous levels of higher integration. The axones of these cells, as has been previously mentioned on a number of occasions, travel out as components of the anterior nerve roots of each thoracic and the first two or three lumbar nerves.

The surface markings and fibre tracts of the white matter have no features deserving of special discussion.

It may be emphasized that the anterior and posterior gray columns are relatively narrow, since there is no great mass of muscle and skin to be supplied such as the extremities provide.

## Sympathetic System

While various portions of the sympathetic division of the autonomic nervous system have entered the previous discussion, a brief review seems justified in the light of past experience with students. A number of points, unconsidered in the other sections, must receive attention also.

The axones of the cells of the lateral gray column, after passing through the anterior nerve root, the nerve trunk and into the anterior primary ramus, leave as a white ramus communicans to travel a short distance to enter the ganglionated chain. Some of the fibres terminate in the ganglion of entrance, while others turn superiorly or inferiorly to pass through a variable number of the paravertebral ganglia prior to termination by synaptic relation with five to seventeen or more postganglionic neurones. Crelin[351] credits each preganglionic fibre with synaptic connection with 100 or more postganglionic neurones. Other preganglionic fibres do not terminate in the ganglionated chain, but rather, pass through without interruption to reach a prevertebral ganglion in the abdominal or pelvic cavity. It is of interest to note that the visceral structures associated with the somatic portion of the body, and those in cranial, thoracic and pelvic cavities are supplied by postganglionic fibres of the paravertebral ganglionic chain. The abdominal splanchnic structures, on the other hand, have their postganglionic cell bodies in the prevertebral ganglia that lie in relatively close relation to the viscera. It will be noted later that there are physiological, as well as anatomical differences, between these postganglionic fibres for abdominal structures and those for other regions of the body.

It is of interest to note that the white rami communicantes are composed of both the myelinated preganglionic fibres, above traced, and also visceral afferent fibres which have returned to the sympathetic chain from the organs in the cavities of the body, to pass through without synaptic relation, to reach their cytones in the posterior nerve root ganglion of Thoracic one to Lumbar two or three, in accordance with the description by Gray[352] and other authors of authority. Because of the location of the cell bodies and the fact that these afferent fibres are indistinguishable from somatic afferent neurones, some neurologists have been constrained to deny the existence of sympathetic afferent fibres, although acknowledging the existence of afferent fibres from visceral structures, but prefering to classify them as cerebrospinal afferents. To avoid confusion in these writings the terms "sympathetic afferent" and "visceral afferent" will be utilized as occasion requires distinction of the fibres from viscera from those of the somatic afferent system.

It is gratifying to note that present day authorities, such as Minckler[353] and Curtis, et al,[354] have classified and discussed these afferent fibres under the heading of visceral afferents, since this seems to serve the purpose of keeping these systems more distinct, clear and memorable.

To quote Gray,[355] "There is no evidence of the existence of any interganglionic association fibres." This, of course, means that, despite the fact that the visceral afferents from the cavities of the body pass through the ganglionated chain, they must enter the spinal cord before synaptic connection may be made with the effector sympathetic neurones.

Some neurologists describe the Dogiel cells of the posterior nerve root ganglia as being connector neurones between sympathetic, or visceral afferent, fibres and somatic afferent fibres to permit the sensations from viscera to be transferred to somatic afferent fibres that these impulses may reach the conscious centres of the brain. This does not appear to receive general acceptance, but as Gray[356] has stated, the majority of the Dogiel dendrites terminate as receptor endings for the reception of stimuli from changes within the posterior nerve root ganglion itself.

It would be well to note Gray's[357] italicized statement before leaving the discussion of white rami communicantes: *"Postganglionic fibres never travel in a white ramus communicans."*

The paravertebral ganglionated chain consists of twenty-two or twenty-three ganglia connected to each other by interganglionic rami. One, or sometimes several, gray rami communicantes unite with each spinal nerve for the distribution of postganglionic fibres to the blood vessels of somatic tissues, to the pilomotor muscles and sudoriferous glands of the skin. Only fourteen or fifteen spinal nerves on each side are able to boast their contribution of white rami communicantes to the ganglionated chain.

The two chains of ganglia, one on each side of the vertebral column, unite inferiorly, immediately anterior to the coccyx, as the ganglion impar.

The superior end of the chain is continued into the cranial cavity as the Internal Carotid Nerve, which passes with the artery through the carotid canal. This nerve divides to help form the internal carotid plexus and both afferent and efferent fibres are distributed to the carotid artery, through the trigeminal ganglion, sphenopalatine ganglion, ciliary ganglion, abducent nerve, tympanic branch of the glossopharyngeal nerve, oculomotor, trochlear and ophthalmic division of the trigeminal nerve. Other fibres are distributed to the ophthalmic, middle and anterior cerebral arteries and their branches. Gray[358] has been imposed upon for the authority for the above description, although it has been greatly condensed.

## Thoracic Sympathetic Ganglionated Chain

The three cervical sympathetic ganglia received considerable discussion in the previous chapter, but the modifications of distribution of the fibres from the thoracic portion of the sympathetic chain are deserving of brief description.

There are ten or eleven ganglia on each side, resting on the heads of the ribs in intimate relation with the pleura anteriorly. Each ganglion provides a gray ramus communicans to one or more of the thoracic nerves for distribution in the somatic structures.

The ganglia associated with the first five thoracic nerves give off fine bundles of postganglionic fibres for distribution to the thoracic viscera, which pass directly into the mediastinum to take part in the formation of the aortic, posterior pulmonary and deep cardiac plexuses. From the remaining thoracic ganglia bundles of preganglionic, medullated fibres unite in the formation of the Greater, Lesser and Least Splanchnic Nerves.

Gray[359] states that the fibres of the Greater Splanchnic Nerve are derived from the first or second thoracic ganglia and those to the ninth or tenth inclusive, but the fibres leave the fifth to the ninth or tenth ganglia only as the named nerve.

This unusual statement from the British edition of *Gray's Anatomy* relative to fibres being derived from the first or second thoracic ganglion down to the ninth does not appear in the U.S. editions consulted nor other available texts, therefore it would appear to deserve disregarding. All authorities do agree on the fifth or sixth to the ninth or tenth ganglia.

These fibres terminate in the Coeliac Ganglion and other collateral ganglia. It must be emphasized that the cell bodies of the fibres of the Greater Splanchnic Nerve are situated in the lateral gray horns of thoracic segments one to ten, but particularly in the fifth to ninth neuromeres inclusive. The axones of these neurones in the more cephalic thoracic segments of the cord leave in the described manner to enter the ganglionated chain via a white ramus communicans, then descend in the chain to escape from fifth to the ninth ganglia as components of the Greater Splanchnic Nerve. It is not until these preganglionic fibres reach the Coeliac or other prevertebral ganglion that they terminate and synapse with postganglionic neurones. Some of these preganglionic fibres fail to synapse and innervate the adrenal gland directly, since embryologically it has a similar formation from the primitive neural crest as the sympathetic ganglia.

The Lesser Splanchnic Nerve is composed of preganglionic fibres that escape from the ninth and tenth thoracic ganglion. These synapse in the Aorticorenal Ganglion.

The Least Splanchnic Nerve is composed of fibres from the twelfth thoracic ganglion with the fibres passing into the renal plexus. This nerve is also formed by preganglionic fibres, whose cell bodies are located in the lateral gray column of the medulla spinalis.

## Prevertebral Ganglia and Plexuses

While the Carotid Ganglion, lying in relation to the internal carotid artery, does not truly belong to the prevertebral group of ganglia, it must receive mention here. A few of the preganglionic sympathetic fibres that enter the ganglionated chain by way of white rami communicantes of the upper thoracic nerves continue through the various ganglia without interruption to leave the superior pole of the superior cervical ganglion as part of the Internal Carotid Nerve. These fibres synapse in the carotid ganglion and with a few scattered postganglionic neurones, whose cell bodies are in the superior cervical sympathetic ganglion, form the Internal Carotid Plexus. In addition to these efferent fibres, there are sympathetic afferent fibres intermingled in the formation of the plexus.

The prevertebral ganglia found in the thorax belong to the parasympathetic division and it is within these tiny ganglia that many of the fibres of the Vagus Nerve synapse. The sympathetic fibres are postganglionic, having their cytones in paravertebral ganglia.

The situation changes drastically in the abdominal and pelvic cavities, for here the ganglia are a mixture of cells belonging to the postganglionic neurones of both the sympathetic and parasympathetic divisions, although most parasympathetic fibres pass into the viscera before synapsing with their postganglionic neurones.

The largest prevertebral ganglion is the Coeliac of the Solar Plexus, situated one on each side of the coeliac artery and subdivided inferiorly into the Aorticorenal ganglion. The Coeliac ganglion is joined by the Greater Splanchnic Nerve of the same side and the Lesser Splanchnic Nerve joins the Aorticorenal ganglion.

The prevertebral plexuses are an intricate network of fibres and scattered ganglia. Vagal fibres are both afferent and efferent, both types being well myelinated. The sympathetic fibres are myelinated preganglionics until they reach a ganglion in which they synapse, then beyond the ganglion are postganglionic, relatively unmyelinated. Of course, there are also medullated afferent fibres in all the plexuses.

The Coeliac Plexus is subdivided into numerous other named plexuses, listed by Gray[360] as the Phrenic, Hepatic, Splenic, Left Gastric, Suprarenal, Renal, Superior Mesenteric, Inferior Mesenteric, Abdominal Aortic, Testicular or Ovarian. Each of these forms a network of fibres on the corresponding artery.

The Phrenic Plexus is joined by additional afferent fibres of the Phrenic Nerve.

The Superior Mesenteric Plexus has an associated ganglion of the same name on each side, deriving preganglionic fibres from the Greater Splanchnic Nerve predominantly.

The Suprerenal Plexus is distinctive in that some of the myelinated preganglionic fibres of the Greater Splanchnic Nerve pass through to the gland without benefit of postganglionic connections. This is the only example of preganglionic fibres innervating tissue directly.

The Renal Plexus is worthy of mention, since the lowest, or Least Splanchnic Nerve from the twelfth thoracic ganglion joins in its formation and a number of scattered small ganglia serve for synaptic connection with the cells of the postganglionic fibres.

The Inferior Mesenteric Plexus is distinctive in that it boasts the Inferior Mesenteric Ganglion, in which preganglionic fibres synapse after having travelled without interruption from the Coeliac Plexus downward through a number of plexuses.

The remaining listed plexuses are deserving of no special mention, other than to point out that the majority of the sympathetic fibres intermingled in these plexuses are postganglionic in type, while the other fibres are myelinated sympathetic afferents, parasympathetic afferents and efferents.

While this is in no manner an exhaustive discussion of these prevertebral plexuses and ganglia, it is hoped that sufficient review has been presented to make the following discussion of the vertebral fixations, or subluxations, understandable.

## Physiological Idiosyncracies

The sympathetic division of the autonomic nervous system presents a number of variations within its functional capacity that bear mention. First, Sachs[361] brings out the information that these sympathetic fibres conduct from 60 to 100 times more slowly than somatic fibres and are much less prone to fatigue.

All preganglionic sympathetic fibres synapse with more than one postganglionic neurone and some activate cells of more than one ganglion. According to Kuntz,[362] the range of possible connections is from two to seventeen postganglionic neurones, depending upon the portion of the system examined.

Further, some of the postganglionic fibres at their terminal endings secrete acetylcholine, e.g., those for the sudoriferous glands, while most secrete adrenaline-like substance, called by some "sympathine," or norepinephrine.

Another point of interest is that all efferent fibres leaving the fourth thoracic ganglion and those above are postganglionic and relatively unmyelinated, while those below this level are postganglionic in the gray rami communicantes, but preganglionic, medullated fibres extending into the cavities below the diaphragm. However, fibres from the ganglia in the lower lumbar and sacral regions revert back to postganglionic fibres from the ganglia to the visceral structures in the cavities, thus further complicating the picture. It seems that there may be preganglionic fibres from these latter ganglia also.

The degree of vasoconstriction, or vasodilatation, present in the skin supplied by the ganglia above and including the fourth thoracic is accompanied by a like condition of the vessels of the mucous membrane of the respiratory system, while the reverse is true for the structures supplied by the ganglia from the fifth thoracic inferiorly. Thus, constriction of the vessels of the skin is accompanied by dilatation of the vessels of the abdominal viscera, according to the findings of Kuntz.[363]

Some of the postganglionic fibres distributed to blood vessels are cholenergic, resulting in vasodilation, but the great majority are adrenergic and vasoconstrictor in type, as described by Kuntz,[364] who also points out that there is no evidence of a general distribution of vasodilator fibres in the skin.

The evidence presented by most neurologists indicates that the sympathetic fibres are important for the maintenance of vascular tone and that an increase in the impulses results in constriction, while a decrease produces dilation, but exceptions to the rule are frequent.

Certainly, these brief remarks about the thoracic portion of the ganglionated chain leave a tremendous volume of factual material uncovered, but suffice for the needs of the moment and the interested reader is referred to any good textbook on the subject, of which there are a multitude.

## Upper Thoracic Fixation

Distortion, subluxation or fixation of one or more of the first four thoracic vertebrae may have far reaching disturbing influences, as the first chiropractic patient demonstrated so graphically. At first blush, it might be considered ridiculous to suggest that an upper thoracic subluxation could possibly disturb the function of the ears, eyes, nose, paranasal sinuses, mouth or teeth. However, a superficial knowledge of neurology should convince the skeptic that such is not only possible, but is probable and that the cranial meninges, as well as the brain itself, may be disturbed by the controlling influence exerted by the sympathetic system over the vascular bed of all the above mentioned structures.

There will never be proof of the exact mechanism by which D. D. Palmer restored the hearing of the first chiropractic patient, Harvey Lillard, by adjusting the fourth thoracic segment. However, there are a wealth of possibilities. The mucous membrane of the Eustachian tube may have been decongested by stimulation of the sympathetic fibres and subsequent vasoconstriction, allowing for normalization of air pressure on the two sides of the tympanic membrane and restoring the freedom of motion of the tympanum. The mucous membrane of the middle tympanic cavity may have been decongested, permitting freedom of motion of the ossicles. The vascular supply of the cochlear nerve via the vasa nervorum may have been normalized providing for normal neural conduction. The nuclei, pathways or superior temporal gyrus of the cerebral cortex may have had the vascularity normalized and hence the function.

The cytones of these preganglionic sympathetic fibres are lodged, especially, in the lateral gray horns of the upper four thoracic neuromeres, although Kuntz[365] states that the lowest source of preganglionic fibres for the influence of the above listed structures is from the seventh thoracic neuromere, extending into the superior cervical sympathetic ganglion. He goes on to mention that the inferior cervical ganglion receives preganglionic fibres from as low as the ninth thoracic segment.

A fixation in the upper thoracic area may disturb the functional capacity of the nerve trunk and the neuromere, as discussed in Chapter XII. Through the abnormal centripetal flow of impulses, the lateral horn cells may be disturbed in their function and send out impulses to the postganglionic neurones in the superior, middle or inferior ganglia to produce the symptom complexes discussed in the latter part of the previous chapter. Space will not be occupied with repetition.

Attention will be directed now to those visceral structures supplied by the upper four thoracic sympathetic ganglia. Sachs[366] has recognized that viscera respond reflexly to mechanical irritation of the somatic structures and it is contended by this writer that the malfunction attendant upon vertebral fixation, or subluxation, is a central response, rather than direct involvement of the nerve trunk by mechanical pressure. The statement has also been made by Sachs[367] ". . . every pathological condition is obviously associated with disturbances in the autonomic nervous system."

From Gray's[368] description of the distribution of the postganglionic fibres from the first five thoracic ganglia, it is found that they supply the visceral structures of the thoracic cavity, viz., the thoracic aorta and branches, pulmonary structures, the heart and its vessels.

Turning to Kuntz,[369] it is found that sympathetic fibres are amply distributed to the tunicae adventitiae and mediae of the aorta and its branches. These fibres serve to maintain the required tone of the muscular layer. In the event that the fixation created an excess of impulses over the fibres, a degree of hypertension could result. Conversely, the fatigue, or central inhibitory state, as a resultant of the fixation, could decrease the tone of any of the vessels supplied within the thorax with the exception of specific branches of the coronary arteries to be discussed later.

Kuntz[370] is utilized again as the authority in determining the response of the bronchial tree to sympathetic impulses. He states that these fibres produce bronchodilation and, of course, vasoconstriction of the vascular bed upon stimulation.

Rasmussen[371] has expressed the view, shared by others, that the antagonistic action of the parasympathetic and sympathetic fibres is more physiological than anatomical. It seems doubtful that the same cells would have a double innervation, as a decrease in quantity of nerve impulses would have the reverse action to increasing the number of impulses. In the instances of the bronchioles, it would seem more reasonable and economical for the increase in sympathetic signals to result in vasoconstriction, due to increased tonus of the muscle fibres of the tunica media, while the corresponding decrease in parasympathetic activity reduces the tonus of the bronchial musculature to result in bronchodilation.

Should the subluxation in the upper thoracic segments occur, resulting in an inhibition of normal sympathetic impulses through the pulmonary plexus, then vasodilation, bronchial constriction, and overactivity of the mucous glands are likely responses, being the symptoms in catarrhal complexes and asthma. These are also the symptoms of overactivity of the parasympathetic system whose fibres are distributed to the respiratory structures.

The three cervical ganglia contribute the Superior, Middle and Inferior Cardiac Nerves, composed of postganglionic sympathetic fibres, to the cardiac plexuses and thence to the heart. Now, to these may be added the fine bundles of postganglionic sympathetic fibres from the superior four thoracic ganglia of each side. These modify the innate ability of cardiac muscle to maintain a rhythmical contraction although devoid of all extrinsic nerve supply.

Sympathetic fibres are given credit by Kuntz[372] for accelerating the rate of contraction of the heart (Curtis, et al)[373] and a greater response when those fibres of the right side are stimulated. Also, the strength of atrial contraction is increased by these fibres, but not the force of ventricular contraction. The fibres from the left side increase the force of ventricular contraction with no atrial influence.

Again, it should be apparent that fixation of an upper thoracic vertebra, especially the relation between the second and third, are of very significant import to the functional aberrations of the heart. The side of greatest irritation of the disrelation is of no minor importance in determining the symptoms that would be expressed. The doctor of chiropractic would be able to add much to his diagnostic ability by keeping clearly in mind the variations of distribution and function of the fibres of the two sides of the spinal cord.

While tacchycardia may lead the doctor of chiropractic to seek first an upper thoracic fixation, he should not be unmindful that an inhibitory spinal lesion involving the Vagus might well decrease this Vagal function, and result in similar symptoms. He would then examine the upper cervical region for an explanatory subluxation, for, as was discussed in the previous chapters, a fixation may result in a central excitatory state in one group of efferent neurones and a central inhibitory state in another group closely associated anatomically or quite distant. Another element that received consideration previously was the effect of fatigue as an inhibitory mechanism. Fatigue of either the pre- or post-ganglionic sympathetic fibres would result in symptoms of parasympatheticotonia, while fatigue of the Vagal fibres would create an illusion of sympatheticotonia with tacchycardia.

Furthermore, the doctor may find subluxations in both regions of the spine, which demand correction for the normalization of the patient's problem. The inhibitory type of upper cervical fixation may have been present for some time, as an example, yet the patient experienced no marked cardiac symptoms until a relatively minor upper thoracic subluxation increased, by irritation, the sympathetic outflow to the heart with resultant tacchycardia, which brought the patient to the office of the doctor with alacrity.

There are those emergency states in which the doctor adjusts according to the severe symptom, rather than in accordance with the usual studied plan of the causative vertebral disrelation. For instance, when the doctor of chiropractic arrives at the bedside of a patient, who has experienced some form of cardiac attack and displays a very low blood pressure and a feeble contraction of the cardiac muscle, the doctor does not wait to reason through the many and varied signs that point to the offending vertebra or vertebrae, but immediately delivers a stimulative form of upper thoracic adjusting. Such a stimulation is helpful in increasing the strength of cardiac contraction. The doctor may deliver stimulatory adjustive moves in the area of the ninth thoracic to stimulate the adrenal glands to further assist in the emergency response.

Once the emergency aspects are under control, the doctor will then begin the total corrective procedure indicated. During all of the care of such a patient, the upper cervical adjustings would be delivered with the minimum of stimulation from sudden movements, deep palpation, or forceful adjustive techniques. This area is gently handled to minimize stimulation. The upper thoracic fixations are adjusted with speed, more force and depth and any palpatory or manipulative techniques of the associated muscles may be deeper, quicker and less gentle to provide additional stimulative effects.

The doctor of chiropractic is cognizant of the needs of each patient generally and of each area of the spine specifically, as he begins the administration of the chiropractic adjusting which may appear to the unskilled to be a routine applied to all in like manner.

In this age of coronary occlusions as a status symbol, it would be negligent not to discuss the influence that the doctor of chiropractic may exert in caring for such conditions. Kuntz[374] has clearly documented the confusion and conflicting evidence relative to the influence of the Vagi and sympathetic fibres upon the calibre and capacity of the coronary arteries. He has stated that the majority of experiments strengthen the theory that the Vagi are vasoconstrictors, while the sympathetic fibres have a dilating influence. This is consistent with the functional influence of these fibres upon the cardiac muscle. As the heart speeds its contractions by sympathetic stimulation, it is to be expected that the coronary arteries would dilate to provide a greater volume of blood to the active myocardium. Conversely, as the Vagi inhibit the rate of the heart and thereby decrease the requirement of the heart muscle for blood, it is to be expected that vasoconstriction would occur.

It is of interest and import that Guyton[375] has brought out the "self-regulation" of the coronary arteries due to the activity of the heart. As the heart increases its activity under sympathetic stimulation, the force of contraction increases the quantity of blood propelled into the coronary arteries and causes dilatation. With a decrease of cardiac activity under parasympathetic influence, the arteries receive less blood and contract.

Experience has established the fact that the administration of chiropractic adjusting is efficacious in handling both the acute and chronic cases of coronary occlusion, but no button has been located either theoretically or clinically, that may be pushed in every patient to make the correction.

Nor is this remark to be taken as an indication that all that is required in every case of coronary occlusion, thrombosis or infarct is the correct spinal adjustment. Such a case must have the complete bed rest and excellence of nursing care required by one treated by drugs. Accessory oxygen supply may be essential and the supportive intake of alpha-tocopherol aids in the utilization of oxygen, etc. The convalescence of such a case must follow much the same procedure and rationale no matter the primary form of therapy. The chiropractic physician influences the heart and its circulatory vessels via the neural system by his skillful adjusting of structures and normalization of the muscular contractions resulting from the visceromotor reflexes, while the allopath seeks to influence these structures via potent drugs. Unfortunately, few of the drugs used are without potential serious complications, as discussed thoroughly by Moser.[376] Rupture of fresh myocardial infarcts tend to occur twice as frequently with the use of anticoagulants, according to Spain,[377] and hemorrhagic pericarditis was three times more frequent.

The doctor of chiropractic must assess each patient and be guided by his knowledge and experience.

One of the greatest contributions the chiropractic profession could make is in the field of prophylaxis against coronary occlusion. Maintaining structural integrity and physiological nerve supply is of prime importance. The chiropractor's knowledge of the importance of nutrition and exercise adds to his armamentarium. Kuntz[378] has quoted the findings of Greene that the coronary circulation is improved by somatic muscle exercise. Chiropractic has the method par excellence for releasing the tensions of somatic muscles occasioned by emotional, or mechanical, stress, as well as the responses to the visceromotor reflexes. The doctor is best able to assess the condition of the individual and prescribe the exercises best suited to his particular needs.

The chiropractic profession has developed the premise of the Pyramidal System of Postural Measurements, the essential instrumentation, the techniques for releasing abnormal myotonic variance and the exercise equipment to employ the necessary principles of postural correction. The research and writings of Johnston[379] provide the knowledge and the methods by which the profession can make an extensive prophylactic contribution both in the field of coronary and cardiac problems, as well as general physical fitness.

## Fifth to the Ninth Thoracic Fixations

Fixations, or subluxations, in the group of vertebrae inclusive of the fifth to the ninth thoracics are quite common and it may be recalled that the seventh and eighth are the transition from a right rotatory scoliosis above to a left rotatory scoliosis below in Carver's Typical Complex Opposed Rotational Scolioses, or in those cases that compensate properly for a lateral tipping of the base. As has been discussed in previous chapters, transitional areas are under mechanical stress and tend to become subluxated more readily under added stress.

However, any thoracic subluxation in this region under discussion may disturb the normal activity of the lateral horn cells and alter the signals passing over fibres of the Greater Splanchnic Nerve for distribution through the postganglionic fibres of the prevertebral plexuses to numerous abdominal viscera. In general, the sympathetic fibres are vasomotor for all abdominal vessels, motor for the sphincters of the gut and, when active, the tone of the general musculature of the gut is decreased, motility and glandular secretion are inhibited.

The research of Kamieth[380] has demonstrated that peptic ulcers demonstrated by x-rays are accompanied by scolioses in the thoracic spine in 86% of cases and disc aberrations in 90%, involving those segments which are embryologically associated with the stomach or duodenum.

There are exceptions and specific influences that the scope of this text cannot cover in detail, but several of particular interest to the doctor of chiropractic and to the development of the present discussion must be mentioned.

Kuntz[381] has established that the sympathetic fibres control the constriction of both the arterial and portal vessels of the liver, decreasing the input and at the same time accentuating the volume leaving the liver. While the production of bile does not appear to be dependent upon nerve supply directly, it is influenced by the volume of blood, thus activity of the sympathetics, as above mentioned, decreases the amount of bile produced. Subluxations that are stimulating to the lateral horn cells of the cord may, thereby, disturb the production of bile and justify the chiropractor's confidence in his ability to restore some degree of normality to this function of the liver.

Gray[382] gives credit to the sympathetic system for the control and regulation of carbohydrate and protein metabolism by the liver, although many authorities place greater emphasis upon the secretions of endocrine glands, especially the suprarenals and Isles of Langerhans of the pancreas. Activity of the sympathetics increases the release of glucose from the liver, while the parasympathetics appear to promote the storage of glucose as glycogen.

It was briefly discussed in the chapter dealing with the general effects of the vertebral fixation that the presence of an optimum quality of glucose in the blood stream is essential for the normal activity of the central nervous system. Here it may be appreciated that a subluxation in this thoracic region, fifth to the ninth, may overactivate the release of glucose from the liver with a hyperglycemia developing and even a demonstrable glycosuria. Hyperglycemia decreases the irritability of the central nervous system and thereby develops an abnormal response to stimuli. Conversely, the fixation may inhibit the sympathetic supply, which is likely to be a response to chronicity with a fatiguing of the reflex pathways, rather than any direct inhibition of the passage of neural impulses resulting from direct mechanical impediment. Furthermore, as has been discussed supra, there are the potentials for stimulation of some reflex pathways with corresponding inhibition of others by the same afferent input to the cord segment.

The sympathetic-parasympathetic balance may be altered with the parasympathetics being in the ascendency, resulting in a hypoglycemia with its disturbing influences upon the irritability of the nervous system generally. Such conditions may result from upper cervical subluxations disturbing Vagal function, or combination of thoracic and cervical subluxations, which is perhaps the more common circumstance. It may be that the symptom complex is established in a much more subtle and involved manner, in that subluxations disturb the nerve supply to essential ductless glands and through this route upset the normal functioning of the liver.

Hypoglycemia or hyperinsulinism has become an important clinical entity with a multitude of symptom complexes that had defied successful treatment. Abrahamson[383] has done much to centre attention upon this clinical entity and made practitioners of all branches of generic medicine more aware of the need for fasting blood sugar assessment of patients and the altered dietary regimen required for best results.

It may be appreciated that the doctor of chiropractic can never be a "button-pusher," for there is no single vertebra to be adjusted for each organ, or symptom complex.

Kuntz[384] has stated that "the stomach also responds reflexly to stimulation of somatic afferent nerves." D. D. Palmer[385] pointed out that the closer the source of stimulation is to the central nervous system, the greater is the response of the nervous system. This peculiarity has been confirmed by authorities, both prior to and since D. D.'s time. It is not unusual that the fixation of vertebral segments should have such marked disturbances as are manifested in distant organs, such as the stomach, embryologically associated with neuromere, or neuromeres, involved by the subluxation.

The thoracic, vertebral fixation may cause local muscular contraction and vasomotor disturbance of the somatic structures and concordantly local vascular constriction of the vessels of the gastric mucosa. The resistance is thereby reduced to the gastric secretions, which are then capable of digesting the mucosa with the formation of an ulcer and the resulting symptoms. Cardiac and pyloric sphincters may be altered in function by an appropriate thoracic fixation with the symptom complexes associated.

While it appears well established that the exocrine and endocrine cells of the pancreas are directly influenced by secretomotor fibres of the Vagus, Kuntz[386] has quoted Richins, who demonstrated that there are about nineteen unmyelinated fibres to each one myelinated fibre passing to the pancreas. The medullated fibres are preganglionic vagal and afferent fibres of the Greater Splanchnic Nerve, according to the same investigator. It has been demonstrated that reducing the blood flow through the pancreas inhibits the production of pancreatic juice, while an increased blood supply results in increased secretion. The role of the vertebral fixation in upsetting the physiology of the pancreas should be obvious to the reader, since the greater ratio of neurones are postganglionic sympathetic for distribution to the blood vessels.

It is of interest to note that Kuntz[387] has stated that splenic function is under the influence of the sympathetic fibres of the sixth, seventh and eighth thoracic nerves with no parasympathetic fibres and the ratio of afferent fibres to efferent fibres is 1 to 20. The postganglionic sympathetic fibres are distributed to both the blood vessels and the unstriated muscle fibres of the splenic capsule and trabeculae and contraction is common in response to sympathetic stimulation.

However, Guyton[388] states that the splenic capsule in man is devoid of muscular fibres, but the stimulation by sympathetic fibres causes vasoconstriction with the stored blood driven into general circulation.

Again, the reader is left to work out the details of the influence of a sixth, seventh or eighth thoracic subluxation as it would influence the function of the spleen.

## Tenth or Eleventh Thoracic Fixation

As has been brought to the attention of the reader previously, some of the sympathetic fibres of the ninth and tenth nerves pass through the corresponding ganglia without interruption to form the Lesser Splanchnic Nerve of each side. These fibres synapse, for the most part, with their postganglionic neurones in the Aorti corenal ganglion of the corresponding side, but many pass without synapsing into the adrenal plexus and reach the gland as preganglionic fibres. Other fibres from as high as the eighth thoracic neuromere are credited by Kuntz[389] with joining in the supply of these important glandular structures. He also points out that, while these glands are primarily controlled by hormones, the medullary substance is greatly influenced by the sympathetics and somatic afferent stimulation may produce reflexly an increased rate of secretion.

Selye[390] has extensively investigated the body reactions to all manner of stress and has revolutionized much of the thinking of allopathic medicine. While his concern has been primarily with endocrine responses and hormonal effects, his findings closely parallel those of the chiropractic profession and it might well be said that chiropractic has been concerned with the anatomy of stress, and Dr. Hans Selye with the endocrinology of stress. He has pointed out that the medullar tissue of the adrenal is not under the control of the anterior portion of the pituitary gland but under sympathetic influence via the splanchnic nerve fibres.

The Alarm Reaction to any nonspecific stressor, as described by Dr. Selye,[391] includes enlargement of the suprarenal glands and in this General Adaptative Syndrome, hyperemia and even hemorrhage of the adrenal cortex is noted. Furthermore, Selye[392] makes clear that "emotional stimuli or localized nervous impulses may influence many organs, thus causing systemic stress." It is suggested that subluxations, or fixations, of the vertebrae related to the neuromeres concerned with the control of the suprarenal glands are of particular significance in disturbing the general function of the human and modifying the subsequent reactions to added stressors.

His experiments demonstrated the marked lowering of resistance to stressors by the removal of the adrenals, which included among the stressors infection, anoxia, trauma, emotion, etc. Adrenal insufficiency produces symptom complexes similar to the shock phase of the Alarm Reaction, which are "hypotension, hemoconcentration, hypoglycemia, hyponatremia, hypochloremia, hyperpotasemia, hypothermia, muscular weakness, gastric and intestinal ulcers." These are the symptoms listed by Selye.[393]

The doctor of chiropractic would, therefore, be well advised to carefully investigate this region of the vertebral column, make such corrections as indicated and eliminate basic distortions which bring mechanical stress to bear upon this area by compensatory distortion, as it plays an important role in the ability of the individual to adapt successfully to nonspecific stress.

## Twelfth Thoracic Subluxation

D. D. Palmer[394] wrote: "I have found the last dorsal to be the one most frequently displaced, as it is not as well braced as are other vertebrae"; and in another portion of this textbook: "A personal examination of hundreds of vertebral columns, usually displays a weak place at the thoraco-lumbar junction."

Furthermore, D. D. Palmer[395] wrote: "For example, in spinal curvature adjust the twelfth dorsal and not every vertebra found awry." Years later, Dr. Fred Illi[396] of Switzerland demonstrated with exactitude the importance of the twelfth thoracic vertebra in spinal distortion and even worked out a method of prognosis of the degree of correction to be expected and the likely time factor to effect the degree of correction by an examination of this vertebra.

Anatomists are agreed that this vertebra is of a transitional type, not completely a thoracic nor a true lumbar in its structure. It is an area of relatively free motion without benefit of strong osseous locks or the limitations of costal support. The twelfth thoracic is the usual and normal transition from the anterior lumbar curve to the posterior thoracic curve. Even in the healthy subject, demonstrating the Typical Complex Opposed Rotational Scolioses, as described by Beatty,[397] it is the apex of a left scoliosis with all the stress of such a location in a distortion. Should the basic distortion of tipping and rotation be exaggerated, the degree of stress and consequent irritation would be magnified proportionately.

In view of these factors, it is justified to devote a special section to this particular segment of the vertebral column. The distribution of many of the fibres of the Least Splanchnic Nerve, derived from the corresponding neuromere, provides added justification. Most of the fibres of the Least Splanchnic Nerve pass into the renal plexus and are joined by fibres from the Lesser Splanchnic Nerve and many postganglionic fibres from the Coeliac Ganglion, as well as some from the superior lumbar paravertebral ganglia.

Kuntz[398] demonstrates that the sympathetic fibres are vasoconstrictors and decrease the renal output. He doubts that there are secretomotor fibres to the kidney. He has mentioned also that cooling of the skin in the lumbar region inhibits renal function, while warming up the skin increases the output. Stimulation of other somatic afferent fibres were shown by the same authority to cause the kidney to be contracted and its output inhibited. Therefore, there seems little reason to argue against the possibility of an irritating subluxation causing a decrease in kidney function, or symptoms of a reverse sign, should a central inhibitory state be established or fatigue effects supervene.

In view of the importance of optimum kidney function to the homeostasis of the body and the frequency of distortion in this portion of the spine, every chiropractor would do well to devote attention to this region.

The influence of the crura of the Diaphragm and the fibres of the Psoas Major muscles attached to the lower border of the twelfth thoracic vertebra frequently produce a relatively local lordosis of the thoraco-lumbar area. This finding should suggest to the chiropractor underlying emotional stress that appears frequently to be associated with an aversion to sexual gratification and is accompanied by anterior nodding of the pelvis to retract the external genitalia. This was a common finding of Wilhelm Reich,[399] a student of Freud.

The lumbar lordosis is increased in compensation for this basic distortion, but the local lordosis is superimposed. Release of the above named muscles and the deep local postvertebral muscles is necessitated to accomplish correction and psychological counselling may be indicated to uproot the true cause of the problem.

With these few examples, the thoracic portion of the spine is to be left for consideration of the lumbar segments.

# CHAPTER XV

# The Lumbar Fixation

THE FIRST TWO or three lumbar neuromeres contain cells of the pre-ganglionic sympathetic system in the form of the lateral gray column. This is, of course, a continuous inferior extension of the same column found in the thoracic region, nor is there any distinguishing feature that marks the transition from thoracic to lumbar segments. The remainder of the five lumbar neuromeres are not blessed with lateral horns.

Gray[400] has stated that the lumbar segments are large, owing to the great increase in size of the anterior and posterior horns. The white matter is relatively less in quantity, as the descending tracts progressively synapse in the gray matter from above downward, becoming successively less massive as they pass through each neuromere, and the ascending tracts increase in size with their upward progression by the addition of fibres in each segment. The two pairs of horns of gray substance are very wide with little difference existing between anterior and posterior masses. The requirements of the lower extremities with the added mass of muscle and the greatly increased area of skin necessitate the increase in volume of cytones.

The paravertebral sympathetic chains of ganglia are continuous inferiorly into the lumbar region. There are usually four ganglia on each side of the vertebral column, closely related to the medial border of the psoas major muscle. (Curtis)[401].

Again, each lumbar nerve receives a gray ramus communicans from one of the ganglia for the distribution of postganglionic sympathetic neurones through the various branches of the spinal nerve, as has been described on several previous occasions.

Only the first two or three lumbar nerves give off white rami communicantes to supply the ganglionated chain with additional preganglionic sympathetic fibres, some of which terminate in the lumbar ganglia of entrance, but most take an inferior course through the chain to synapse in the lower lumbar ganglia, sacral ganglia and the ganglion impar.

The distribution of fibres within the abdominal and pelvic cavities from the lumbar ganglia is more straightforward than those thoracic sympathetic neurones discussed in the previous chapter. Most of these sympathetic fibres are postganglionic and take part in the formation of the abdominal aortic, common iliac, external iliac, internal iliac, and hypogastric plexuses.

## The Hypogastric Plexus

The plexuses mentioned in the above paragraph are primarily concerned with vasomotor control and space will not be occupied with a discussion that may be read in the standard books by authors of authority. The hypogastric plexus is of interest in the development of the theme of vertebral fixation, thereby justifying a succinct coverage.

This plexus, lying in the angle of bifurcation of the aorta, between the common iliac arteries, is an inferior continuation of the aortic plexus and divides into the right and left pelvic plexuses for the supply of pelvic viscera.

It is necessary to mention that Gray[402] has stated that sympathetic fibres are derived from the first two sacral sympathetic paravertebral ganglia to join the pelvic plexus in addition to those from lumbar ganglia and even from the lower thoracics. The two bundles of preganglionic parasympathetic fibres derived from the second and third sacral nerves enter in the formation of the pelvic plexus of the same side. These fibres will receive more detailed consideration in the next chapter.

The visceral structures supplied by the subdivisions of the pelvic plexus are the rectum, urinary bladder, prostate gland, seminal vesicles, testicle and penis of the male, or the uterus, vagina and ovary of the female.

Kuntz[403] has mentioned that most of the preganglionic sympathetic fibres of the urinary bladder synapse in tiny ganglia of the vesical plexus, although postganglionic fibres are present also as extensions from the lumbar ganglia.

The distribution of sympathetic and parasympathetic fibres within the bladder wall are not agreed upon by authorities, but Kuntz[404] claims the sympathetics inhibit the muscular wall, close the apertures of the ureters and pull them toward the mid-line and cause contraction of the internal urethral sphincter. Curtis,[405] et al, give credit to the sympathetics for vasoconstriction, ejaculation of semen, inhibition of peristalsis of the sigmoid colon and rectum.

Fixation of a lumbar vertebra, more particularly the first, second or third, may well disturb the urinary bladder function, resulting in symptoms which bring the patient to the office of the doctor of chiropractic. While bladder problems may suggest upper lumbar distortion, it must not be overlooked that the lower thoracics are concerned, as are the second and third sacral neuromeres, with the innervation of the bladder. Difficulty always exists in the determination, on a neural basis only, of the location of the offending subluxation in any symptom complex. Arriving at a diagnosis is merely one-half of the doctor of chiropractic's concern prior to ministering to the patient. He must then make a careful structural analysis. The diagnosis has its greatest importance in determining those cases of pathology that may require more radical care than the chiropractor is equipped to render, such as surgery. The structural analysis provides the information upon which this specific case may have the chiropractic technique selected that is in keeping with the needs of the distortional complex, for each patient presents an individual challenge to the doctor of chiropractic.

While the influence of the two divisions of the autonomic nervous system upon the functions of the uterus is not clear to the authorities quoted by Kuntz,[406] clinical experience in chiropractic offices indicates that the premenstrual colic and menstrual cramps can, most frequently, be relieved by adjusting the fifth lumbar vertebra only. When the patient presents a problem of excess menstrual flow, the adjusting of the second lumbar usually brings the condition under control. These findings suggest that the proximity of the fifth lumbar to the sacral parasympathetic neurones may result in afferent impulses coursing down to these fibres from the site of the fixation. Overactivity may result in contractions of the musculature of unnatural severity, resulting in pain. Guyton[407] credits the sympathetic afferents with conducting the impulses of abdominal pain due to dysmenorrhea, through the hypogastric nerves.

The other possibility is that the adjusting results in stimulation of the parasympathetic neurones, which may have an inhibitory influence upon the cervix uteri. Relaxation of the cervix and contraction of the body of the uterus permits the escape of the menstrual fluid from the uterus proper without undue pressure contractions and the distress of colic.

Adjusting the second lumbar for haemorrhagic tendencies also presents two reasonable explanations in keeping with the description of the innervation presented by authorities. The patient may have a vertebral kinetic aberration that has resulted in a lack of normal neural impulses to the vascular bed of the uterus either through the mechanism of fatigue of the reflex pathway or via the central inhibitory effect, since it may be anticipated that the muscular tension responsible for the vertebral disrelation demands increased blood supply, hence vasodilation as a result of decreased sympathetic supply to the tunica media of the arteries. The sympathetic neurones to the visceral vessels may experience inhibition also, perhaps through the connections of Renshaw cells. The decrease of tone of the vascular bed to maintain optimum supply may result in the congestion and excess loss of blood. The stimulation of the adjustive technique may cause the lateral horn cells to increase the rate of impulse transmission with a resultant vasoconstriction of the uterine vessels. While the explanation is of purely academic interest, both chiropractor and patient are pleased with the results achieved by correct adjusting of the vertebral segment indicated by the symptom picture and the spinal analysis.

There is a need to discuss briefly the terminal portion of the colon and the rectum, in view of the number of patients the average chiropractor sees, who present problems in this region of the digestive tract. Generally speaking, the musculature of the entire colon is activated by parasympathetic impulses, while the sympathetics control the vascular bed and the sphincters of smooth, or involuntary, muscle.

The proximal half of the colon, perhaps as far as the splenic flexture, is supplied by Vagal fibres, while the remainder is influenced by the sacral parasympathetic fibres. While the physiological activities of the two divisions of the autonomic nervous system are not clear-cut and distinct and there appears to be overlapping of activity under varying circumstances, certain observations may be made from the chiropractic clinical investigation. As in most organs, the colon has an intrinsic rhythmical activity which is merely modified by the nerve supply and brought into functional harmony with the needs of the total body in its response to the external and internal environment.

Many cases coming to the attention of the doctor of chiropractic, show a spastic descending colon and flaccid caecum, ascending colon and perhaps even the transverse colon is atonic. This condition suggests hyperirritability of the parasympathetic fibres associated with the second and third sacral neuromeres. Distortion of the sacroiliac articulations would be suspected, but it may prove to be fixation of one of the lower lumbar vertebrae. In the latter instance, the afferent fibres, irritated by the subluxation, enter the spinal cord via the posterior nerve root, divide into ascending and descending branches, as previously described. The descending branches would enter the sacral neuromeres and synapse with internuncial fibres, which then stimulate the lateral horn cells of the sacral parasympathetic outflow. The distal portion of the colon may then express the symptoms of spacticity, if it has been the cytones of the fibres of supply to this organ that were influenced by the above mentioned descending fibres.

Other organs, supplied by sacral parasympathetic fibres, may express disturbed function and the final efferent response is determined by the relative threshhold of irritability of the cell groups concerned with the neural supply of the viscera, the intimacy of synaptic relation of the afferent pathway with the parasympathetic efferent component of the reflex arc, and the degree of responsiveness of the splanchnic cells. The irritability of neural cells has been discussed at considerable length in a previous chapter, and it should suffice to mention that vascular supply and drainage, nutrition, oxygen availability, etc., are a few of the basic modifying influences.

The intimacy of synaptic relation is not constant between one afferent pathway and all efferent neurones of the neuromere in which it synapses. The utilization of a particular reflex pathway, canalized by the process of neurobiotaxis, makes for the passage of a weaker stimulus over the facilitated chain of neurones. Hence, afferent impulses travel the path of least resistance, which may be to the colon of one patient but the urinary bladder of the next, etc.

There is not uniformity of the calibre of the colon, since the proximal half or more receives parasympathetic neural supply via the Vagus Nerve, which is unlikely to be disturbed by a fixation of a lumbar vertebra to create spasticity of the proximal portion of the colon. Another reason for the atonic state of the proximate portion and attendant spasticity in the distal portion may be the simultaneous stimulation of sympathetic neurones by the ascending branches of the same afferent fibres from the tissues of the lumbar fixation. Activation of this component of the nerve supply of the colon is associated with decreased tonus of the muscular fibres and a vasoconstriction of the supplying arterial vessels.

Gastro-enterologists, such as Alvarez,[408] have shown that a locus of irritation in the colon is followed by spasticity distally and flaccidity proximally. Thus, were the subluxation to result in even a contraction of a segment of the distal portion of the large intestine, spasticity to the terminal end would develop, accompanied by the more flaccid state of the more proximal portion.

Another problem that commonly occurs is constipation with very tight anal sphincters. The internal sphincter is influenced primarily by the sympathetic fibres from the first two or three lumbar segments. This is rarely a condition developing from a single lumbar fixation, creating excess neural supply. Such a condition is most commonly associated with a generalized sympatheticotonia in a so-called "nervous, high-strung, emotionally upset" individual. Such a one demonstrates a general atonic digestive tract, including the entire colon. The sphincters of the gastro-intestinal tract may all be relatively hypertonicized. If into such a symptom complex is introduced an upper lumbar fixation, the internal anal sphincter may be further activated and add to the difficulties of elimination. Such a patient benefits from the chiropractic techniques, designed to normalize the balance of the nervous system. If anal dilation is added to the regime, gratifying relaxation of the somatic musculature and improved colonic function are experienced by most patients.

## Sympathetic Connections

The lumbar area of the spine produces more chiropractic patients than any other region. Thousands of other sufferers from low back problems would benefit from the skill of doctors of chiropractic were the public better informed of the efficacy of this profession's "techniques" of caring for this common disturbance. Perhaps more occupational injuries occur in this region of the vertebral column than in any other single portion of the body. In no other area of the human structure is such an amount of force and weight sustained by such a structure of limited size.

Many of the reasons for the inherent predisposition to injury and stress have received previous consideration, but a brief review may not be time wasted. The weight of almost two-thirds of the entire body comes to bear upon the junction of the fifth lumbar and sacrum and the long lever of the remainder of the spine applies force at this area that is almost unbelievable.

The lower lumbar vertebrae, especially the fifth, are more prone to developmental anomalies than any other. Spina bifida occurs in a considerable number of the populace. Gray[409] states that spondylolisthesis occurs in five percent of the spines examined, a condition which may permit the body of the vertebra to shift anteriorly, separating from the posterior arch.

Other investigators agree with Gray as to the occurrence of such abnormalities, and Hollingshead[410] has established that a sixth lumbar vertebra occurs in about 3.5 percent of columns, which accentuates the leverage brought to bear at the lumbosacral junction.

Such developmental mistakes are due to the failure of ossification to follow the normal pattern. This potential structural weakness may be quiescent until middle age, when the muscular activity is decreased for a more sedentary way of life and posture begins to deteriorate. An excessive or unguarded lift may then result in the separation of centrum from posterior arch with pain, muscle "splinting," and incapacitation. It may be appreciated that the intervertebral disc, the anterior and posterior longitudinal ligaments are subjected to a great deal of stress by this structural abnormality. The extreme case of spondylolisthesis will tax the skill of even the chiropractor and in instances only two-man techniques and very localized forms of traction are successful in reducing the gross displacement.

The importance of the unilateral and bilateral sagittal facing of the inferior facets of the fifth lumbar and superior facets of the sacrum have been recognized and reported in recent years as culprits in some cases of almost intractable lower lumbar discomfort with recurrent exacerbations of acute pain. These facets normally transmit some of the superimposed weight to the sacrum. In the instance of sagittal facing, there is an instability created with a tendency for one or both lumbar articular processes to be forced anteriorly. If the condition is unilateral, the holding elements, particularly the joint capsule of the affected side, suffer unnatural strain and bombard the spinal cord with nociceptive impulses that are experienced as pain, as well as producing considerable muscle "splinting."

In the event that the condition is bilateral and extreme in degree, the fifth lumbar vertebra may be forced anterior with the articular processes passing between those of the sacrum. This is another serious problem for anyone to correct and it may be an impossibility to bring sufficient force to bear in the desired manner to re-establish the correct position of the fifth lumbar vertebra.

Fusion and partial fusion of one or both transverse processes of the fifth lumbar with the sacrum creates mechanical problems and added stress to the area, to which it reacts with pain, aching, muscle tension, and increasing distortion.

The basic distortion of anterior nodding of the sacrum or pelvis brings added strain on the lumbosacral junction, since it is the transition from a posterior sacral curve to an anterior curve in the lumbar region. This junction is also the apex of any scoliotic curve resulting from tipping of the sacrum.

234

In sacroiliac subluxation, in which the innominate is relatively posterior nodded in relation to the sacrum, the pull of the iliolumbar ligament tends to pull posteriorly upon the transverse process of the fifth lumbar and to a lesser degree the fourth lumbar, causing them to rotate toward the side of ligamentous pull. The iliolumbar ligament seems to receive its sensory nerve fibres from the first lumbar nerve, judging by the referred pain. Therefore, the pain experienced is usually felt in the lower abdominal, inguinal and upper medial thigh regions. A "trigger point" that increases the pain upon deep pressure, slightly lateral to the posterior superior iliac spine on the inner border of the ilium, is a reliable confirmation of the cause of the pain.

Faulty posture has been demonstrated by Johnston[411] to be an important factor in the symptom complex of the low back disability in some sixty-eight percent of cases. By the posterior shift of the weight of the superimposed structure in relation to the fifth lumbar, great stress is brought to bear upon the facets and even upon the spinous processes and interspinous tissues of this area.

Judovich and Bates[412] have recognized that many cases of segmental pain and tenderness respond to correction of faulty posture and Goldthwait[413] made a valiant attempt to impress the importance of posture in both health and disease upon his profession.

In discussing the treatment of lumbo-sacral strain and spondylolisthesis, Mennell[414] advocated postural training as a necessary adjunct following manipulation.

All of these factors, and many more, account for the very high percentage of the population who suffer from low back discomfort. While this portion is to be devoted to the somatic problems, it must be emphasized that despite the fact that no cells of the autonomic system are contained in the fourth or fifth lumbar neuromeres, the proximity of the sympathetic neurones above and the parasympathetic neurones below provide opportunity for visceral disturbance in response to a vertebral kinetic aberration of one of the lower lumbar segments.

The fourth and fifth lumbar nerves contribute extensively to the formation of the sciatic nerve, while the second, third and fourth contribute the fibres for the formation of the femoral nerve. Thus, the chiropractor seeks the cause of painful symptoms of the lower extremity in the lumbar and sacral regions, having long recognized that reflex pain may be manifested far from the site of actual irritation. "It is commonly known that back pain is usually derived from the spinal column. It is not so commonly known, however, that such pains may be felt in other localities, equally commonly," states Fahrni,[415] Judovich and Bates[416] in more recent years, discuss the possibilities of reflex pain from somatic irritation being interpreted in consciousness as arising distal to the primary site of irritation in structures supplied by the same neuromere which receives the noxious stimulus.

Problems of the anterior and medial aspects of the thigh lead the doctor to seek the causative factor in the upper lumbar area of the spine. Pain, experienced in the posterior thigh or in the leg and foot, directs the investigator to the fourth and fifth lumbar segments and the sacrum. Sir Thomas Lewis[417] expressed surprise at the distance pain may be referred by a locus of muscle contraction as the source of noxious impulses.

Lewis[418] investigated the contraction of muscle in response to visceral irritation and spinal muscle irritation and concluded that each source was equally potent and could not be distinguished one from the other. He observed that localized muscular contraction could not be produced by irritation of the skin. Injury to the lumbar articulations and associated muscles in the form of a fixation, or subluxation, may express itself in a variety of forms, as has been discussed for the other regions of the spine.

Walshe[419] has established that it is not the sensory nerve fibre that is stimulated that determines the final effect, but, rather, the synaptic connections that are open to it and the central excitatory state within the spinal cord or higher centres. Hence, some patients with a lower lumbar fixation may have pain and muscle spasm in the lower extremity, while others may have more symptoms indicative of an overactivity of the parasympathetic innervation of a pelvic viscus, and yet others may experience symptoms that indicate disturbance of the sympathetic supply of a specific organ or part.

The chiropractor is cognizant of the fact that not all pain in the lower extremity is of this simple reflex type from a fixation of a vertebral segment. Many painful conditions develop which are vascular in origin, due to involvement of sympathetic neurones. It may become necessary then to seek the structural problem at a higher level than the site of the painful symptoms may dictate, even into the lower thoracic region.

Any lumbar or lower thoracic fixation may send noxious impulses into the spinal cord that may reach the levels of the lateral horn cells to make synaptic connection and thereby alter the vasomotor control of the vessels in the lower extremity. Judovich and Bates[420] suggest that the paravertebral trunks may be involved directly by structural disrelations, but it would appear that the reflex involvement of the preganglionic fibres is a more likely source of the disturbance.

As has been brought to the attention of the reader earlier, lumbar fixations beyond those associated with neuromeres containing sympathetic elements, may evoke alterations in function of visceral tissues which may, or may not, be predicated upon vascular modification. Wolff and Wolf[421] have shown that an unremitting, burning pain occurs from anoxia of a nerve and such a condition may be the source of sciatic pain. In such an instance, the lumbar fixation would send noxious impulses into the spinal cord via the posterior nerve root and these fibres would ascend to the level of the sympathetic cytones in the lateral horns. Either by collaterals or by connector neurones the preganglionic sympathetic neurones responsible for the vasomotor control of the vessels of the sciatic nerve might well be stimulated. From the cells the axones would escape from the spinal cord in the usual way to descend in the paravertebral sympathetic chain to the level of the ganglia whose postganglionic fibres are to form the gray rami communicantes of the fourth and fifth lumbar and first three sacral nerves. These fibres travel in the large nerve and its branches and some of them are distributed to the arteries which, in turn, supply the sciatic nerve. Overactivity of these sympathetic neurones could then result in vasoconstriction and relative ischemia of the nerve. The anoxia produced would then be sufficient stimulus to create the acutely painful syndrome of sciatica.

Again, attention is directed to the extensive capillary plexuses that are embedded in the endoneurium of each nerve, as described by Wyke,[422] running longitudinally in the nerve and responsible for the nutrition to a considerable degree of the axones via the Nodes of Ranvier. Hence, vasoconstriction of the branches from muscular arteries have the potential of producing a degree of ischemia of the neurones.

It should be clarified that the pain response to the vascular disturbance may not follow a pattern of distribution consistent with the dermatome or any definite nerve. This phenomenon is due, of course, to differences of sensitivity of the various sensory fibres to anoxia, to the lack of involvement of the complete nerve, and to the fact that the nerve is composed of fibres derived from a number of neuromeres.

Another phenomenon that is not confined to the lumbar area only, but is more prone to be discovered in relation to the developmental defects occurring in this region, is the hyperalgesia of a dermatome. This increased sensitivity of the skin supplied by a specific posterior spinal nerve root is indicative of a viscerosensory reflex, involvement of the radicles, ganglion, posterior nerve root or nerve trunk by some direct form of irritation. Such an irritation may occur as a result of herniation of the nucleus pulposus of an intervertebral disc, by osseous growth encroaching upon the nerve trunk, distortion of the segment to the point of direct irritation which may be permitted by abnormal development, or inflammatory conditions involving any of the neural structures above mentioned.

Lewis[423] explains hyperalgesia as being due to a constant irritation over a period of time, which results in antidromic impulses coursing from the site of irritation down the fibres to the various terminal branches. These antridromic impulses appear to cause a chemical change and sensitize the receptor endings. Such involved receptors become exquisitely sensitive and pain may be elicited by a relatively minor stimulus. Volleys of neural signals are sent up the centripetal fibres into the cord and traverse the fibres to reach the conscious centres in the cortex to be interpreted as pain.

Rasmussen[424] has given two other possible explanations for hyperalgesia. First, the source of irritation has established an irritable focus within the neuromere which lowers the resistance to stimuli from the receptors of the skin, which, under normal conditions, would be inadequate to cross the synapses to reach the postcentral gyrus and consciousness. Second, that the sensory impulses entering the cord from the primary centre of irritation causes reflex discharges of efferent sympathetic impulses which do actually alter the condition of the skin. This disturbance of the integrity of the skin serves to increase the sensitivity of the receptors.

The lumbar region of the spinal column may be more prone to demonstrations of hyperalgesia, due to the frequency with which associated viscera are disturbed and the higher percentage of developmental abnormalities and postural faults that place the somatic musculature under serious strain. This region of the spine is more subject to herniation of the nucleus pulposus of an intervertebral disc, bringing direct mechanical irritation to bear upon the nerve trunk.

Burns, Chandler and Rice,[425] reporting for the osteopathic research group, have demonstrated that a vertebral subluxation or fixation by disturbing the range of motion of a vertebra, interferes materially with the vascularity of the vertebral body and thereby interferes with the nutrition of the intervertebral disc, predisposing it to herniation.

One last point of interest has been made by Sachs,[426] who has demonstrated that the viscero-sensory reflex, or referred pain, is more extensively distributed in the back than in the anterior. While this applies in all regions, the frequency with which the chiropractor is faced with patients suffering from lumbar pain suggests the importance of careful investigation of the organs embryologically associated when hyperalgesia of the skin is discovered.

This discussion would seem adequate to demonstrate some basic facts and principles relative to the lumbar subluxation and the stimulus to further extend the study of this highly important and complex area of the vertebral column.

# CHAPTER XVI

# Sacral Distortion

THE SACRUM AND coccyx will be dealt with as a unit. Much has been previously presented relative to the sacrum as part of the pelvis and base of the spine, which modifies the superstructure in response to any distortional relationships assumed by the base. Furthermore, it is impossible to discuss the lower lumbar nerves or the pelvic plexuses of nerves without involving the sacral nerves.

The nerve trunks and the escape of the primary rami have received considerable discussion in a previous chapter, and the contribution of the first, second and third sacral nerves to the formation of the sciatic nerve entered the presentation of the previous chapter. However, a few ends remain to be brought into the picture to complete the complex problem of spinal fixation, or subluxation, and distortion.

The sacroiliac articulation has been the centre of much disagreement by anatomists over many years. In the early days it was classed as a synarthrosis, or an immoveable joint; later, it was shifted into the amphiarthrodial classification with credit for slight movement; in more recent years it has been promoted to the diarthrodial category as a freely moveable articulation with a joint cavity, synovial membrane, and synovial fluid. The confusion is compounded by the latest edition of Gray,[427] contradicting his classification on the same page. First, calling the sacroiliac articulation a synchondrosis and then a few lines later, states: "In a considerable part of their extent, especially in advanced life, they are separated by a space containing a synovial fluid, hence the joint presents the characteristics of a gliding joint."

The movement of the sacrum in relation to the innominate has never been doubted by the chiropractic profession, and any experienced doctor of chiropractic can recognize a sacroiliac fixation in a person walking the street in front of him. Dr. Fred Illi,[428] in his early research, devised a number of methods of determining and analyzing the sacroiliac problem with accuracy. Later, his extensive dissections of human sacroiliac articulations produced considerable helpful information for the understanding of the function of this articulation, and the problems to which it is subjected. In recent years, his cineradiography of this region established without question many of the contentions previously advanced. Many other chiroprac-

240

tic authorities had recognized the importance of these two articulations to the integrity of the entire vertebral column.

It is doubtful that any mechanical genius could devise a better, more efficient, stronger base of support for the spine than has been provided. Here is to be found a triple wedge-shaped bone, tapering from above inferiorly both in its lateral width and anteroposterior thickness, in addition to being wedged from anterior to posterior. Its auricular facets are uneven and provided with osseous locks to add both stability and limitation of motion.

Illi,[429] after extensive dissection of cadavers at the National College of Chiropractic, described an intra-articular ligament that had not previously received consideration. For all its stability, the sacroiliac motion is essential for graceful, efficient locomotion. Fixation or subluxation may be productive of structural problems in the vertebral column above, but is a causative factor for many local somatic and visceral disturbances with which this chapter must concern itself.

Gray[430] recognizes the posterior nodding of the innominates in relation to the sacrum that may occur during pregnancy and, if not properly seated at the time of involution, may cause increasing pain as the ligaments shorten in their return to normal. He suggests manipulation to correct this problem, but gives no indication that he recognizes the possibility of such a disrelation occurring in any age group of both sexes under other circumstances.

In the writings of Hackett,[431] mention is made of his findings of more sacroiliac ligament relaxation than lumbosacral, although these two areas account for 80% of all low back problems in his practice. Although he mentions finding "slight displacement" at the sacroiliac articulations, no indication of manipulative correction prior to fibro-osseous proliferation is to be found.

In discussing the movement of the sacroiliac joint, Bourdillon[432] makes mention of the fact that the range is very limited and even this and its importance are a source of disagreement among authorities. However, all who concern themselves with human structure and, especially those skilled in correction by manipulation or adjusting, recognize subluxations or fixations and confirm these by x-ray visualizations.

Unfortunately, this writer has not been able to find any description of the levels of the spinal cord which distribute afferent fibres to the ligaments of the sacroiliac region, and it must be assumed that the recurrent spinal nerves and twigs from the posterior primary rami of the sacral nerves are responsible. Some of the pain symptoms that occur from irritation of the sacroiliac ligaments suggest that the source of afferent fibres for distribution to the more superficial fibres, are derived from upper lumbar segments.

## Somatic Symptoms

Fixation of a sacroiliac articulation may be seen as the individual walks. The affected side of the pelvis appears to move anteriorly as a unit with each forward step of the corresponding foot. The slight, normal posterior nodding of the innominate does not take place. This latter movement cannot be observed through clothing, but the former is quite apparent.

Sacroiliac articular fixation may not cause any seriously painful symptoms if the distortion does not bring undue strain upon the ligamentous structures. However, through the application of Hilton's Law,[433] the afferent impulses returning to the neuromeres from the ligamentous holding elements may cause hypertonicity of those fibres of the longissimus muscles, that Favill[434] lists as being supplied by the posterior primary rami of the first, second and third sacral nerves, and the Multifidus, as mentioned by Gray.[435]

Muscular contraction may be observed or detected by palpation. Other muscles, supplied by the same neuromeres, may experience increased tonus of those fibres innervated, but are difficult to detect, due to the complexity of development of the muscles of the lower extremity.

Hackett[436] shows an illustration of the pain distribution down the postero-lateral thigh and leg from posterior sacroiliac ligamentous strain that varies from a true sciatic distribution.

More serious distortion causes greater strain, or even injury to the fibres of the ligaments, and may arouse serious pain and muscle "splinting." Many of these problems are reflex pain over the distribution of some of the branches of the sciatic nerve. The conscious centre in the cerebral cortex has misinterpreted the source of noxious impulses, because the noxious impulses entering the spinal cord by way of the fibres of the posterior nerve root have activated the second order neurones that normally conduct impulses from the region of the lower extremity supplied by the sciatic nerve.

Due to the shape of the sacrum and its auricular articulating facets, the distortion created at the sacroiliac articulation results in a relative anterior-inferior disrelation of the sacrum. The innominate is relatively posterior nodded in comparison to the sacrum. Other distortions, such as anterior nodding of an innominate, carry the sacrum into similar distortion. Many pelvic problems are seen in patients but the actual, true sacroiliac fixation is the one described above.

The disrelation created at the sacroiliac articulation has the possibility of creating hypertonicity of the piriformis muscle, which takes origin from the anterior surface of the second, third and fourth sacral segments, and is supplied by fibres of the first and second sacral nerves, according to Gray.[437] The piriformis muscle escapes from the pelvis through the greater sciatic foramen in company with the superior gluteal nerve and vessels above and the sciatic, posterior femoral cutaneous, pudendal and muscular nerves from the sacral plexus, along with the inferior gluteal and internal pudendal vessels below.

The hypertonicity of the piriformis coupled with the tension exerted by the sacroiliac distortion upon the sacrotuberous and sacrospinous ligaments, which form the posterior boundary of the greater sciatic foramen, may bring unusual pressure to bear upon these sensitive structures above listed. From the clinical manifestations, the nerves and vessels, more particularly the sciatic nerve, escaping below the piriformis are affected. Thus, the doctor of chiropractic seeks to correct the sacroiliac articulation and release the tension of the piriformis in instances of sciatica. Of course, many such cases are associated with lower lumbar fixations, either alone or in company with sacroiliac problems. It cannot be stressed too often, or too strongly, that each case must be considered on its own merit and not handled in a routine manner lest the most important causative feature be overlooked and neglected with disappointing consequences.

It would seem superfluous to review the neurological involvement productive of piriformis and postvertebral muscle hypertonicity to establish the problem cited above. However, to avoid confusion or the criticism that any critical facet of the discussion has been omitted, the mechanism will receive brief coverage. Stress, strain or tearing of the sacroiliac ligaments concomitant with the sacroiliac subluxation produce a volley of neural signals that return to the sacral segments over fibres of the posterior nerve roots, especially the first, second and third. These noxious impulses are transferred, either by collaterals of the afferent fibres or by connector neurones to the efferent neurones of the anterior gray horns. The axones of these latter fibres leave the spinal cord as components of the anterior nerve roots, pass through the nerve trunks and enter either the anterior or posterior primary rami. The fibres that pass through the posterior primary rami cause the hypertonicity of that portion of the post-vertebral musculature which they supply, while the fibres that aid in the formation of the anterior ramus have a similar effect upon the piriformis and others may extend into the sciatic nerve or other branch of the sacral plexus to result in like problems in muscles of the extremity.

Another peculiar symptom complex appears with stress upon the posterior sacroiliac ligaments, which causes the patient to experience pain down the postero-lateral portion of the hip and thigh in a pattern atypical of that of sciatica. The distribution of this pain may extend well down into the leg and suggests that the more superficial portions of the posterior sacroiliac ligaments have been derived embryologically from the mesoderm of the lumbar segments below the first and the latter, apparently, gives rise to the ilio-lumbar ligament. Afferent fibres from the corresponding neuromeres are stimulated by ligamentous strain, or injury, and the pain is referred to distant areas. In the case of the ilio-lumbar ligament irritation, the pain is experienced in the inguinal area and antero-medial thigh of the homolateral side. Hackett[438] has thoroughly discussed and illustrated the differential diagnosis of the referred pain from the ilio-lumbar ligament and divisions of the posterior sacroiliac ligaments.

While those engaged in the manipulative arts may not be in agreement with Hackett, who credits a very high percentage of the articular pain, especially of the lower vertebral column, to ligamentous relaxation and has reported outstanding success with his treatment method of fibro-osseous proliferation, it must be recognized that he has mapped out the areas of referred pain in a most commendable manner. Dr. Hackett does not emphasize the neurology of the problem, but does suggest that the relaxed ligaments "induce pain by overstimulating the sensory nerves which do not stretch."

This writer would have the temerity to disagree with the eminent surgeon, and suggests that the osseous disrelations result in ligamentous tensions, strain and the stimulation of receptor nerve-endings imbedded between the ligamentous fibres, which are most numerous at the fibro-osseous junctions. The concentration of the receptor endings in the osseous attachments of ligaments accounts for the location of many of the so-called "trigger points."

The application of corrective adjustive techniques is efficacious in removing the tension from the strained ligaments and reducing the stimulation of pain receptors. Proliferation techniques may destroy receptors, as well as encourage the formation of scar or fibrotic tissue within the ligament. Such would both remove the pain and strengthen the ligament to withstand the stress of faulty osseous relationship.

There are instances of serious need for the rationale of Hackett but this should follow osseous correction of any existing disrelationship. Severe trauma or long continued strain upon ligaments as a result of neglected osseous disrelation present patients to the doctor of chiropractic, whose osseous structure will not "hold" a corrective adjustment, and the same subluxation recurs time after time. These would seem to be prime candidates for the proliferative treatment administered by a proficient orthopaedist or such other conservative methods as may be devised to strengthen and shorten the damaged ligaments.

The referred pain from strain of the superior portion of the posterior sacroiliac ligaments is to the postero-lateral region of the buttock and thigh supplied by the second and third lumbar nerves and beyond the knee to the postero-lateral aspect of the leg supplied by the fourth, fifth lumbar and first sacral nerves, although the distribution of the pain pattern does not correspond completely to the dermatomes.

The referred pain of strain to the inferior portion of the posterior sacroiliac ligaments is more centrally located in the buttock, thigh and leg in the posterior aspect supplied by sacral nerves one to three.

It must be admitted that no authority, such as Gray or Arey, can be quoted for this suggestion of the development of the ligamentous structures from embryological segments above their location in the adult, but the pattern of pain suggests that such must be the situation and the development of the limb-bud in this region of the embryo gives further credence to the supposition. If such is not true, a very glaring exception from the standard pattern has been created by the nervous system, which is most unlikely.

## Sympathetic Connections

The sacral nerves receive postganglionic sympathetic fibres from the ganglionated chain in the form of gray rami communicantes, at least one for each nerve, but none of the sacral nerves, or the coccygeal nerve, provide white rami communicantes for the sympathetic chain. The preganglionic sympathetic fibres leave the first two or three lumbar neuromeres and a variable number of the lower thoracic segments to descend in the sympathetic chain to the sacral ganglia and the ganglion impar, where the synaptic connections are made with the postganglionic neurones.

It may be appreciated that the afferent fibres of the posterior nerve roots of the sacral nerves must be related either directly, or indirectly, through interculated neurones, with these sympathetic neurones to modify their activity in accordance with the needs of the tissues supplied by the sacral nerves.

Such intimate relationship with the cells of the lateral gray column, may, under appropriate conditions of irritability or strength of the stimuli, involve fibres destined for the supply of visceral structures associated with these lumbar or lower thoracic neuromeres. Function may be disturbed by such a sacroiliac distortion in organs that would not be suspected of being related to the sacral nerves. Another example of the difficulty of arbitrarily listing vertebrae to be adjusted for a given set of symptoms or the normalization of the nerve supply for a stated viscus.

## Parasympathetic Outflow

The second and third, or third and fourth, sacral neuromeres are the only spinal segments that contain cells of the preganglionic parasympathetic class, aggregated into a lateral gray column. The axones of these cells leave the sacral segments much the same as white rami communicantes, but fail to join the ganglionated chain. They enter the pelvic plexus of the homolateral side and synapse with postganglionic neurones, either in small scattered ganglia of the plexus or within the walls of the visceral structures to be supplied.

As has been discussed by Kuntz,[439] some of the ganglia of the pelvic plexus and its subdivisions are associated with the sympathetic system, deriving preganglionic sympathetic fibres from the tenth thoracic to the second lumbar neuromeres. Some postganglionic fibres are derived from the sacral portion of the ganglionated chain as well. Afferent fibres accompany the sympathetic and parasympathetic fibres back to the spinal cord and form a considerable proportion of each plexus.

Disturbances of relationship of the sacroiliac articulation arouse afferent impulses which return to the sacral segments from the holding elements and may well alter the neural outflow of the parasympathetic fibres, thereby adversely influencing the function of one or more pelvic viscera. It is possible that afferent impulses may be conducted cephalad within the spinal cord to disturb the lateral horn cells of the sympathetic system in the lower thoracic and upper two lumbar segments in keeping with the mechanisms previously discussed on several occasions.

The unit structure of the sacrum does not obviate the segmental function of the sacral portion of the spinal cord, since the sacrum developed from five segments and each segment is associated with a pair of spinal nerves. While the articular discs and the intra-articular joint spaces have been obliterated by ossification and the joint capsule and interspinous and intertransverse ligaments have ossified also, the massive size of the sacroiliac joints requires afferent fibres from the nerve trunks and are the source of as much, if not more, noxious stimuli as the supporting tissues of true vertebral segments. This nociceptive bombardment is capable of the usual reflex disturbances within the neuromeres to produce muscle contraction, referred pain, visceral dysfunction, etc. The presence of parasympathetic neurones in two sacral segments adds a further possibility of visceral functional aberrations as a response to sacroiliac fixation.

It must be conceded that the foramina of the sacrum are not subject to change in size and some of the suggested mechanisms by which the nerve and the neuromeres are disturbed in other regions of the vertebral column cannot apply to this area.

### Coccygeal Nerve

The last of the thirty-one pairs of spinal nerves is the coccygeal nerve of each side, which has descended from the sacral hiatus on the posterior surface of the coccyx, to pass around the lateral border of the coccyx below the rudimentary transverse process. The Coccygeus Muscle is pierced and the nerve takes part in the formation of the coccygeal plexus, consisting of a branch from the fourth sacral, the anterior ramus of the fifth sacral and the coccygeal nerve. This plexus is concerned with the supply of the Levator Ani and Coccygeus Muscles and has a small cutaneous branch to the skin over the coccyx.

Injury occurs to the coccyx quite frequently. In the child and young adult, falls may drive the coccyx anteriorly in true subluxation. After fusion of the coccyx to the apex of the sacrum, a similar injury may fracture the coccyx. Either condition may produce a great deal of pain, tenderness and even difficulty in walking, since the action of muscles attached in that region create a pull upon the traumatized tissues. Defecation is a painful experience in the acute stage of coccygeal injury, as the proximity of the lower rectum and anal canal results in pressure upon the sensitive coccyx as the faecal bolus passes.

After the acute stage has subsided, the patient may experience continuing difficulty when protracted sitting is required. Some patients develop distressing symptoms at each defecation, such as sweating and faintness, even tacchycardia which alarms them. The explanation of this peculiar symptom complex would appear to rest upon the location of the ganglion impar, where the two sympathetic chains join anterior to the coccyx. This ganglion, which supplies a gray ramus communicans to both coccygeal nerves, is carried anteriorly by the coccygeal distortion and is, therefore, subjected to pressure as the faecal bolus is passed. This appears to have a widespread stimulatory influence upon the sympathetic nervous system, thereby increasing the activity of the sudoriferous glands, the rate of contraction of the heart, and the activity of respiration. In some, the distribution of blood may be disturbed with the decrease in circulation to the brain and the sensation of bordering upon a faint.

The extensive and pronounced reaction of the nervous system to disturbances to the ganglion impar has long been known and utilized in the form of anal dilation, as an emergency measure to stimulate failing heart or respiratory action.

Distortion of the coccyx has frequently been found to be an important contributory factor in constipation. Several mechanisms may be involved in disturbing the eliminative activity. The afferent impulses returning to the cord from the holding elements under stress could activate the parasympathetic fibres of the second and third sacral segments to increase the tonus of the walls of the rectum and descending colon, creating the condition of spastic constipation.

The other possibility is that the irritation creates a hyperactivity of the sympathetic fibres concerned in the control of the internal anal sphincter with a relative decrease in parasympathetic signals to the walls of the gut and the hypotonia interferes with the normal propulsion of faecal matter from the colon.

No doubt, other symptom pictures result from distortion in this terminal region of the vertebral column, but it is anticipated that the reader has developed the ability to reason out the neural connections and the disturbances to be expected.

As in every area of the body, the response to somatic disrelations are predicated upon the condition of the nervous system, the activity of higher brain centres, psychic influences, and the chemical balance extant in the effector tissues. It is impossible to arbitrarily prognosticate the functional disturbances to be expected when a given vertebra is subluxated, or fixated, a given degree. Nor can the exact vertebra that is in a state of dysfunction be determined with absolute accuracy from a set of known symptoms. Usual, average and expected conditions may be suggested with a degree of accuracy by an experienced practitioner that may astound those unfamiliar with the nervous system, but there are always the exceptions to the rule.

The doctor of chiropractic concerns himself with a thorough case history, which gives much information as to the experience of the nervous system, thus the channels that are expected to be canalized and the localized irritability to be anticipated. He determines the symptom complex, both subjective and objective. He makes such examination, laboratory and x-ray investigations as may be indicated and from all of this information arrives at a diagnosis. He also analyzes the spine and general somatic structure of his patient to determine the basic distortion, compensatory distortion, distortion that does not fit into the pattern of compensation, and segmental fixations or subluxations. Such analysis is performed by inspection, palpation, measurements, the use of various instruments, including the x-ray and all standard diagnostic aids.

With these two sets of findings the doctor may co-relate the two and provide the patient with the answer to his health problem. Also, the two sets of data serve to check each other and assure the doctor of the accuracy of his findings, or the need to recheck in certain areas.

D. D. Palmer[440] wrote in his textbook: "In making a diagnosis it should be the Chiropractor's business, first of all, to determine the nature of the disease by learning what functions are abnormally performed; what part of the body is affected. Then take into consideration the nerves which ramify the diseased portion in which they are likely to be impinged upon, and lastly, not the first of all, examine the locality where he has decided the luxation exists which by its displacement impinges upon those nerves. To examine 'the 300 articulations of the skeletal frame first of all,' would be to leave out the diagnosis."

And from the same page of Dr. Palmer's book: "Why not make a diagnosis and determine therefrom which vertebra is displaced?"

It is doubtful that there exists a more important area of the vertebral column than the sacrum for the determination of the true cause of the average patient's health problem. For here is the base and as the base goes, so goes the superimposed spine. The necessity for compensation for basic distortion creates areas of stress within the spine, which tend to give way under added stress that would be insufficient to overcome the inherent resistance of a normal spine. Furthermore, these areas of stress along the spine, created by compensation, pre-determine the segments likely to suffer fixation and consequently the organs that are most probable to suffer dysfunction.

The diagnosis, as suggested by D. D. Palmer, provides highly sug-gestive evidence of the location of the segmental fixation or subluxa-tion responsible for the neural disturbance which underlies the visceral malfunction. The chiropractic analysis should utilize every method to confirm, or disqualify, the local segmental fixation as the cause of the symptom complex, but then proceed to determine the primary cause of such fixation. A large percentage of segmental fixa-tions are largely secondary to a basic distortion, but the conscienti-ous doctor of chiropractic will not be content until the primary cause, or causes, of his patient's health problem has been revealed, removed or corrected.

The doctor must not lose sight of the possibilities of external irri-tations, mechanical, chemical or mental, being the true cause of the problem. These may be difficult to isolate and eradicate. It may even be necessary for both doctor and patient to recognize that the causa-tive factors cannot be eliminated and the structural distortion cannot be completely corrected, as a result. The best that can be expected under such circumstances is for the chiropractor to keep the patient functional by continuous, regular care, and this may be a very real and important contribution. To prevent the degeneration of a patient's condition may be a marked victory, even when correction and cure are out of all reason.

# CHAPTER XVII

# Applied Embryology

A REVIEW OF the embryology of the central nervous system prior to embarking on its detailed study will greatly assist the student's understanding and make the material much less of a challenge to memory and recall. Crelin's[441] monograph would be found very helpful. Space will not be devoted here to such duplication.

Presuming then that the reader has a knowledge of embryology, or will review the subject, these pages are to attempt to pull together many of the practical aspects without attention to detail or exhaustion of the topic. Nor will the subject of teratology be undertaken, as gross developmental defects are seldom the concern of the primary health care provider.

## Cranial Structures

Concern is justified over infections of the scalp, root of the nose, middle ear, etc., since the venous network of the exterior is joined with the venous sinuses internally by the emissary veins which pass through the skull, draining the diploic veins in their course.

The Olfactory (I Cranial) Nerve is a diverticulum of the primitive telencephalon while the olfactory membrane of the roof and upper walls of the nasal cavity are reported by Allan[442] to have been derived from the ectoderm of nasal placodes which become pits and then sacs and sink into the tissues to become the receptor organ of smell. The actual first order neurones develop by differentiation from cells of this epithelium. These bipolar neurones whose axones pass through the foramina of the cribriform plate of the ethmoid and enter the olfactory bulb synapse with cytones that are second order neurones with their axones forming the olfactory tract.

Since bulb and tract are an outgrowth from the medial aspect of the telencephalon, the pia and arachnoid layers of the meninges form the supporting and limiting outer walls. It is of import to recall that the olfactory impulses are the only afferents that do not pass through the thalamic nuclei on their way to the cortex.

Again, infections in the nasal cavity are particularly dangerous due to the thin roof of the nasal cavity with possibility of spread into the olfactory bulb and thence to the general meninges to establish meningitis.

It should be noted that the blood vessels of the mucosa of the nasal cavity are supplied by postganglionic sympathetic fibres whose cells are in the superior cervical sympathetic ganglion. These cells receive stimulation via the preganglionic fibres from cells of the lateral horns of T.1 to 4, especially. Thus, upper thoracic adjusting may influence the vascularity of this mucosa. The reader is reminded that Kuntz[443] established that ischemia of the mucosa provides the milieu for the filterable virus associated with colds and these, in turn, prepare the way for microbial infection.

The Optic (II Cranial) Nerve is a diverticulum from the medial surface of the primitive prosencephalon, which enlarges at its terminal end to form the optic bulb. It should be noted that the cavity of this diverticulum is continuous with that of the ventricle. The growth of the nerve fibres fills and obliterates the lumen as the optic nerve is formed. The optic bulb invaginates and forms a double layer, the external one thin and pigmented, while the inner thickens and differentiates into a photosensitive (rods and cones) layer, bipolar neural, ganglion, and sustentacular cells, later to become the retina and other structures. The outgrowth of the diverticulum carries the meninges along and the dura mater forms the outer coat of the optic nerve and the sclera of the eyeball. The arachnoid and pia maters ensheath the nerve and modify to become the choroid coat of the eyeball. The subarachnoid space and cerebrospinal fluid continue to the posterior wall of the adult optic bulb, hence increased intracranial cerebrospinal fluid pressure may be transmitted to eyeball and cause the optic disc to bulge into the interior which can then be visualized with an ophthalmascope as a diagnostic sign of increased intracranial pressure.

It should be recalled that the dilator pupillae, a portion of the levator palpebrarum, and the Muller Muscle of the orbit, as well as the dilator pupillae muscle and the arteries of the eyeball and adnexia are supplied by postganglionic sympathetic fibres from the superior cervical ganglion with the outflow from T.1 to 4. Upper thoracic adjusting may be expected to influence the eye and its associated structures through these sympathetic pathways. Also, traumata, such as the so-called "whiplash," of the cervical column may injure the Longus Capitis and Longus Colli muscles and the swelling or hematoma may either irritate or inhibit the cells of the ganglia of the sympathetic system lying on the surface of, or very close to, these muscles. A dilated pupil and exophthalmic appearance is indicative of hyperactivity of the sympathetics.

The Oculomotor (III Cranial) Nerve, Trochlear (IV Cranial), and Abducens (VI Cranial) are motor to the extrinsic muscles of the eye with little consideration necessary. The muscles that are supplied with these nerve fibres have blood vessels under the control of the sympathetic system, again from superior cervical ganglion and T.1 to 4. The Oculomotor Nerve has preganglionic parasympathetic fibres for supply of the lacrimal gland, constrictor pupillae and ciliary muscles.

The Trigeminal (V Cranial) Nerve is complex, both externally and within the central nervous system, but requires little consideration from an embryological view. It is of interest that the anterior two-thirds of the tongue is derived from the mandibular arch and receives fibres of common sensation from this nerve. The cells of the sensory ganglion of the Trigeminal were derived from the neural crest in the same manner as posterior nerve root ganglia.

Pottenger's[444] statement that tooth decay and atrophy of the half of the tongue corresponding to pulmonary tuberculosis is, in his opinion, a trophic reflex involving the Vagal afferents from the lung and the Trigeminal and Hypoglossal Nerves as the efferent limb.

The Facial (VII Cranial) Nerve has been credited by Pottenger with being the efferent limb of a trophic reflex arc that causes atrophy of the facial muscles, derived from the hyoid arch, in response to the low grade irritation of vagal afferents by chronic tuberculosis. Also, via the parasympathetic fibres of this nerve excessive mucus from the nose may be a response to chronic tuberculosis of the lung. There may be an excess of salivary activity as well, and may occur, also, in instances of angina pectoris and gastric distress. The sensory ganglion cells of the VIIth are derived from the neural crest, too.

The Auditory (VIII Cranial) Nerve is an afferent nerve of special sensation and, like the sensory fibres of all cranial and spinal nerves, these fibres develop within the ganglia formed from the neural crest. Both divisions, chochlear and vestibular, retain the bipolar cytones of the developing afferent neurones.

The two divisions have practical chiropractic significance. The first chiropractic patient, Harvey Lillard, regained his hearing following the adjusting by D. D. Palmer of the fourth thoracic vertebra and a new school of generic medicine was born. The mechanism of the neurological response to the first adjusting, restoring the lost hearing, was discussed briefly under the heading of Upper Thoracic Fixation in Chapter XIV. There are a number of possibilities and it will never be known which is the correct explanation.

While the adult structure of the ear may appear to be at some distance from the superior cervical sympathetic ganglion, it should be recalled that the middle ear and Eustachian tube were derivatives of the pharynx with postganglionic sympathetic fibres modifying the calibre of the lumen of the vascular bed of the endothelial lining of these structures. Further, similar fibres are contributed to the various cranial nerves for distribution to appropriate tissues. Again it must be emphasized that the vascular system, especially the arterial side, supplying almost all tissues from scalp to soles, is under regulation by the sympathetic system. Thus, those who attempt to ridicule D. D. Palmer's initial discovery display their own limited knowledge and appreciation of the nervous system. The sympathetic supply to Eustachian tube and middle ear may be readily accepted, since these are an evagination of the endoderm of the primitive pharynx with a continuous vascular bed. This continuity of tissue makes for ease of spread of inflammation or infection from pharynx to middle ear (otitis media) and from there to involve the lining of the mastoid air cells (mastoiditis).

Prior to the advent of antibiotic drugs, chiropractic physicians successfully cared for some patients with these conditions. The hospitalization of the patient and treatment by antibiotics and/or chemotherapy are the choice of almost all physicians at present.

The Vestibular complex, concerned with sensing and reporting alterations of the position and movements of the head in space, has extensive connections with the centres for modification of muscular tone and balancing of the body weight around the gravity line. As has been brought to the reader's attention previously, the position of the head modifies the cotour assumed by much of the vertebral column from above downward.

A subluxation of occiput on atlas, or atlas on axis, may cause the skull to be posteriorly or anteriorly nodded, tipped right or left, or rotated right or left, or any combination of these. The afferent impulses from the vestibular mechanism, interacting with the proprioceptive impulses from the supporting tissues of the area of subluxation, may cause a compensatory increase or decrease of the anterior curve of the cervical area, or a minimal rotatory scoliosis, or some combination to level the head and normalize the afferent input from the two vestibular organs as well as the visual complex.

Fear of falling and fear of a loud noise seem to be the two fears inherited, all others are learned. The response to fear is flexion — a tendency to return to the embryological position. The "chronic" fear (anxiety) dictates that attention be paid to the flexor muscles when structural correction is being undertaken, since this is such a common emotion as to be practically ubiquitous in patients.

The Glossopharyngeal (IX Cranial) Nerve is in part responsible for the excess salivary secretion as mentioned under the Facial Nerve discussion. Its sensory ganglion cells are derived from the neural crest.

The Vagus (X Cranial) Nerve has the most extensive distribution of any of the cranial nerves. Since the heart, lungs, and part of the primitive gut had origin in the cervical area, they acquired neural fibres from the Vagus and as migration occurred, the Vagal fibres were elongated, maintaining supply to the developing organs as far as the transverse colon.

The Vagus, being afferent, somatic and visceral efferent, is responsible for many of the viscerosensory, visceromotor, and viscerovisceral reflexes. Further, the Trigeminus seems to have very intimate reflex association with the Vagus and is said by some neurologists to be an afferent root of the Vagus.

The gag reflex involves Trigeminus (afferent) and Vagus (efferent), as well as somatic muscles being recruited. The oculocardiac reflex is another involving the same nerves.

Irritation to the gastro-intestinal mucosa (Vagus) may cause nausea and vomiting which requires both parasympathetic (Vagal) efferent activity and somatic (spinal) stimulation of the muscles of the abdominal wall, etc. This is a combined viscerovisceral and viscerosomatic reflex response coordinated by a vomiting centre in the medulla.

An example of the viscerovisceral reflex, utilizing only Vagal fibres, is in instances of dilatation by overeating or accumulation of gas in the stomach that triggers angina pectoris or an asthmatic seizure in patients with either problem. The trophic reflexes, where the Vagus acts as the afferent limb of the arc, were mentioned above. All of these may be expanded considerably. In fact, most symptoms are expressions of one or more reflexes.

The primitive heart and lungs have developed in the neck area of the embryo with the septum transversum, later to be the central portion of the diaphragm, caudal to them. It is, therefore, not a great distance for the Vagus to grow into the various tissues of this area, including the primitive gut. As the structures enlarge and migrate, the Vagus is elongated to continue the supply of larynx, pharynx, trachea, lungs, heart, and much of the gastro-intestinal tract, with both afferent and efferent fibres.

The stomach developed as a posterior bulge of the primitive gut with the anterior border later becoming the lesser curvature and the posterior border the greater curvature. As enlargement takes place, a turning occurs and the right surface with the right Vagus as major supply becomes the anterior wall of the stomach. Of course, the posterior wall is supplied mostly by the left Vagus.

The heart turns also, bringing the right atrium and ventricle to the anterior, although the greater size of the left ventricle causes it to form a part of the left anterior surface, especially at the apex. The formation of superficial and deep cardiac plexuses decreases the limitation of nerve supply to one section of the heart, as does the specialized form of neural supply via sino-atrial, atrio-ventricular nodes, and Purkinje system.

The intimate development of these structures with a common nerve supply facilitates the viscerovisceral reflexes from one to the other. Thus, it should not be surprising that a serious disorder in one, e.g., myocardial infarct, etc., may cause symptoms reflexly in another organ, e.g., nausea and vomiting. The patient with a developing myocardial infarct may have diarrhea and nausea several hours before the onset of pain. Vomiting may occur and then the precordial and left arm pain. This pain may radiate to the medial or ulnar side of the right arm, into the neck, angle of the jaw, and the upper pharynx.

Pottenger[445] explains in detail the various reflex effects that may occur from inflammation of pulmonary tissue to any musculature or glandular tissue supplied by the Vagus. Therefore, diagnosis is not the straightforward science that is desired. The signs and symptoms which cause the patient to consult the physician may be secondary to the real problem.

The Spinal Accessory (XI Cranial) Nerve is atypical as either a spinal or a cranial nerve, being composed of fibres from both the spinal cord and the medulla, but these are atypical, also. The somatic efferent fibres arise from cytones in the anterior horns of the first five cervical neuromeres, but exit on the lateral surface of the segments between anterior and posterior roots, turn upward to enter cranial cavity through the foramen magnum. Within the cranium the spinal root is joined by a cranial root which is in reality composed of Vagal fibres. The XIth nerve exits through the jugular foramen and, almost immediately, the fibres of the two roots separate with the Vagal fibres returning to the Vagus Nerve for distribution. The somatic efferent fibres enter the mass of mesenchyme at the base of the future occiput, which differentiates to form the Trapezius and Sternocleidomastoideus muscles. The afferent fibres for the Sterno-cleidomastoideus are derived from the second cervical and those for the Trapezius from C.3 and 4.

Reflex response in these two large muscles which migrate over such a distance, may confuse the picture of the location of the primary source of the problem. From the afferent fibres of the Trigeminus, which descend as the Spinal Tract into the superior three or more cervical segments, impulses may reach the efferent neurones of the spinal root of the XI cranial nerve. Afferents of the Phrenic Nerve, or afferents from the supporting tissues of the upper cervical segments in the area of subluxation may be primary sources of hypertonicity or trophic changes in these two large muscles.

The Hypoglossal (XII Cranial) Nerve is the motor nerve of the intrinsic and extrinsic muscles of the tongue, which are derived from the occipital myotomes and migrate ventrally. The glossal atrophy in chronic pulmonary disease has been previously noted.

The sympathetic postganglionic supply to the vascular bed of tissues supplied by some of the cranial nerves has not been repeated, but it is essential for the chiropractic physician to be cognizant and mindful of the fact. The potential for influencing these tissues by adjusting vertebral segments can be explained most readily by considering the sympathetic distribution. The more complex explanation with very few authoritative references is via the influence of afferent pathways ascending from spinal cord to alter the outflow of neural impulses from the cranial nerve nucleus at issue.

## Structures of the Neck

A surprising number of important visceral structures begin their developmental history in the area of the cervical region of the conceptus. Some of these have received mention previously, but, in the interest of order, will receive additional consideration.

The vertebral segments develop from the scleroderm of the segment, surrounding the notochord and gradually differentiating into centra of vertebral bodies while the discs form and the residue of notochord remains as nucleus pulposus of each disc. It is important to remember that the vertebral column developed as a continuous column of tissue with the osseous portions progressing from mesenchyme, through the stages of scleroderm, chondrification, and finally ossification. The portion destined to be a disc fails to progress to ossification, but becomes fibrocartilage with a definite laminal structure, lamina fibrosa, retaining the nucleus pulposus more or less in the centre.

The vertebral column was not assembled, and the discs are not separate structures that are capable of slipping and sliding. From the earliest stages the discs and vertebral bodies were merely modifications of cells of a continuous column which continues throughout life as a functional unit. No doctor of chiropractic should be guilty of using the erroneous term, "slipped disc."

As the process continues, the neural tube is surrounded, pedicles, laminae, spinous process, articular processes, and transverse processes take form, but ossification is not complete until years after birth. It is of interest that a costal process is differentiated for each vertebra, but the future in each area differs drastically.

In the cervical region the costal processes remain very small and short, being the anterior portion of the transverse processes and anterior boundary of each of the foramina transversarium. In some instances the costal processes for the seventh and, even, sixth cervical may continue growth to become cervical ribs. These may produce no symptoms until well into adult life when poor posture and muscle tension contribute to the problem and irritation of the brachial plexus and/or interference to the subclavian artery and vein may produce extensive symptoms. Structural correction and improving posture may be too demanding a challenge for the patient and surgery offers the easy way.

The atlas and axis development into atypical vertebrae, provide opportunity for many abnormalities that are thoroughly discussed in other texts.

The musculature offers many interesting developmental peculiarities, but it will be called to the reader's attention that the deep postvertebral muscles arise from the myotomes, while others, lying more superficial, arise from the limb bud and migrate into this area, then overlying all are the sternocleidomastoideus and trapezius derived from the ocipital myotomes. The segmental nerve supply indicates the level of primitive development, e.g., the Platysma, being the most superficial of the anterolateral muscles, is supplied by the Facial (VII Cranial) Nerve and is, therefore, derived from the hyoid or second branchial arch.

The tubular endoderm, surrounded by the musculature and supporting tissue derived from mesoderm, becomes the gut. From the foregut in the cervical or neck region, many important structures differentiate. The cephalic end becomes the pharynx continuous with the oesophagus and this, in turn, with the stomach and then part of the duodenum. The laryngotracheal diverticulum of endoderm is an evagination from the primitive pharynx and buds to develop into bronchi and lungs. Another pouch from each side of the primitive pharynx aids in the development of a middle ear, the endoderm lines the Eustachian tubes and middle ears. There are other diverticula from which thyroid, thymus, and parathyroid glands are developed. Another diverticulum just beyond the developing stomach grows into a portion of the septum transversum and the liver and ducts begin to take form. The capsule and supporting tissue of the liver is derived from the mesenchyme of the septum and is supplied with afferent fibres from the Phrenic Nerve.

The heart and diaphragm arise in this area, also, as has been previously mentioned. It is interesting to note that the fibres of the Phrenic Nerve (C.3-4-5) grow into the mesochymal tissue from which the fibrous pericardium, mediastinal pleura, and central diaphragmatic pleura arise. Also, many fibres of the Phrenic are motor for the Diaphragm.

These viscera, developing in the cervical region, receive Vagal fibres and with growth, modified shape, and migration, the Vagal fibres are elongated to assume the complex adult form. Nor is it surprising that viscerovisceral reflexes are common between such viscera.

Those structures supplied by afferents of the Phrenic Nerve (fibrous pericardium, mediastinal and central diaphragmatic pleura, capsule of the liver, etc.), may cause a viscerosensory reflex with pain at the base of the neck and shoulder. Visceromotor reflexes may involve muscles supplied by the third, fourth and fifth cervical segments, but most of these muscles have a number of segments of supply, thus a portion of a complex muscle may show altered tone. The segmental muscles may contribute to the hypertonicity at the site of subluxation, helping cause or perpetuate this dysfunction.

A final point relative to the heart should be made. Each of the three pairs of cervical sympathetic ganglia contribute a bundle of postganglionic sympathetic fibres to the heart and its vessels, a pair of Superior, Middle and Inferior Cardiac Nerves. The cells of the preganglionic fibres are part of the lateral horns of the upper thoracic neuromeres and other fibres synapse in the upper four, or more, thoracic ganglia which contribute additional postganglionic fibres to the heart. It is to be anticipated that subluxations of the upper thoracic region may have an adverse effect upon the sympathetic supply to the heart. Further, the afferent fibres accompanying the sympathetic fibres enter the upper thoracic segments of the cord, especially T.2, but some authorities note that a few of these afferent fibres may enter the cord as low as T.7. However, the viscerosensory reflex of pain due to myocardial ischemia is expressed not only in the precordial area, but down the ulnar side of the left arm, forearm, little and ring fingers. It may be appreciated that these impulses have irradiated by way of the fibres ascending several segments, thus involving second order neurones in the eighth cervical neuromere.

## Thoracic Area

There is much less interest in this area than in the cervical region.

The vertebrae are typical with relatively minor modifications from above downward. The costal processes do not fuse with the vertebrae, but form the ribs and costal cartilages. The sternum forms from two separate bars which fuse from above downward. Ossification is not complete until well into adult life with the ensiform or xiphoid process being the last to ossify and sometimes remaining bifid.

The musculature offers points of interest, since the Trapezius, as the most superficial of the muscles of the back, has attachment to all thoracic spinous processes and supraspinous ligaments of the thoracic vertebrae. This muscle receives its motor supply via the Spinal Accessory (XI Cranial) Nerve and afferent fibres from cervicals three and four with no thoracic fibres other than sympathetic for vascular control.

The Latissimus Dorsi under the inferior tapered end of the Trapezius has origin, in part, from the spinous processes and supraspinous ligaments of the lower six thoracic vertebrae and the nerve supply from cervicals six to eight, indicating that this muscle was derived from the arm limb bud. Many of the other muscles that lie on the thorax (pectorales, serratus anterior, etc.) have a similar origin, with nerve supply from the brachial plexus.

The intercostal muscles are the most clearly defined of those derived from a single myotome with a single spinal nerve of supply.

The parietal pleura and peripheral portion of the diaphragmatic pleura are supplied by fibres of the anterior primary divisions of the thoracic nerves, thus inflammation of the lower parietal or diaphragmatic pleura may refer pain and muscle hypertonicity into the abdominal area to be confused with abdominal disease. Appendectomies have been performed quite frequently with a normal appendix and pneumonia the reward. The symptoms and laboratory findings in an early pneumonia have not pinpointed the source of the trouble, but rather confused the location.

The mediastinal and central diaphragmatic pleura, as well as the fibrous pericardium, received consideration previously as to the referral of pain to the base of the neck and shoulder.

## Abdominal Region

The lumbar vertebrae in the posterior wall of the abdomen are more massive to support the superimposed weight and are subject to frequent developmental abnormalities of importance to the doctor of chiropractic, but receive little attention here, since much has been written by more competent authors.

Spondylolisthesis, occurring most frequently at the fifth lumbar, is due to the failure of ossification to fuse the posterior arch and centrum. Although this is a developmental abnormality, it is usually quiescent until well into adult life, then as posture degenerates, an increased lumbar lordosis develops, the deep postvertebral muscles respond to Davis' Law,[446] and a careless use of the spine in lifting, all contribute to the separation of centrum from posterior arch. The common techniques of chiropractic may not be very successful in restoring the apposition of the segments. The more powerful techniques, as described by Beatty,[447] utilizing the Traction Swing or two-man Incline Plane methods, may be required and, although good relationship may be restored, the two portions of the vertebra will never fuse, thus the potential for recurrence remains. Minimizing the risk of a similar happening requires postural correction with release of the tense, shortened postvertebral muscles and the iliopsoas, balancing of the tone of the muscles of pelvis and thighs to restore the correct facing of the pelvis, training in proper lifting, as well as forbidding attempts to lift any heavy object. Such a condition may require surgical fusion, if the full cooperation of the patient is not forthcoming.

The Iliolumbar Ligament seems to have migrated from a higher level in the embryo, since afferent fibres seem to return to the twelfth thoracic and first lumbar neuromeres. Due to its attachment along a section of the inner lip of the iliac crest and to the transverse processes of L.4 and 5, relative posterior nodding (rotation around a transverse axis) of the innominate causes excess tension and irritation of the ligamentous fibres, perhaps even tearing of some fibres. The referred pain is into the groin and superomedial aspect of the thigh. This may be confused with symptoms of inguinal hernia, ureteral calculus, appendicitis, oopheritis, or strain of inguinal tissues. Goading of the iliac attachment accentuates the pain, and, coupled with the signs of disrelation of the innominate, settles the diagnosis without the need for extensive laboratory tests.

It is of interest that the transverse processes are derived from the costal processes embryologically; are relatively long and slender, and should be avoided as contact points for a thrust from posterior to anterior. The mamillary processes are much more stable, although not offering as much leverage. In a small percentage, the costal processes greatly enlarge for L.5 and may fuse on one or both sides to the sacrum — sacralization, forming a sixth sacral segment and decreasing the number of true lumbar vertebrae to four. Other oddities are not uncommon, but are not within the scope of this text.

The most superficial muscle of the lumbar area is the Latissimus Dorsi which had its embryonic origin in the limb bud and retains attachment (adult insertion) to the shaft of the humerus with nerve supply from cervicals 6 to 8. Thus adjustive influence for this muscle must be directed to the lower cervical spine.

The muscles attached to the bodies of the lumbar vertebrae, Psoas Major and Crura of the Diaphragm, have quite different embryological origins, the first mentioned from the limb bud mesoderm for the leg and the latter from the mesoderm of the primitive lower thoracic region. The import of these muscles is the effect of combined hypertonicity that may be responsible for the short lordosis in the thoracolumbar area of some patients, which involves two or three vertebrae. Hypertonicity of the postvertebral muscles of the same area contributes, also, by approximating the posterior arches. Trophic changes of the skin and superficial fascia are likely to be accompanying findings, decreasing the thickness of the tissue and accentuating the apparent lordotic area.

The abdominal musculature is derived, for the most part, from the anterior (hypaxial) portion of the myotomes of the lower thoracic region, thus deriving nerve supply from the T.5 to L.1 neuromeres. The parietal peritoneum, lining the abdominal musculature, receives afferent fibres from the same segments. It should be appreciated by chiropractic students that these abdominal muscles are of considerable importance in providing support for the anterior portion of the

262

pelvis. Loss of tone results in anterior nodding of the pelvis and is very common in the adult, since the sedentary habits of the present day tend to encourage decreased tone with the effect seen upon total posture and vertebral column compensation.

The various abdominal viscera may produce reflex responses in the abdominal wall through the common neuromeres of supply. Acute appendicitis may have, as one sign, the flexion of thigh on pelvis. This would seem to be the result of afferent impulses returning in company with the postganglionic sympathetic fibres to pass through the ganglionic chain without synapse, through white rami communicantes, through the posterior nerve roots, into the spinal cord segments T.12 and L.1. The descending collaterals pass down into several lumbar neuromeres and reflex response of the motor pool in L.2 and 3 results in contraction of the Iliopsoas muscle of the same side. The Quadratus Femoris has a similar supply and could be involved, as well as the hypertonicity in the area of McBurney's Point of the abdomen (T.12).

## The Pelvis and Content

The sacral segments lose most of the characteristics of true vertebrae, although each is present in rudimentary form. The costal processes of the sclerotome expand greatly in the first three sacral segments to form the main mass of the lateral portion.

It is of interest that the intervertebral foramina are within the sacrum and the anterior and posterior foramina seen on the surfaces permit the passage of the anterior and posterior primary rami of the nerve trunks, due to the ligamentous tissues of the true vertebral segments ossification, forming the boundaries of the foramina.

The viscerosensory reflex of the prostate or uterus may involve the tenth and eleventh thoracic distribution and the second and third sacral. Thus, pain may be experienced in a band around the body at the level of the umbilicus and slightly lower. The sacral distribution will involve the lower gluteal, posteromedial thighs, and the posterior ankles, as well as the soles of the feet. The uterus has an even broader area of referred pain. The urinary bladder refers pain to the area of the symphisis pubis, over the sacrum, and a limited area of the upper posteromedial thighs.

The testicles and ovaries have a higher level of embryological development and, therefore, a higher segmental nerve supply. The T.10 dermatome is involved for the ovary, and T.11 and 12 for the testicle.

The kidney (T.10 to L.1) and the ureter (T.11 to L.4) refer pain to a broad area of the back, over the upper lateral thigh, pelvis, and the anterior wall from umbilicus down into medial thigh.

These would seem to be the embryological associations of most import.

## Limb Buds

At approximately the fifth week the conceptus shows the beginning of the limb buds for the upper extremity and several weeks later those for the lower limbs appear. Into these condensations of mesenchyme, covered by ectoderm, grow the nerve fibres from the neuromeres of the area. Thus, the cephalic buds receive fibres from C.5 to 8 and T.1 with a few from C.4 and T.2, and the buds for the legs derive fibres from L.2 to 5 and S.1 and 2.

The extremities develop with thumb and big toe superior and the palm or sole facing anterior, therefore, these derive nerve supply from the corresponding segments, e.g., thumb from C.6, middle finger from C.7, ring and little finger from C.8, etc.

The illustrations by Chusid[448] provide excellent coverage of the dermatomes, muscles, and bones supplied by fibres from each neuromere.

The important viscerosensory reflex from the heart to the ulnar aspect of arm, forearm, hand, and fingers received consideration previously, as has the pain and circulatory disturbance of cervical ribs. The scalenus syndrome which produces similar symptoms to the cervical rib, is more frequently a problem developed after birth, or from a birth injury.

Those viscera of the pelvis that receive parasympathetic supply from the second and third, or third and fourth sacral segments, also have afferent fibres that conduct impulses back to these same segments and there may then be viscerosensory and/or visceromotor reflexes into the leg(s) as symptoms of inflammation or pathology. This was described briefly above for several of the structures.

Visceromotor reflexes, involving the muscles of the lower extremities, do not appear to be diagnostically significant.

## Peculiarities of the Sympathetic System

While no embryological explanation can be provided, it is of note that the distribution of the sympathetic fibres to viscera differ above and below the diaphragm.

First, it should be mentioned that all sympathetic fibres to the somatic areas for blood vessels, sudoriferous glands, and erector pilii muscles are relatively the same in arrangement. The myelinated preganglionic fibres leave the spinal cord as part of an anterior nerve root of T.1 to L.3, leave the trunk or anterior ramus as a white ramus communicans, synapse with cells of the ganglionated chain. The axones of these latter cells return to the spinal nerves as unmyelinated postganglionic fibres, forming a gray ramus communicans (at least one for every spinal nerve) for distribution through the spinal nerve and its branches.

## Above the Diaphragm

Those structures within cavities above the level of the diaphragm also receive postganglionic sympathetic fibres from the cells located in the paravertebral ganglia. These fibres merely leave the ganglia and, for the most part, follow the course of blood vessels to the viscus to be supplied. The three pairs of Cardiac Nerves from Superior, Middle, and Inferior Sympathetic Ganglia are unique, but are the axones of cells of the ganglia and are postganglionic, unmyelinated, or poorly myelinated fibres.

## Below the Diaphragm

Some of the preganglionic sympathetic fibres that enter the paravertebral ganglia from the fifth to ninth thoracics pass through without synapsing to form the Greater Splanchnic Nerve. Those of the tenth and eleventh thoracics travel through to form the Lesser Splanchnic Nerve, and others pass through the twelfth thoracic ganglion to form the Least Splanchnic Nerve. These nerves are paired, of course. Synaptic connection is made in the prevertebral ganglia, such as the coeliac, aorticorenal, superior and inferior mesenteric, etc. The postganglionic fibres continue on from their cell bodies in these prevertebral ganglia to supply the vascular bed and sphincters of the abdominal viscera.

The pelvic visceral structures receive postganglionic sympathetic fibres mostly from the paravertebral ganglia, but some from the prevertebral ganglia as well. Thus, their supply is a mixture of the two types.

The last unusual development to be noted is the medulla of the adrenal gland which is, in fact, a derivative of the primitive neural crest and rather than differentiating into neural cells of a prevertebral ganglion developed glandular characteristics that secrete norepinephrine and epinephrine. This is the only structure that receives nerve impulses directly from preganglionic sympathetic fibres.

## The Subluxation

The old Meric system of chiropractic attempted to systematize analysis and adjusting on an embryological basis with simplicity being the goal. From the broad knowledge present-day students must master and the pages that have gone before in this text, it must be obvious and disappointing that the science and art of chiropractic will never be simple. There can never be one vertebra to adjust in every spine to influence the same viscus, nor will each set of symptoms be corrected by the adjusting of the same vertebra in different patients.

A knowledge of embryology assists in the understanding of gross anatomy, the interrelations of reflexes, symptoms, and the various vertebral areas to be considered in each case.

While the structures in the head and face are supplied by cranial nerves, it must not be forgotten that all of their blood vessels are under the influence of the postganglionic sympathetic fibres whose cell bodies, for the most part, are in the superior cervical ganglia and these receive the impulses from the sympathetic outflow of the upper four thoracic neuromeres. Subluxation in that area of the spine is to be anticipated when symptoms occur in the structures of the head. On the other hand, upper cervical subluxations may be involved and these disturb the cranial nerve function through reflexes from the site via afferent fibres and connector or intercalated neurones within the cord and brain stem.

Subluxations in the upper cervical area may adversely influence the Trapezius and Sternocleidomastoideus, but so may irritation to fibres of the Trigeminal Nerve.

Irritation of the pericardium, mediastinal or diaphragmatic pleura may produce the motor action of muscles to subluxate C.3, 4 or 5. A subluxation of one or more of these vertebrae may alter diaphragmatic function. Since afferents from the diaphragm and peripheral diaphragmatic pleura return to the lower six thoracic neuromeres, a subluxation in this region may have adverse reflex influences upon the motor function of the diaphragm, e.g., hiccoughs may not respond to mid-cervical adjusting, but be eliminated by correction of one or more of the lower thoracics.

Although the heart derives a large percentage of its sympathetic impulses from the cervical ganglia, it is the upper thoracic segments, especially T.1-4, that is the outflow and the location to be examined for subluxation. It is these cord segments that receive the afferent fibres from the heart.

Again, the lower cervical vertebrae must be examined in instances of problems of muscles as far removed as the Latissimus Dorsi, Serratus Anterior, Pectorales, etc.

In the following chapter, attention is directed in more detail to the afferent fibres returning to the neuraxis from specific visceral structures.

It is to be appreciated that viscerovisceral reflexes may disturb the function of an embryologically associated secondary viscus and the afferent impulses from the second viscus may summate in an area of the spine under stress from a number of other sources, e.g., hereditary weakness, compensatory stress, afferent bombardment due to chemical irritation of another viscus, psychologically induced muscle hypertonicity, etc., thus becomes the final factor in the production of a subluxation.

The subluxation, due to other causes, may contribute adverse effects to the secondary viscus involved in a viscerovisceral reflex, thus increasing the disturbance of function.

From this sketchy coverage of the subject, it is hoped that the reader may be motivated to refresh his memory of embryology and give to the subject a new appreciation of its practical value.

CHAPTER XVIII

# Afferents, Time and Trophic Function

IN THE PRECEDING pages little has been said relative to the time factor, as it relates to the subluxation, nor has the trophic function of the nervous system received the consideration it deserves. There are also many points relative to the afferent side of the nervous system which require further elaboration to bring such a dissertation as this closer to completion. In this chapter an attempt will be made to cover as many aspects of the problem as possible to stimulate the interest of the reader in further research into the many interesting possibilities of disturbance by the fixation.

D. D. Palmer recognized full well the importance of the nervous system in its controlling and integrating activities, but went beyond this in his recognition of the necessity for normal neural activity to maintain the integrity of the cellular elements of the entire human structure. This latter activity he relegated to the supervision of "Innate Intelligence," an arbitrary name to designate a peculiar functional capacity of the nervous system, more recently called homeostasis.

First, he recognized a superhuman, infinite force, "Universal Intelligence." God, Cosmic Law, etc., etc. Within each individual he visualized a tiny segment of that Universal Intelligence. Furthermore, an infinitesimal spark of Innate resides in each living cell. Thus, each cell "knows" how to acquire nutrition, eliminate metabolites, reproduce, function according to a plan, and react to environmental conditions, both normal and adverse.

Many have skoffed at the use of the term "Innate Intelligence," but, as utilized by D. D. Palmer, it possesses the explanatory significance few other terms boast. Unfortunately, the term has been abused and utilized as a subterfuge to disguise ignorance, intellectual laziness or frank intellectual dishonesty. There seems little reason to discard such an expressive term and no apology should be made by the chiropractic profession for the utilization of this portion of the heritage in proper context.

Another arbitrary term coined by the founder of chiropractic is "Educated Intelligence," which conforms to the understanding of the layman and psychological student of the term "intelligence." He recognized that intelligence, in its usual connotation, is dependent upon Innate Intelligence and cannot be separated one from the other, except for descriptive purposes. Furthermore, he suggested that the autonomic division of the nervous system, which he called the sympathetic system in accord with one nomenclature popular in his day, was more concerned with the vegetative functions of the body and therefore, a useful tool of Innate Intelligence; while the Educated Intelligence utilized the cerebro-spinal division for the volitional expression of its function. Another method of classifying the activities of these two divisions of intelligent function is under the headings of "subconscious" for Innate's activities, and "conscious" for Educated Intelligence's performance. D. D. Palmer was acutely aware that these classifications were artificial and served a useful purpose for description, rather than a true and complete outline of the functions.

Utilizing some of the quotations from D. D. Palmer's book, the above intricate picture, as visualized by the founder, may be painted in his own words. These have been taken piecemeal from numerous sections of his book, but the reference numbers will permit the reader to locate with ease the pages from which these remarks have been gleaned.

"Intelligent Life — Force of Creation is God. It is individualized in each of us." [449]

"The soul is intelligent life — life guided by intelligence. It resides thru-out the body wherever life is manifested." [450]

"Innate, spirit, vital force, runs the material body as long as it is habitable — as long as its structure is capable of transmitting impulses and placing them in action. When, by any means, the channels of communication become useless, because of necrosis (softening), or sclerosis (hardening), functions cease and death ensues." [451]

"I think I have fully shown that there is a system of nerves known as the sympathetic nervous system; that Innate, thru this system, controls all the vital functions; . . ." [452]

"As the sympathetic, the visceral division of the nervous system, is dependent upon and is a part of the cerebro-spinal system, so the intellect is subject to and is a part of Innate's mind. Innate stores all the information and knowledge gleaned during a lifetime." [453]

"Innate Intelligence, known, also, as Nature, intuition, instinct, spiritual and subconscious mind, has duplicate senses in Educated Intelligence. While the former looks after the material corporal body night and day, as long as the bond of union — the soul — continues to exist, the latter cares for the outward needs; each has its special work to perform." [454]

"The impulses of Innate are transmitted over the sympathetic, ganglionic, nervous system, the nerves of organic life which ramify the viscera of the four cavities of the body; whereas, the mental impulses are of the mind, under the control of Educated; they go to the somatic portion of the body over the anterior and posterior branches of the spinal nerves. It will be seen that the impulses of Innate and those of Educated (the mind) have different origins, are each transmitted over their special nerves, the splanchnopleure to the inner or visceral portion and the somatopleure to the body wall. It will be readily seen that these two classes of impulses, destined for different portions of the body, over entirely different divisions of nerves, the one voluntary, the other involuntary, the former devoted to animal life, the latter to organic, ought not to be thrown into one indiscriminate lot, as Innate mental impulses." [455]

"Do not forget for one moment that every physical function of the body is managed by Innate thru the nervous system. Even nerve-sheaths and the walls of blood-vessels are covered by a complete network of nerves to facilitate the transportation of sensation, motion, transudation and circulation." [456]

"The intellectual functions do not run the vital functions. . . . Vital functions are those essential to life. Animal functions belong to the encephalon; they are functions of the Intellect — the mind." [457]

"The Chiropractor looks upon the body as more than a machine; a union of consciousness and unconsciousness; Innate's ability to transfer impulses to all parts of the body — the co-ordination of sensation and volition; a personified immaterial spirit and body linked together by the soul — a life directed by intelligence uniting the immaterial with the material." [458]

"The mind governs the intellectual functions. Innate directs the vital actions, those of the vegetative functions of the animal economy. . . . The mind, like other functions, is dependent upon Innate and the condition of the nervous system. . . . Innate, the spiritual, has the power to conceive, judge and reason on matters which pertain to the internal welfare of the body." [459]

While these quotations may appear somewhat disjointed, since they have been lifted out of context and arranged in an orderly sequence to express the total thought of the founder, it is hoped that the reader may experience little difficulty in grasping the depth of perception of D. D. Palmer. His thoughts may not be in agreement with those of the reader, but they form a rational hypothesis relative to a field of knowledge as obscure to the best minds of our times as to those existing seventy-odd years ago, when D.D.'s book was written. It is doubtful that the next sixty years will present the world with a complete, factual explanation of the things called "Life," "Soul," "Conscious," and "Unconscious," as well as many of the other hidden mysteries of the functioning of the animal body.

The founder of chiropractic made every effort to seek out and utilize the available knowledge of anatomy and physiology to build a solid foundation for chiropractic and never sought to disguise gaps in his knowledge by an involved barrage of discussion of Innate Intelligence, nor did he hesitate to reveal anatomical facts inconsistent with his general theory, but made every effort to bring his general explanation parallel to the facts. This remains a challenge for the chiropractors of the present and the future to maintain the explanation of chiropractic in conformity with newly discovered factual data, being constantly brought forth by the research workers in the biological sciences.

The use of those erudite sounding terms, such as homeostasis, subconscious, superego, etc., etc., are no more revealing of the true facts of the body's function than are the terms used by D. D. Palmer in 1910 to attempt to convey the functions observed but not understood or explainable.

## The Afferent System

Since the days of D. D. Palmer, chiropractic literature has devoted its attention to the efferent subdivision of the nervous system with a relative dearth of consideration of the centripetal fibres which the previous chapters have emphasized in relation to the vertebral fixation and the mode of disturbing function in both somatic and splanchnic structures. In the chapters devoted to the causes of vertebral disrelations, the afferent fibres received consideration in part. It is fitting that a large portion of one chapter should be devoted to the afferent side of the nervous system to attempt to tie in any thoughts left in limbo.

These neurones outnumber the efferent fibres in a ratio of about five to one, according to Freeman,[460] and as Gray[461] has stated, this ratio is three to one for the spinal nerves. It may be appreciated that many of the large cranial nerves, such as the olfactory, optic, trigeminal and auditory are almost exclusively sensory and others are mixed, both afferent and efferent, thereby increasing the ratio of total fibres to the five to one mentioned.

In view of the numerical superiority of this division of the nervous system, justification for more detailed investigation of its functional significance should be obvious. It has been well established by the authorities that the afferent impulses from the exteroceptors and interoceptors are of the utmost importance in determining the efferent outflow at any given moment. It is hoped that the case for the chiropractic fixation as an additional source of modification of the efferent outflow, primarily on a local basis, has been established in the previous pages.

Little additional needs to be said about the somatic afferent fibres relative to their mode of return to the spinal cord from the structure supplied. It is easily comprehended that most peripheral nerves are mixed, efferent and afferent. As the nerves return to a plexus, such as the brachial plexus, the components of the individual nerve trunks separate and become distinct as a mixed bundle belonging to a single neuromere. Upon entering the vertebral canal, the nerve trunk divides into a posterior nerve root, which is sensory, and an anterior nerve root, which is motor, or efferent. Each root joins the cord as a number of fine bundles of fibres, called radicles. The distribution within the cord has been covered a number of times and will not be repeated.

The afferent return from visceral structures is not always so clear and simple and, thus, requires some further elucidation under a number of subdivisions.

## Afferents from Somatic Arteries

The arteries, veins and other tissues associated with the somatic tissues, but under the controlling influence of the sympathetic division of the nervous system are well supplied with afferents, whose course back to the spinal cord offers no peculiarities worthy of extensive discussion. The structure of these fibres presents no differences from ordinary somatic neurones either. The cell bodies of such afferent fibres are located in the posterior nerve root ganglia and are unipolar in type, resembling in every detail ordinary somatic efferent cytones.

The connections made within the gray matter of the spinal cord present no peculiarities worthy of the attention of neurologists or special mention in this treatise.

## Cranial Afferents

In addition to the afferent fibres of common sensation and the specialized receptors of vision, taste, smell, hearing, etc., the arteries supplying the structures of the cranium have afferent fibres, whose course is particularly involved and deserving of consideration at this point. Cobb[462] mentions the wealth of nerve fibres distributed to the meninges and vessels of the cortex itself, many of which are afferent in type.

It must be recalled that the common carotid artery and the vertebral artery received postganglionic sympathetic fibres from the cervical sympathetic ganglia, especially the superior, to form a plexiform network on the external surfaces. Kuntz[463] established that intermingled in these plexuses are afferent fibres and with each division of an artery, both efferent and afferent fibres continue on the surface of each new vessel to its final terminal branches.

Tracing these afferent fibres back to the spinal cord, it is established that they enter the superior cervical sympathetic ganglion, travel down the sympathetic chain to leave in white rami communicantes, especially those for the first four thoracic nerves. These fibres then become integrated into the nerve trunk, the posterior nerve root, with their unipolar cells in the posterior nerve root ganglion. Upon entrance into the cord, they are distributed according to their type, influencing primarily the lateral horn cells, but having the potential of disturbing somatic neurones of the anterior gray horn, or establishing synaptic connection with second order neurones of the sensory pathway from a somatic structure. Such an arrangement, as the latter, permits modification of the vascular bed of the structure in which the afferent fibres were stimulated; alteration in vascular response in tissues supplied by the same neuromere; somatic muscle hypertonicity; referred pain into a somatic structure neurologically associated with the afferent fibres from the cranial structure.

Much of the afferent nerve supply of the meninges of the cranial cavity is received from the Trigeminal Nerve, especially fibres of the ophthalmic and maxillary divisions, although the mandibullar division contributes also, as does the Vagus, according to Cunningham.[464] It is of interest that the tentorium cerebelli and posterior third of the falx cerebri are supplied by fibres of the ophthalmic division, as well as contributions from this division to the dura of the middle cranial fossa. It would appear significant that the nociceptive fibres of the ophthalmic descend in the Spinal Tract of the Trigeminal to the lowest level in the spinal cord (C.3) before synapsing. This provides an explanation for some of the headaches resulting from upper cervical subluxation. The afferent impulses returning from the supporting tissues of the subluxated segment enter the cord, radiate to the second order neurones whose cytones are part of the substantia gelatinosa which normally receive impulses from the ophthalmic fibres. These conduct to the thalamus and third order neurones and then third order neurones to the cortex where the interpretation is pain in the occipital area.

It is likely that the headaches of vascular origin are accompanied by nausea and even vomiting due to the irritation of Vagal fibres with involvement of the vomiting centre in the medulla.

## Thoracic Visceral Afferent Fibres

The tissues of the thoracic cavity are not supplied with afferent fibres in identical fashion and must be separated to a degree for description. It is also necessary to include some of the abdominal structures in this phase of the discussion to avoid further duplication.

The pericardium, mediastinal pleura, central area of the diaphragm with attached diaphragmatic pleura, the capsule of the liver and the hepatic ligaments all receive afferent fibres from the Phrenic Nerve and return impulses to the third, fourth and fifth cervical segments, especially the fourth cervical neuromere. It may be expected and is well established clinically that irritation of these above mentioned structures may demonstrate reflex involvement of the somatic tissues supplied by the same cervical neuromeres. Referred pain to the base of the neck and shoulder is common, as are other somatic symptoms.

The parietal pleura, lining the thoracic cage, and the peripheral portions of the diaphragmatic pleura are supplied by afferent fibres of the thoracic nerves with no peculiarities worthy of note. The peripheral diaphragmatic pleura refers pain to the abdomen, because of its being supplied with afferents from the sixth to the twelfth thoracic segments. Thus, inflammation of this portion of the pleura may present a symptom complex which would lead the diagnostician to believe that he was dealing with an acute abdominal crisis. Care must be exercised to avoid serious mistakes in diagnosis, as was previously discussed.

The truly visceral tissues, such as the heart and lungs, receive afferent fibres in company with the sympathetic and parasympathetic components of the cardiac and pulmonary plexuses. Those of the sympathetic division pass back from the heart by way of the middle and inferior cardiac nerves to the middle and inferior cervical sympathetic ganglia, while others return to the upper three thoracic paravertebral ganglia. Those that have entered cervical ganglia descend in the sympathetic chain and are accompanied by those of the corresponding thoracic ganglia through the white rami communicantes to the thoracic nerves and thence into the segments of the cord via the posterior nerve roots. It should be noted that these afferent fibres do not synapse within the ganglionated chain and their cytones are in the posterior nerve root ganglia.

Rasmussen[465] has expressed doubt that any afferent fibres return from the heart in the superior cardiac nerve of the superior cervical ganglion and has mentioned also that afferent fibres from the heart enter the left side of the spinal cord mostly and some fibres may enter as low as the seventh thoracic segment.

The afferent fibres from the heart and the lungs, which are components of the Vagus Nerve, have their cell bodies in the Nodose Ganglion of the Vagus and upon entering the medulla oblongata terminate in the sensory portion of the Dorsal Nucleus of the Vagus, according to Gray.[466] Sir Thomas Lewis[467] has established that there are no pain fibres from the heart contained in the Vagus Nerve. Thus, the sensation of pain experienced from cardiac disease is dependent upon the pathways to the thoracic neuromeres.

Rasmussen[468] and other authorities have concluded that afferents from the lungs return with the sympathetic fibres, pass through the sympathetic ganglia and white rami communicantes to enter the first five thoracic neuromeres. While Pottenger[469] agrees with the other authorities as to the neuromeres entered by afferent fibres from the lungs, he emphasizes that these fibres synapse with connector neurones which effect reflex connections with neurones of the mid-cervical region. Hence, the greater proportion of viscerosomatic reflexes in response to pulmonary disease occur in the tissues supplied by the third, fourth and fifth cervical neuromeres.

## Gastro-Intestinal Afferents

The gastro-intestinal tract will receive consideration in its entirety even though the distal part is located in the pelvic cavity and receives sacral afferent nerve fibres, after which attention will be directed to the genito-urinary system.

Rasmussen[470] lists the afferent fibres of the stomach as being associated with the sixth to the ninth thoracic neuromeres, more particularly the right halves of the seventh and eighth segments. These afferents return to the ganglionic chain as components of the Greater Splanchnic Nerve, pass through the sympathetic ganglia without interruption, through the corresponding white rami communicantes, nerve trunks and posterior nerve roots to enter the neuromeres. The same pattern continues to apply to the remainder of the abdominal viscera.

It must not be overlooked that the Vagus contains afferent fibres for all of the digestive tract as far distal as the splenic flexure. Again, it should be mentioned that none of these latter neurones are concerned with pain and they terminate in the sensory portion of the Dorsal Nucleus of the Vagus, as stated above. However, should the stimuli over Vagal afferents be sufficiently strong or the conditions of irritability be propitious, the impulses may "spill over" or "irradiate" to the tracts of the trigeminal nerve and be experienced as referred pain. As Kuntz[471] has explained, nausea and vomiting are common symptoms of irritation of these afferent fibres of the Vagus, but the pain is a viscero-sensory reflex appreciated in some somatic structure.

The small intestine and most of the colon receive afferent fibres from the eighth to the twelfth thoracic segments, as well as Vagal afferents. What has been said relative to the Vagus continues to apply throughout the digestive tract. The afferents, that accompany the preganglionic sympathetic fibres back to the spinal cord, assist in the formation of the Splanchnic nerve to reach the paravertebral ganglia, through which they pass without synaptic connection, through the white rami communicantes, the nerve trunks and the posterior nerve roots.

The liver, gall bladder and pancreas are supplied with afferent fibres from the sixth to eleventh thoracic segments. Both the Vagus and the Phrenic nerves contribute afferent fibres to these structures. Rasmussen[472] has established that gall stones cause referred pain especially on the right side in areas supplied by the tenth thoracic segment, although the ninth to the eleventh neuromeres are involved.

The spleen, although not a digestive organ, is supplied with afferent fibres from the left side of segments six to eight, as well as Vagal afferents.

The vermiform appendix is associated afferencially with the eleventh and twelfth thoracic and first lumbar segments on the right side. It boasts also of Vagal afferent fibres, which are associated with frequent symptoms of nausea and vomiting when the appendix is inflamed.

Afferent fibres for the sigmoid colon are derived from the first and second lumbar segments. This portion of the colon is beyond the reach of the Vagus and, therefore, derives centripetal fibres from the Nervi Erigentes of the second and third sacral nerves, as described by Gray.[473] Such fibres are concerned in their distribution with the descending colon and approximately the distal one-third of the transverse colon and splenic flexure.

Sacral nerves two, three and four appear to distribute the greater proportion of sensory fibres to the rectum and demonstrate the reflexes in response to rectal irritation. Although Rasmussen[474] did not indicate afferent fibres returning to the first and second lumbar segments of the cord, this is to be anticipated in view of the general pattern of the nervous system by which afferents accompany both sympathetic and parasympathetic efferents. The reflexes in response to rectal irritation are expressed most predominantly through the sacral segments.

It may be well to state at this point that the pelvic viscera, including the rectum, have very well defined reflex connections with the vomiting centre in the medulla oblongata and it is presumed that a series of neurones conduct the impulses up the entire length of the cord and into the medulla oblongata. However, such a tract has not been anatomically demonstrated. Furthermore, headaches and other symptoms have been aroused regularly by irritations of these viscera. For instance, the symptoms of constipation were long ascribed to auto-intoxication and it remained for Alvarez[475] to demonstrate that packing the rectum with sterile gauze results in the same symptom complex, suggesting that irritation to the receptors in the rectal wall is of greater import than the toxic material reabsorbed from faecal matter.

## Uro-Genital Afferents

The segments of the spinal cord from the tenth thoracic to the first lumbar receive afferent fibres from the pelvis of the kidney. This structure receives Vagal afferents also.

The ureter derives its sensory fibres from thoracic eleven to lumbar three, more particularly lumbars one and two. That portion continuous with the pelvis of the kidney may also have Vagal afferents, while the distal portion, associated with the bladder, derives afferents in association with the pelvic splanchnic nerves of sacral two and three.

The urinary bladder is shown by Rasmussen[476] to have rather an involved sensory distribution. The main bulk of the bladder receives fibres from the first to the fourth sacral nerves, while the outlet of the bladder receives fibres from the first and second lumbar nerves. The urethral sphincter and most of the urethra contribute afferent fibres to the first four sacral nerves. Kuntz[477] has shown that there are important reflex centres in the first and second lumbar seg ments, which must receive afferent information. The afferent fibres that may return with the postganglionic sympathetic fibres to the sympathetic chain turn upward in the chain to reach the lower white rami communicantes, which would be those associated with the first, second, and perhaps, the third lumbar nerves. It is through these rami that the sensory fibres gain entrance to the nerve trunks and the neuromeres. Lockhart, Hamilton and Fyfe[478] have established that these sympathetic afferents carry sensations of fullness from the bladder and are a pathway of pain as well as the pelvic afferents.

Kuntz[479] states that the ovary receives sympathetic efferent impulses from the tenth thoracic neuromere, and it is, therefore, reasonable and consistent that the afferent fibres should return to this same segment as Rasmussen[480] listed them.

The fallopian tube has both sympathetic and parasympathetic innervation, and Kuntz[481] suggests that the sacral parasympathetic fibres are the most numerous, but the reflexes appear to be most prominently displayed through the twelfth thoracic neuromere. There is some variance between Kuntz[482] and Rasmussen[483] as to the segments which receive these afferent fibres. The former says the twelfth thoracic and upper lumbar segments, while the latter lists the tenth, eleventh and twelfth thoracic neuromeres.

Rasmussen[484] has listed the afferent fibres from the body of the uterus as being derived from the tenth thoracic to the second lumbar nerves, while the cervix receives its afferents from the second, third and fourth sacral nerves. Kuntz[485] claims that in the human the afferents return to the eleventh and twelfth thoracic neuromeres and he does not differentiate between the body and cervix. However, he does point out the intricate network of fibres concerned with the innervation of this viscus and there is little doubt that the lower thoracic, upper lumbar and the sacral segments mentioned are contributors to the supply of efferent fibres and would be expected to receive afferent neurones in return. Both of the authorities are, no doubt, correct, but their experiences or methods of investigation have differed.

The testicle provides ease of testing and has been shown to return afferent impulses over sympathetic afferent fibres to the level of the tenth thoracic, and even as high as the fifth thoracic as reported by Lockhart et al.[486]

The testis, according to Rasmussen,[487] sends its afferent fibres back to the tenth, eleventh and twelfth thoracic segments. Kuntz[488] agrees with the above, but states that Mitchell found afferents returning to the cord as high as the sixth thoracic neuromere.

Kuntz[489] is not specific as to the spinal cord segments to which afferent fibres of the prostate gland return, but Rasmussen[490] states that the tenth and eleventh thoracics, as well as the second and third sacral segments, are the sources of these fibres.

These are the viscera most frequently involved in health problems and the brief discussion of their afferent nerve supply should be of aid to both student and practitioner.

## Visceral Reflexes

Having reviewed the levels of sensory supply to many of the viscera, attention may now be turned to the varied reflexes that may be initiated by centripetal impulses originating in one of these organs. The past few pages may seem to have had little significance to this consideration of the vertebral fixation, but such is not a true fact. The reader may find in the future a great need for the information provided in these pages and discover more value, for practical application, than the bulk of the writing to this point.

Exogenetic irritants to any of the viscera can be traced to the spine and the most likely vertebral fixation prognosticated, thus permitting the doctor of chiropractic to conserve time and utilize applied psychology for the patient's benefit. By telling the patient beforehand in which area of the spine the subluxation is likely to be found and then proceeding to demonstrate its presence, is dramatic proof that the doctor knows his business and is a technique employed and advocated by D. D. Palmer. D. D. Palmer[491] said: "In making a diagnosis it should be the Chiropractor's business, first of all, to determine the nature of the disease by learning what functions are abnormally performed; what part of the body is affected. Then take into consideration the nerves which ramify the diseased portion in which they are likely to be impinged upon, and lastly, not the first of all, examine the locality where he has decided the luxation exists which by its displacement impinges upon those nerves. To examine 'the 300 articulations of the skeletal frame first of all,' would be to leave out the diagnosis."

The founder of the chiropractic profession was cognizant of the importance of having this phase of neurology at the fingertips of every doctor of chiropractic. Unfortunately, much time may be consumed by attempting to search through the standard, authoritative textbooks, in which this practical, chiropractic data are obscure all too frequently.

Any irritant introduced into a viscus, such as the lung or stomach, adequate to stimulate the receptor nerve endings, sends impulses back over the splanchnic afferent fibres to the spinal cord segments, as previously elucidated. Synaptic connection is effected with the anterior horn cells, resulting in somatic muscle hypertension, especially significant to the doctor of chiropractic, since postvertebral muscle fibres are involved. The degree and extent of muscle contraction is dependent upon many factors, such as the strength of the irritant, the local condition of irritability of the viscus, the state of irritability of the cells and synapses of the neuromeres, etc. This somatic muscle reaction to a visceral irritation has received the descriptive name of "Visceromotor Reflex" from neurologists and "Motor Reaction" from Willard Carver.[492]

That D. D. Palmer[493] was cognizant of the importance of the visceromotor reflex as a causative factor in the production of vertebral fixations or subluxations is demonstrated by the following quotation: "Poisons taken into the system in food and water that is polluted or by breathing noxious effluvia from decaying vegetable or animal matter, or by the outrageous practice of the M.D. who injects vaccine poison into a healthy person, affects nerves, which act on muscles sufficient to displace vertebrae and impinge nerves, causing derangements which we name disease."

### Viscero-Sensory Reflexes

The Viscerosensory Reflex has received previous mention, but is deserving of repetition. As the sensory impulses arrive in the neuromere, they are transferred to second order neurones which, under normal conditions, subserve somatic structure. The resultant stimulation of an area of the postcentral gyrus causes a misinterpretation of the sources of the centripetal impulses and the conscious centre believe the pain to have originated in some somatic structure, rather than in a viscus.

Sachs[494] has established that the Viscerosensory Reflex causes more extensive pain in the back than in the front, and Pottenger[495] has demonstrated that disease conditions of the posterior portion of a lung tend to demonstrate somatic reflexes in the tissues of the back, while a similar involvement of the anterior portion of a lung has a somatic response in the anterior tissues.

While referred pain is one of the most important of the Viscerosensory Reflexes, hyperalgesia is a concomitant and is symptomatic, if not pathognomonic, of irritation of a splanchnic structure. Therefore, the discussion of the neuromeres to which the afferent fibres from a given viscus return gives the required information as to the dermatomes which would experience the hypersensitivity or hyperalgesia. By eliciting cutaneous hyperalgesia, the doctor of chiropractic can be reasonably certain that he is faced with an organic problem, rather than one of somatic structure or a simple functional disorder of a viscus. In the instance that a patient consults him relative to "neuralgia" of the left arm, the history, causes of exacerbations, distribution of the pain, and vertebral fixations may all point to a diagnosis of angina pectoris, but the finding of hyperalgesia of the skin of the medial side of the arm and forearm would provide the additional confirmation necessary for such a diagnosis and justify instrumental investigation of the heart's function by means of cardiograms.

The mechanisms by which hyperalgesia is produced are not agreed upon by neurological authorities. Some feel, as Rasmussen[496] and Pottenger,[497] that the visceral irritation lowers the synaptic resistance at the junction between the first order somatic afferent neurones from the skin and the second order neurones which conduct the impulses to the higher brain centres. Thus, minor cutaneous stimulation is sufficient to arouse unpleasant awareness. The muscles may experience a degree of hyperalgesia also, which Kuntz[498] ascribes to the hypertonus resulting from the visceromotor reflex and states that the hypersensitivity persists as long as the hypertonicity.

Another theory advanced by Sinclair and quoted by Kuntz[499] is that afferent neurones branch, with one division going to a viscus and another to skin, or somatic muscle. Irritation of the splanchnic branch would thereby lower the levels of the strength of an irritant applied to the other somatic branch necessary to evoke a passage of impulses to the centre of awareness. This would be an instance of summation of impulses. Or, the impulses from the viscus might pass down the somatic branch, as antidromic impulses, to cause a secretion at the terminal endings that sensitize the receptors, making them responsive to stimuli that would be normally inadequate. No anatomical basis has been established for this latter theory.

Judovich and Bates,[500] among others, suggest that the afferent impulses entering the cord from the viscus disturb the lateral horn cells and sympathetic impulses alter the vascularity of somatic structures and consequently their sensitivity. Kuntz[501] reports that Wernoe demonstrated that cutaneous ischemia coincides with the area of hyperalgesia, another factor suggestive that the lateral horn cells are involved in the reflex.

It must not be taken for granted that the visceral reflexes are the only method available for a viscus to inform the psychical centres of problems and irritations within its structure. As has been expressed by White and Smithwick,[502] the viscera have the capacity of creating the sensation of pain localized in the organ itself, especially when inflammation lowers the resistance of the receptors. Wolff and Wolf[503] bring out very clearly the increased irritability of receptors in viscera by inflammation, as do many other investigators.

The viscerosensory reflexes, the hyperalgesia, and the visceromotor reflexes are all of very real significance to the chiropractor and he, of all practitioners of healing, should be acutely conscious of these manifestations of neural function. These should be utilized daily in the differential diagnosis of nearly every case, and not kept locked away in the deeper crypts of memory to be paraded only upon special occasions, when the need to impress an audience requires a show of acumen and erudition.

Prior to leaving the viscerosensory reflexes, it must be appreciated that the cutaneous distribution of the lower thoracic nerves is at a lower level than might be expected and, hence, the viscerosensory reflexes are not to be found at a level with the vertebra corresponding to the neuromere into which the afferents enter. As Pottenger[504] and any standard anatomy text indicate, the tenth thoracic neuromere is concerned with the skin over the first lumbar vertebra posteriorly and the area which includes the umbilicus anteriorly, while the twelfth thoracic supplies the skin over the fourth lumbar vertebra posteriorly and just above the inguinal ligament anteriorly.

## Viscero-Visceral Reflexes

Another extremely important reaction of the nervous system to visceral irritation and one of no small import to the skillful and learned doctor of chiropractic, is the Viscero-Visceral Reflex which Pottenger[505] credits with being the "basis of normal physiological integration." In disease, the viscero-visceral reflex may confound diagnosticians and compound the problems of accurate diagnosis. Simply stated, irritation of one viscus may, through the connections made within the spinal cord and brain stem, disturb the nerve supply of another organ supplied by the same segment, resulting in symptoms from the second splanchnic structure which may be even more distressing than those from the viscus primarily involved.

One of the examples used by Kuntz[506] is gastric distress in response to gall bladder irritation. In such an instance the afferent impulses would return from the gall bladder to thoracic segments six to eleven, and, either by collateral fibres or internuncial neurones, establish a reflex arc with those lateral gray horn cells concerned with the sympathetic supply of the stomach from thoracic neuromeres six to nine. Increasing the sympathetic innervation of the stomach tends towards constriction of the vascular bed, increased tonus of the sphincters, cardiac and pyloric, and a general decrease in tonus of the muscular wall, inhibition of the secretory activity of the glands. Such a state may well result in the retention of ingested materials, faulty digestion, fermentation, flatulence, and other problems. These may be the symptoms which the patient presents to the doctor, rather than frank gall bladder symptoms. To treat the stomach would be a mistake, but adjusting the vertebral segments could create beneficial responses of the gall bladder, even though the diagnosis may be quite erroneous. The correct vertebral analysis and application of chiropractic technique often results in correction of problems, whose diagnostic name has been falsely chosen.

This same viscero-visceral reflex might well be applied in another manner. An atlas fixation may disturb the nerve supply to the gall bladder by way of the Vagus, upsetting its function. From the gall bladder afferent impulses may return to the thoracic neuromeres, as above listed, to disrupt the normal sympathetic supply of the stomach. It is self-evident that the atlas subluxation should be adjusted, but the visceromotor, viscerosensory reflexes and the hyperalgesia may make the thoracic problem stand out in apparent importance. Were the doctor to overlook the upper cervical disrelation, his patient might well experience considerable relief, but be afflicted with recurrences of this distress.

The reverse is well within the realm of possibility also. A thoracic fixation may upset splanchnic function and the afferents of the

Vagus carry the impulses back to the medulla oblongata and through connector neurones stimulate the anterior horn cells of the upper cervical cord segments to result in hypertonicity of the occipital muscles and fixation or subluxation or disrelation of the attached segments, whichever term best suits the terminology of the reader. In such an instance, adjusting the upper cervical disrelation would not be to correct the primary problem, and the results might well be disappointing to both patient and doctor.

It must not be assumed that the viscero-visceral reflex is operative only between viscera whose neural cytones are contiguous. Such is not the case. The nausea and vomiting that may occur in the female with a uterine problem is an example, cited by Kuntz,[507] Pottenger[508] and others. The afferent impulses from the uterus return to the lower thoracic, upper lumbar and sacral neuromeres and through connector neurones travel up the remainder of the cord and into the medulla oblongata to activate the vomiting centre in the reticular formation. Such reflexes are not the exception, but, rather, form the basis for the symptom complexes presented in most, if not all, disease conditions.

## Somato-Visceral Reflexes

While the neurological authorities do not appear to have concerned themselves with the Somatovisceral Reflexes to an appreciable degree, these are the basis of the chiropractic contention that vertebral fixation or subluxation, if you prefer, create disturbed neural supply to splanchnic tissues. Much of this book has been devoted to discussion of such reflexes acting upon the viscera. Kuntz[509] does mention the important influence stimulation of the skin has upon visceral function, especially the vascular supply and says: ". . . it must be apparent that many visceral disorders, particularly of the gastro-intestinal tract, may be influenced beneficially by appropriate stimulation of the corresponding cutaneous area." Pottenger[510] has pointed out that a continuous stream of somatic afferent impulses pass by connector fibres to neurones supplying viscera and that these are essential for visceral function.

Sachs[511] states: "The essential characteristic of visceral reflexes lies in the response of the internal organs to some mechanical irritation of the surface of the body."

Despite such recognition of the importance of these reflexes, little investigation seems to have been conducted to determine the influence of such mechanical irritations in health and disease.

## Psycho-Visceral Reflexes

One last type of reflex relative to splanchnic function that appears to be assuming greater significance in the present day literature of all the healing arts is the Psychovisceral Reflex. This mechanism is behind the psychosomatic problems, of which so much is presently being written. Cobb[512] cites worry as being an accepted etiological factor in gastric hyperacidity and ulceration, as well as constant emotional strain resulting in arteriosclerosis. Kuntz[513] states: "Indeed, every visceral function is subject to influence exerted by psychic and emotional states through the autonomic nerves."

Freeman[514] makes the statement that visceral structures are disturbed in function even in normal individuals subjected to chronic emotional tension.

White and Smithwick[515] demonstrated that an intense emotion causes a general response of the sympathetic division of the nervous system, which is, of course, the fight-flight mechanism described in every physiology textbook.

Sachs[516] has suggested that the psychovisceral reflexes may result in visceromotor, viscerosensory and viscerovisceral reflexes, thereby complicating materially the symptom picture.

Curtis et al[517] devote about eight pages of description to what they call the Emotional Brain with the input from the various afferent sources, the complex circuits, the influence of the hypothalamus upon the varied nuclei. Fibres are reported to extend from the hypothalamus down through the lateral portion of the recticular formation and the length of the spinal cord with both sympathetic and parasympathetic influences. The effects via the sympathetic fibres to the adrenal medulla are the most potent, since epinephrine and norepinephrine decrease blood flow in the periphery, with an increased flow internally, increased rate and force of the heart, as well as the conversion of liver glycogen to glucose for the accompanying muscular contraction.

The majority are aware of diarrhea in time of severe emotional stress, and Guyton[518] credits the parasympathetic overactivity with the responsibility for excessive mucous secretion and motor activity of the terminal colon and rectum.

Guyton,[519] furthermore, discusses at some length the influence of the hypothalamus upon the autonomic system and the pituitary gland in response to emotion, as well as the increased or decreased somatic muscle tone. Increased tone has a proprioceptive feedback to the reticular activating areas of the brain stem, maintaining alert-

285

ness and insomnia.

He describes the generalized effect of overactivity of the sympathetic division and more localized ill-effects of parasympathetic hyperactivity, e.g., hyperacidity and gastric ulcer, or constipation, etc.

Prior to leaving this phase of the topic, the writer would like to drop a word of caution to chiropractic students and practitioners not to become "caught up" in a popular trend, the psychosomatic "kick" of the present. While there has never been a question in the minds of doctors of chiropractic who have built their knowledge of chiropractic upon the foundation of D. D. Palmer's principles that the mind is an important contributory factor in the cause of disease, the somatic and visceral states also have important predisposing influences upon the mind and the emotions. The human is a unit of structure and function; what disturbs structure, disturbs function; what disturbs the body, disturbs the mind; what disturbs the mind, disturbs the body. The human can be compartmentalized for purposes of discussion and description only, but never for purposes of function.

Experience and neurological facts should convince the chiropractor that the somato-psychic response of the body is of equal importance and stands upon a similar plane with the psycho-somatic reflexes. There is need on occasion for the application of mental catharsis as the first and major therapeutic agent. However, every mental problem has its reflection in the somatic structure and many are the instances when the problems of the soma are reflected into the psychic realm, making the somatic disturbance the primary source of trouble. Chiropractors should not underestimate the potency of their own technical armamentarium for normalizing structure as a means of reaching and eliminating the psychic dysfunctions.

The ever-advancing knowledge of the Reticular System into which all sources of afferent information are fed has shown that this system is responsible to a great degree for sleep, wakefulness, concentration, attracting attention, and influencing emotion. This gives further evidence of the inter-relation of body and mind.

The encouragement of patients to freely discuss the causes of their emotional distress should form a part of the health care of the average chiropractic patient. The empathy established between chiropractor and patient in the course of the chiropractic ministration encourages the revelation of intimate personal history that should be utilized for the patient's benefit. A small mouth and large ears are requisites for the truly efficient doctor of chiropractic. "Let the patient talk!" should be a motto found hanging at the head of every chiropractic adjusting table for the doctor to constantly see before his eyes. Thus, the combination of somato-psychic and psycho-somatic approaches would be merged into an efficacious technique for the betterment of the patient.

## Trophic Function

Marcus Singer[520] reported experiments that had been conducted to determine the influence of nerve fibres in the regeneration of body parts. It was found that the type of neurones present was unimportant, but the number was critical. It was presumed, although not proven, that the nerve fibres provide some chemical substance essential to growth. The sciatic nerve of a frog was implanted in the stump of its amputated foreleg and a new leg grew. Singer suggests that it is proper for the nervous system, which integrates and controls the thoughts and actions, to subserve tissue repair. Such a contention as the latter, has been held by chiropractors since the days of D. D. Palmer.

Not only is neural function important to growth and repair, but plays an essential role in the functional aberrations and the cellular alterations of disease. There is a growing recognition of this important influence of the nervous system in the literature of the healing arts.

The trophic function of the nervous system is little understood at present, but is recognized as a proven fact. It has long been appreciated that, if the cells or the axones of motor neurones are destroyed, those muscle fibres associated in the composition of the Motor Units will undergo disintegration. This is not the atrophy of disuse, but true dissolution with the loss of ability to be stimulated by any means and the loss of cellular integrity.

Studies in recent years since the advent of electron microscopy, have demonstrated the neurotubules and Minckler[521] credits these with the axoplasmic flow from trophic centre to the formation of vesicles in the terminal buttons of the fibres. It is hypothesized that the release of chemical substances influence the trophic activity.

Sachs[522] has quoted the experiments of a number of researchers who have demonstrated that the capillaries are dependent upon the development of the cerebral cortex; that any failure of the cortex to develop into the normal adult state results in a primitive form of capillary bed being carried over into the adult life.

The newborn brain of 200 to 300 grams of weight has the vast majority of its cells present, but, as Feldenkrais[523] has established, the growth and increased weight to 1,360 to 2,300-odd grams in the adult is dependent upon the growth of the processes and the myelination of the fibres. He credits this immaturity of the central nervous system with the tremendous plasticity of the human to learn new reactions to a stimulus and also the many modifications of structure in response to the functional patterns imposed by this developing and experimenting nervous system.

Kuntz[524] has pointed out that, especially between the eighth and fourteenth years, many automatic ganglion cells develop many new dendrite processes, greatly increasing the sources of stimulation and the complexities of reaction.

Feldenkrais[525] mentions that habitual patterns of activity can modify both the bone structures in accord with Wolf's Law and the muscles, thus, the habit of faulty posture may result in fibrous deposits in articular cavities that have been exaggerated, shortening of some ligaments and muscles, while other muscles increase in strength and size, and others weaken and atrophy. These somatic responses are dependent upon the learning by the nervous system of a faulty postural habit.

Davis' Law states: "If the origin and insertion of a muscle are moved further apart for some time, the muscle loses tone and becomes relaxed. If they are approximated the muscle contracts or becomes contractured." It may be appreciated that the changes in muscles resulting from the alteration in the tension exerted and the element of time, result in trophic changes that may be observed or palpated by the trained student of human mechanics.

Feldenkrais[526] has credited Miss P. Localtellis as having shown that the neural components are the "primary factor" concerned with the development of the tissues of the embryological segment. It would seem that the nervous system, even in the early developmental stages, is in command and remains as the correlating, integrating, and modifying factor that controls the responses of the body to the exteroceptive and interoceptive stimuli both in health and disease.

Cobb[527] has demonstrated that stimulating the anterior group of nuclei of the diencephalon results in a discharge of impulses over the Vagus, that, if continued for a variable time, produces ulceration and hemorrhage of the mucous membrane of the stomach, as well as other aberrations of body function. He demonstrated that chronic worry may be the precipitating cause of gastric ulceration.

That every pathology is associated with alterations in the neural supply of the autonomic division of the nervous system is becoming better recognized by neurologists, such as Sachs,[528] if not by the authorities in the field of pathological investigation, who are enamoured with micro-organisms and filterable viruses.

It should be obvious that the distortion of vertebral structure and the subsequent bombardment of afferent impulses cannot but have a disturbing influence upon the neurones of the associated neuromeres. Such alteration of neural integrity influences adversely the trophic activity of the effector cells and has a deleterious effect. These cells may demonstrate structural change or their resistance altered to make them more prone to the infliction of cellular trauma by such agents as micro-organisms, viruses and noxious chemical compounds.

## The Time Factor

Sherrington[529] pointed out that time is a most important factor in considering the function of the nervous system. A mild stimulus must be suddenly applied, if it is to cause either a sensation or a reflex response. However, many mild stimuli do not reach either consciousness nor produce a noticeable reflex action, yet they are not without their influence upon the nervous system. If these impulses are just below the threshhold level required to overcome the resistance of a synapse and follow sufficiently close, one upon the other, summation may occur and a reflex discharge be effected. However, more minimal impulses are not without their influence at both the central termination and throughout the various branches of the afferent fibre. It has been shown that these weak stimuli do have an influence upon the synapse, by which the resistance is lowered to permit another stimulus of less than the usual minimal requirement to prove adequate to cross the synapse, Facilitation, as discussed by Curtis et al.[530] The antidromic impulses that course down each branch of the afferent fibre seem to sensitize the receptors to permit milder stimuli to be adequate for the activation of the receptor mechanism. There appears to be, in addition, an influence upon the local capillary bed, resulting in greater permeability with extravasation of the plasma into the tissue spaces. Such a condition is, of course, the forerunner of trophic disturbance of the cells, since this tends to balance the chemistry of the intracellular fluids, thereby interfering with the vital exchanges of nutrition and metabolic end-products.

The continual bombardment of nerve cells by afferent impulses results, as Pottenger[531] reports, in injury to the sensory cell bodies and the neurones with which synaptic connections are made, disturbing the normal reflex arcs and resulting in trophic changes in the tissues with which the efferent paths are associated. Pottenger[532] utilizes the chronic pulmonary diseases to illustrate the trophic changes which occur in the somatic soft tissues in response to long continued bombardment of the mid-cervical neuromeres by afferent impulses which enter the upper four thoracic segments, but create the trophic changes in the tissues supplied primarily by the fourth cervical segment and have been described by Rasmussen[533] also.

Pottenger[534] carried the investigation still further to demonstrate that there is a degree of selectivity of the trophic disturbances. He showed that chronic pathology of the anterior portion of the lung results in trophic changes in the somatic tissues anteriorly distributed, while the posterior lung causes alteration in the somatic tissues of posterior distribution.

It is one of the peculiarities of neural function that the strong stimuli result in very pronounced responses, such as muscle contractions and pain, but the minor irritations, prolonged over a considerable period of time are much more detrimental to the integrity of the structure, due to the dystrophic changes which occur. It is submitted that the vertebral fixations, whose irritation is insufficient to bridge the numerous synapses to reach conscious awareness, are a potent source of minimal irritation, and when prolonged over a long period of time, are adequate for the production of dystrophic changes in some of the tissues supplied by the neuromere with which the vertebra is associated. The adverse influence of the vertebral subluxation upon the neuromere disturbs the trophic function of cytones and the tissues with which they are functionally related. The mechanisms of such disturbing influences have been discussed at some length in previous chapters.

In the event that the irritation is not sufficient in strength to overcome the resistance of the synapse, Kuntz[535] and other investigators, have demonstrated that axone reflexes may occur. In such an instance, the nerve stimulus aroused at one branch of the axone spreads over the entire fibre, including its collaterals and causes a local response in the end-organs, with increased permeability of the capillary bed, extravasation of plasma and a tendency for the intracellular and extracellular chemistry to balance, thereby interfering with cellular function, as previously mentioned. "It is the delicate balance of electrolytes and water that serves to maintain the constancy of the internal environment, the importance of which Bernard was the first to emphasize. For the preservation of this constancy the mechanism of homeostasis has been evolved," states Boyd.[536] Deviations from the normal cellular environment results in fluctuations from optimum cellular function.

The subluxation or vertebral kinetic aberration may prove of sufficient disturbance to the nerve fibres passing through the intervertebral foramen that a similar problem may be triggered at the terminal endings of some of these fibres, for it is well established that any irritation, viral or other, to the posterior nerve root ganglion results in trophic changes in the tissues supplied. This latter problem is commonly called herpes zoster, or shingles.

Once the process of inflammation and tissue breakdown in a viscus commences, the toxic products liberated serve as adequate irritants to receptor end-organs and begin, as Pottenger[537] has observed, to manifest in somatic tissues as reflexes of the motor, sensory or trophic types.

Selye[538] has demonstrated that any number of agents which threaten the integrity of the tissue produce a high protein concentration in the tissue spaces, directly associated with the escape of plasma from the capillaries, whose permeability has been increased. The cells take in sodium chloride, calcium and water, eliminating potassium and phosphoric radicles. The intracellular and extracellular fluids thus tend to equalize.

It may be appreciated that subluxation of a vertebral segment may have been caused by mechanical force sufficient to injure the tissues of the holding elements, even to a minor degree, but sufficient to create the release of histamine-like products, which dilate the capillaries and increase the permeability with the results above mentioned. Nerve endings are irritated by this process and subsequent tissue swelling, thus begins the bombardment of the neuromere to activate a sympathetic neural response which directs additional blood into the area to create an active hyperemia and further accentuates the response to tissue injury. The afferent impulses entering the lateral horn of gray matter are not without disturbing influence upon other sympathetic fibres of more distant distribution. Thus, a fixation of the sixth thoracic vertebra might well disturb some of the sympathetic fibres destined for the stomach, resulting in trophic changes, thereby laying the foundation for ulceration and other aberrations of function.

Speransky[539] used many forms of irritation, mechanical, chemical, bacteriological and electrical, to irritate nerve trunks and finer filaments within muscles. In many instances he was able to duplicate symptoms and tissue changes that had previously been credited to the invasion of pathogenic micro-organisms. By injecting potassium iodide solution into a muscle eczema, baldness, papules, blisters, erosions and ulcers were produced on the side of injection first, then in a symmetrical distribution on the other side and, after some lapse of time, a spread of the process was noted. The reader might note that these dystrophic changes in the skin tend to follow Pflueger's Laws for muscle contraction in response to sensory nerve irritation.

It was emphasized by Speransky[540] that irritation of the nerve creates a dystrophy on the homolateral side and increasing the strength of irritation results in the spread of the process to the opposite side and then more distally. Furthermore, he demonstrated that chronic irritation of the nerve or its receptors, results in morphological changes within the nervous system and the type of irritant is not the important factor. He emphatically states that no differences in the reaction to irritation by micro-organisms and chemicals could be demonstrated.

There would seem to be little reason to doubt that the chronic vertebral subluxation is an adequate source of irritation and closely associated with the central nervous system, which the authorities, such as Speransky,[541] agree makes an irritation more potent, to result in dystrophic changes both of some cells of the associated neuromere and the tissues functionally dependent upon these cytones. Clinical evidence amassed since 1895 confirms this concept. Any source of chronic nerve cell bombardment is injurious and may have permanent detrimental effects, as has been established by Pottenger.[542] Why then should vertebral fixation not be accepted as such a source of chronic irritation?

Furthermore, the generalized state of nutrition, toxicity, and additional sources of irritation play an important role in determining the stability of neurones and their capability of withstanding prolonged bombardment. This latter point has been made by Pottenger,[543] and Charcot is quoted by Speransky[544] as having shown that dystrophic changes occur in response to nerve irritation, rather than to decreased neural supply.

Nor was D. D. Palmer[545] unmindful of the detrimental influence of the overactivity of the neurones, for he stated emphatically time after time: "The cause of nearly all diseases is an over-supply of nerve force"; and again: "The most of diseases are because of too much energy; not because nerve force is 'shut off'."

Pottenger[546] considers that the trophic reflexes of parasympathetic origin are more difficult to recognize than those of sympathetic derivation which tend to manifest themselves in somatic tissues, but the parasympathetic reflexes are probably more of a disturbing influence to the resistance of tissues to the invasion of pathogenic micro-organisms. Thus, an upper cervical segmental fixation may well involve the parasympathetic fibres of the Vagus, distributed to the pharynx or other portion of the respiratory tract, thereby lowering resistance and predisposing the tissues to infection. Certainly, no departure from the facts established by neurological authorities is required to buttress this contention, and clinical evidence supports this view. Associated with an upper thoracic subluxation, which disturbs the vasomotor control of the vessels supplying the same area, which further interferes with normal resistance, the possibilities of a predisposition to infection becomes magnified.

Speransky[547] demonstrated that irritation of a nerve directly or the receptor endings, was equally efficacious in the production of structural changes within the neurones of the central nervous system. Again, there seems little evidence to deny that vertebral fixation can be an adequate source of irritation to receptor endings of centripetal fibres, which, if prolonged for an adequate period of time, may have detrimental influences upon both structure and function of the neural cells.

Speransky[548] has established also that dystrophic processes are not dependent upon irritation of a nerve trunk or ganglion only, but may occur with equal facility when the irritant is applied to receptor endings, "skin, cellular tissues, muscles, etc."

## Infectious Diseases

The above heading may suggest that the theme of the chapter has been forsaken. Such is not the case, as should be evident upon reading the following paragraphs. There is an intimate relationship between Time-Trophic Function and Infectious Disease.

Chiropractors have been castigated frequently for emphasis upon the condition of the host, rather than the importance of micro-organisms as the etiologic factor in disease with which micro-organisms are associated. Laymen frequently say to a doctor of chiropractic, "Well, you don't believe in germs, do you?" Nothing could be further from the truth. The student of chiropractic, after spending several hundred hours studying the subject of bacteriology from the standard textbooks and in the laboratory, is not prone to deny the existence of micro-organisms which he has cultured, fixed on slides, stained and examined under the microscope.

The doctor of chiropractic is well aware of the presence of bacteria and concedes that these minute organisms play a role in many diseases. He would, however, emphatically deny that micro-organisms are *the* cause of the disease with which they are associated, for, if this were true, everyone would be riddled with infection, since bacteria of a pathogenic nature are, like the poor, with us always.

It has been reported by Dubos[549] that potentially pathogenic micro-organisms are carried by the human throughout life and some change must take place before disease is manifested. He considers that biochemical disturbance is "far more important than immunological factors" in converting infection to disease. Also, he writes: "The present-day scientific literature dealing with problems of infection often has a quaint mid-nineteenth-century flavor. It describes disease as a conflict between two opponents. . . ."

"The failure of present-day doctrines to explain any of the aspects of chronic infection is so obvious as to require no comment. Indeed, it is plain that the microbiological diseases for which there is no explanation whatever of immunity mechanisms far outnumber those where susceptibility and resistance can be explained in terms of recognized immunological reactions — cellular or humoral," is another of his observations.

D. D. Palmer[550] did not write extensively about micro-organisms, but did state: "Chiropractors consider the micro-organism a scavenger — not the cause."

Haggard[551] stated in his book: "Most of the symptoms of disease can be counterfeited by the influence of the nervous system upon bodily function."

Selye[552] brought to the attention of his colleagues the interesting discovery that many of the serious symptoms of infectious disease may be present in a patient with no demonstrable pathogenic bacteria.

Selye[553] demonstrated the symptom complex and pathological changes of infectious purpuras by means of hormone injections and without associated micro-organisms.

Selye[554] showed, furthermore, that the toxins of bacteria "trigger" widespread tissue changes that are common to the "Alarm Reaction" in response to stressors of divers form. He concluded that the

"Disease of Adaptation" to the stress of bacterial toxins was commonly out of all proportion to the tissue injury produced by the micro-organisms. This immediately suggests to the chiropractor the probability of a neurodystrophic process at work.

The same authority has investigated thoroughly the reaction of the organism to stressors of most types, mechanical, mental and chemical, including micro-organisms, and has concluded that the nervous system plays an important role in both the Alarm Reaction and the General Adaptative Syndrome. Much emphasis has been placed upon the role of the endocrine glands and the anterior lobe of the pituitary as the master control in both complexes above mentioned.

While the neural influences upon the anterior lobe of the hypophysis cerebri have not been clearly defined, the doctor of chiropractic should have little difficulty in visualizing that a fixation of an upper thoracic vertebra, by its disturbing influence upon the preganglionic sympathetic cells of the lateral horns, could modify the impulses conducted into the sympathetic chain. These fibres then ascend the chain to the superior cervical ganglion, from which the postganglionic fibres aid in the formation of the carotid plexus and follow each branch of the artery. Hence, altered nerve supply to the arteries of the pituitary may confuse the glandular function, resulting in abnormal responses to stress, in this instance the stressor being infection by micro-organisms.

The adrenals are credited by Selye[555] as being very important to the ability of the body to resist all forms of stress, including infection. A kinetic aberration in the area of the sixth to ninth thoracic region through fatigue or central inhibitory effects may decrease the neural stimulation of the adrenals with resultant decrease of "Resistance."

Extensive experimentation in Russia, reported by A. N. Gordienko et al,[556] has shown that the mechanisms for antibody production is unexplained and that the opinion that antigens directly stimulate certain cells to produce antibodies cannot be confirmed by experimentation. Cells of the spleen deprived of neural impulses produced no antibodies. They demonstrated that the nervous system was essential for the reception of the stimulus of the stressor of antigen nature, rather than the blood stream. The nervous system was demonstrated to be the important intermediate system in the process. The autonomic division and the Vagus Nerve give evidence of being the controlling system for immunity.

The claim of the chiropractic profession that the condition of the nervous system of the host is a more salient factor in the development of disease in the presence of micro-organisms than the germs themselves, is born out by eminent researchers, such as Selye, Speransky, and many others.

The profession of chiropractic has long recognized the import of hygiene, sanitation and public health measures to prevent the spread of pathogenic micro-organisms. This profession approves the quarantine of patients and the avoidance, by apparently healthy persons, of contact and needless risk of infection. It is impossible to determine the degree of resistance possessed by an individual and, therefore, foolhardy to expose him to the possibilities that the bacteria may be the added stressor necessary to set in motion a violent reaction of the nervous system, called disease.

Issue has been taken with artificial immunity, the false sense of protection and the risks of neuro-dystrophic processes being initiated, which may be productive of tissue changes more detrimental than the disease itself. The decline of the rate of many infectious diseases has paralleled the introduction of adequate sanitation. Diphtheria has been seen by this writer to recur when the sanitary system breaks down, despite the immunization of the troops.

The eminent scientist, Hans Zinsser,[557] has established a strong case for hygiene and adequate housing in the prevention of typhus by the extermination of the louse and flea, rather than by the injection of foreign matter into the human in an attempt to produce immunity.

Selye[558] has demonstrated that the production of specific resistance is at the expense of lowered resistance to other forms of stress. This being the case, the patient immunized against smallpox may be relatively protected against a form of microbe that he is unlikely to meet in modern civilized countries, but is less resistant to streptococcus, staphylococcus, etc., which are constantly in the environment.

Gordienko is not the only scientist who appreciates the neural regulation of immunity, for Kuntz[559] stated: "The data set forth above regarding the autonomic nervous influences in the distribution of leukocytes and the permeability of the vascular endothelium strongly suggest that immunity and bodily resistance, in a large measure, are determined by the functional condition of the autonomic nervous system. The results of experimental studies also show that specific immune reactions are subject to nervous influences and they may be initiated by specific reflex stimulation."

Speransky[560] strikes out vehemently against the inoculation and skin tests employed, especially for children. It is his contention that these introductions of foreign protein into the tissues serve as a source of nerve irritation to produce the neuro-dystrophic process. No adverse symptoms may be noted for weeks or months. The local irritation results, first, in local changes within the nervous system, which then gradually spread further afield within the nervous system. Such lays the groundwork for a reaction of the nervous system to another minor insult, such as germs, which are then condemned as the cause of the violent reaction or disease.

In the words of Speransky,[561] "Consequently, the clinic, and especially the children's clinic, should accurately estimate the real need for skin tests and all sorts of inoculations, and become quite clear as to the reality of their harmlessness; otherwise, the so-called achievements of science (?) may easily be converted into one of the methods of crippling humanity."

While much more could be added to the argument for the doctor of chiropractic's point of view, the above will suffice to demonstrate that the convictions held by the profession are not the machinations of "crack-pots," but have sufficient basis in neurological research to warrant caution in the use of artificial immunity and increased confidence in the conservative armamentarium of the profession for the normalization of the nervous system.

The extensive experimentation of Gordienko[562] established that stimulation of the Vagus increases the titer of antibodies, the number of leukocytes, phagocytic activity, as well as decreasing total serum protein and altering its fractions. Thus, chiropractic has the ideal method of stimulating the Vagus with no known risk of ill-effects. Unfortunately for the public, chiropractic has been denied by law in most jurisdictions the right to care for infectious or contagious disease without any investigation as to the efficacy of its methods. Allopathic medicine has succeeded in laying claim to many conditions without being required to prove the superiority of its methodology. By eliminating the competition, controlling the statistics, and public relations media, the public has been successfully taught to think or accept the single immunological approach of allopathic medicine as divine revelation.

It does not appear that the public will obtain the facts and demand proof of efficacy of the methods that are mandated for them with little opportunity for free choice. There is a broad field of usefulness permitted by law for the doctor of chiropractic, but the public is being denied the benefit of many forms of primary health care that may be more effective and fraught with few iatrogenic risks. The challenge for the young chiropractic physician to break this monopoly and acquire the earned position of a primary health care provider is great, but the needs of the public demand that the effort be continued.

With the broad understanding of the cause of all disease as being any and all chemical, mechanical and mental irritants sufficient in strength to overcome the tissue resistance, produce structural distortion capable of interference with normal nerve transmission, which disturbs cellular function and structural integrity, the chiropractor need have no qualms about standing in the company of scientists. The clinical proof of the truth of D. D. Palmer's principles and methods provide the necessary confidence for the doctor of chiropractic to stand tall in the company of clinicians of all schools of healing. In the broad field of prophylaxis chiropractic has no peer. It remains for the chiropractic profession to educate the general public to the availability of such a complete and encompassing mode of health care.

# Conclusion

IN ATTEMPTING TO conclude this entire treatise in a few succinct paragraphs one through seems to be uppermost, "How limited has been the coverage of such an important subject!"

A few of the quotations of D. D. Palmer have been utilized, but, it is hoped, sufficient to demonstrate each of the basic principles propounded by the founder of the chiropractic profession.

Neurological authorities have been quoted to demonstrate the wisdom enunciated by D. D. Palmer, some of the anatomical facts that run counter to the simplistic explanation of the mechanism of the subluxation, and presently known facts to substantiate the synthesis attempted by the writer. These references have been classified in the bibliographical index in their order of appearance and the page number provided for ease of reference out of deference to students and practitioners whose time is at a premium.

A richer list of bibliographical references would add little new or important material. While additional references could have been culled from the report of 1975, *The Research Status of Spinal Manipulative Therapy*, NINDS Monograph Number Fifteen, little would have been added and little change required in this hypothesis. The emphasis of those participating scientists was upon pressure upon the nerve trunk or radicles without any evidence of investigation of the possibility of the subluxation, fixation, vertebral articular kinetic aberration, or osteopathic vertebral lesion having the capacity, in fact, of causing pressure upon the neural structures of sufficient degree to warrant the elaborate research that has been undertaken. The results appear to strengthen the doubt that the subluxation, or fixation, or lesion, causes the varied symptoms and tissue changes by simple nerve pressure.

It is hoped that this sketchy presentation may stimulate others to amass additional facts that may buttress the chiropractic contention that the mechanical, chemical and mental irritations produce vertebral subluxation and interference to nerve transmission, resulting in the aberrations of function and cellular integrity, known as disease.

Perhaps this may serve as a stimulus to increase the interest of all chiropractors in the afferent components of the nervous system, which outnumber the efferents five to one and are deserving of much more attention in the future than received in the past.

The doctor of chiropractic should have no hesitation in holding his head high and claiming proud allegiance to the "fish peddler," as D. D. Palmer has been disdainfully called by the opponents of the profession he founded. Only in recent years have the outstanding scientists of our time been proving the truth of many of D.D. Palmer's principles. The future augurs well for the continued proof of his contentions and the recognition that chiropractic is a method without equal in the correction of the majority of visceral and somatic health problems.

May the challenge of chiropractic survival be accepted by the neophytes as enthusiastically as it was by the pioneers, and may chiropractic continue to expand upon the sound foundation of scientific fact and method to the betterment of the health of humanity and the renown of a self-educated humanitarian — D. D. Palmer.

For the practitioner who actively applies the principles and art of chiropractic, the admonition of Young and Barger[563] should aid in keeping us humble and mindful that our efforts are puny in comparison to the ability of the body, "In modern medicine we are prone to think of recovery from a disease or surgery as coming from the beneficial influences and measures instituted by man himself through therapy. . . . We forget, however, to give credit to the body's own inherent ability to overcome disease or injury or at least to put up a fight for its own existence. A surgeon may remove an organ or part whose existence is a threat to life, but he cannot heal the wound that results; this is the exclusive property of the tissue cells."

The chiropractic physician, through his most astute structural analysis, may locate the problem and with great skill restore the function of an articular kinetic aberration, but the response of the nervous system is beyond his power to influence in the manner desired, and the end-result rests exclusively with the neural response.

# Bibliography

1. Palmer, Daniel David: *The Science, Art and Philosophy of Chiropractic:* Portland, Ore., 1910: Portland Printing House Co.: Page 18
2. Weiant, C. W.: *Medicine and Chiropractic* — 5th Ed.: Hluckstadt, Germany, 1975: J. J. Augustin: q.v.
3. Palmer, D. D.: *The Science, Art and Philosophy of Chiropractic:* Page 16
4. Ibid.: Page 228
5. Ibid.: Page 137
6. Ibid.: Page 15
7. Castiglioni, Arturo: *A History of Medicine* — 2nd Ed.: New York, N.Y., 1973: Alfred A. Knopf: Page 914
8. Flexner, Abraham: *Medical Education:* New York, N.Y., 1925: The Macmillan Co.: Page 41
9. Ibid.: Page 41
10. Palmer, D. D.: Page 10
11. Flexner, Abraham: Page 42
12. Spain, David: *Complications of Modern Medical Practices:* New York, N.Y., 1963: Grune & Stratton: Page 4
13. Palmer, D. D.: Page 20
14. Ibid.: Page 36
15. Swanburg, Harold: *The Intervertebral Foramina in Man:*
16. Burke, Gerald L.: *Backache from Occiput to Coccyx:* Vancouver, B.C., 1964: W. E. G. MacDonald: Page 30
17. Mennell, James: *The Science and Art of Joint Manipulation:* London, Eng., 1952: J. and A. Churchill Ltd.: Page 14
18. Palmer, D. D.: Page 39
19. McDowell, R. J. S.: *Handbook of Physiology and Biochemistry* — 41st Ed.: Philadelphia, Pa., P. Blakiston Co.: Page 526
20. Best, Charles Herbert and Taylor, Norman Burke: *The Physiological Basis of Medical Practice* — 3rd Ed.: Baltimore, 1943: The Williams & Wilkins Co.: Page 1321
21. Zoethout, Wm. D. and Tuttle, W. W.: *A Textbook of Physiology* — 7th Ed.: St. Louis: C. V. Mosby Co.: Page 133
22. Mennell, James: Page 14
23. Piersol, George A.: *Human Anatomy* — 7th Ed.: Philadelphia, Pa.: 1919: J. B. Lippincott Co.: Page 142
24. Mainland, Donald: *Anatomy:* New York, 1945: Paul B. Hoeber, Inc.: Page 659
25. Palmer, D. D.: Page 109
26. Mainland, Donald: Page 659
27. Palmer, D. D.: Pages 399 and 699
28. Ibid.: Page 197
29. Ibid.: Page 110
30. Ibid.: Pages 15, 39, 58, 70, 71, 109, 110
31. *Gray's Anatomy* — 28th U.S. Ed.: Philadelphia, Pa., 1972: Lea & Febiger: Page 1015
32. *Cunningham's Textbook of Human Anatomy* — 8th Ed.: London, Eng., 1944: Oxford University Press: Page 1015
33. Piersol, George A.: *Human Anatomy* — 7th Ed.: Page 1278
34. Sherrington, Sir Charles: *The Integrative Action of the Nervous System:* Cambridge, Eng., 1947: Cambridge University Press: Page 160

302

35. Crelin, Edmund S.: *Development of the Nervous System:* Summit, N.J., 1974: Ciba Corp.: *Clinical Symposia,* Volume 26, Number 2: Page 21
36. Guyton, Arthur C.: *Textbook of Medical Physiology* — 5th Ed.: Philadelphia, Pa., 1976: W. B. Saunders Co.: Page 768
37. Palmer, D. D.: Pages 35, 36, 57, 66, 68, 96, 105, 109, 141
38. Ibid.: Page 36
39. Ibid.: Page 275
40. Ibid.: Page 335
41. Ibid.: Page 276
42. Ibid.: Page 416
43. Ibid.: Page 298
44. Ibid.: Page 847
45. Ibid.: Page 730
46. Ibid.: Page 876
47. Ibid.: Page 828
48. Ibid.: Page 970
49. Ibid.: Pages 446, 56
50. Trever, William: *In The Public Interest:* Los Angeles, Calif., 1972: Scriptures Unlimited: Pages 47-59 plus documentation
51. Kervran, Louis: *Biological Transmutations:* New York, N.Y., 1972: Swan House: Pages 2-3
52. Palmer, D. D.: Page 359
53. Ibid.: Pages 379
54. Ibid.
55. Beatty, Homer G.: *Anatomical Adjustive Technic:* — 1st Ed.: Denver, Colo., 1939: author: Page 18
56. Selye, Hans: *Stress:* Montreal, Que., 1950: Acta Inc.: g.v.
57. Sachs, Wulf: *The Vegetative Nervous System:* London, Eng., 1936: Cassell and Co., Ltd.: Page 24
58. Guyton, Arthur C.: *Textbook of Medical Physiology* — 5th Ed.: Philadelphia, Pa., 1976: W. B. Saunders Co.: Page 6
59. Pottenger, Francis Marion: *Symptoms of Visceral Disease:* St. Louis, Mo., 1944: C. V. Mosby Co.: Page 194
60. Goldthwait, Joel E.; Brown, Lloyd T.; Swaim, Loring T.; Kuhns, John C.: *Essentials of Body Mechanics in Health and Disease* — 4th Ed.: Philadelphia, Pa., 1945: J. B. Lippincott Co.: Page 6
61. Hilton's Law — A nerve trunk which supplies a joint also supplies the muscles which move the joint and the skin over the insertions of such muscles.
62. Pflueger's Law — If the stimulus received by a sensory nerve extends to a motor nerve of the opposite side, contraction occurs only from the corresponding muscles, and if the contraction is unequal from the two sides, the stronger contraction always takes place on the side which is stimulated.
63. Lowman, Charles L.: *Postural Fitness:* Philadelphia, Pa., 1963: Lea & Febiger: Page 177
64. Kraus, Hans; Rabb, Wilhelm: *Hypokinetic Disease:* Springfield, Mo., 1961: C. C. Thomas Co.: Page 29
65. Kennedy, President John F.: As guest speaker at a sports banquet: New York City, Dec. 5, 1961
66. Scott, M. Gladys: *Analysis of Human Motion:* Crofts and Co.: Page 122
67. Johnston, Lyman C.: *The Theory and Practice of Postural Measurement:* Toronto, Ont.: by the author
68. Feldenkrais, M.: *Body and Mature Behaviour:* New York, N.Y., 1949: International University Press: Page 69

303

69. Carver, Willard: *Carver's Chiropractic Analysis* — 4th Ed.: Oklahoma City, 1922: Dunn Printing Co.: Page 143
70. Beatty, Homer G.: *Anatomical Adjustive Technic:* Page 73
71. Johnston, Lyman C.: *The Theory and Practice of Postural Measurement:*
72. Davis' Law — If the origin and insertion of a muscle are moved further apart for some time, the muscle loses tone and becomes relaxed. If they are approximated the muscle contracts or becomes contractured.
73. Krieg, Wendell, J. S.: *Functional Neuro-Anatomy* — 2nd Ed.: New York, N.Y., 1942: The Blakiston Co., Inc.: Page 30
74. Sherrington, Sir Charles: *The Integrative Action of the Nervous System:* Cambridge, Eng., 1947: The Cambridge University Press: Page 160
75. Pflueger's Law — When the excitation of a sensory nerve elicits reflex action involving both halves of the body, and the action is unequal on the two sides, the side of stronger contractions is always that homonymous with the seat of application of the stimulus.
76. Carver, Willard: *Carver's Chiropractic Analysis:* Page 158
77. Beatty, Homer G.: Page 78
78. Johnston, Lyman C.
79. Palmer, D. D.: Page 211
80. Hilton's Law: See No. 61
81. Hackett, Geo. Stuart: *Joint Ligament Relaxation Treated by Fibro-osseous Proliferation:* Springfield, Ill., 1956: Charles C. Thomas: Page 62
82. Fahrni, W. Harry: *Backache Relieved Through New Concepts of Posture:* Springfield, Ill., 1966: Charles C. Thomas: Page 27
83. Davis' Law — See No. 72
84. Goldthwait, Joel E. et al: *Essentials of Body Mechanics:* Page 173
85. Hilton's Law — See No. 61
86. Pflueger's Law — See No. 62
87. Pottenger, Francis Marion: *Symptoms of Visceral Disease:* Page 166
88. Sherrington, Sir Charles: *The Integrative Action of the Nervous System:* Page 160
89. Ibid: Page 160
90. All-or-None Law — The magnitude of the impulse set up in any single nerve fibre is independent of the strength of the exciting stimulus, providing the latter is adequate. The individual muscle fibre does not respond at all if the stimulus is weak; it responds maximally (for the prevailing environmental conditions) when the stimulus rises to threshhold; the contraction is not increased if the stimulus strength is further raised. Stronger stimuli, however, progressively bring more muscle fibres into action.
91. Palmer, D. D.: Page 39
92. Pottenger, F. M.: *Symptoms of Visceral Disease:* Page 191
93. Ibid: Page 169
94. Ibid: Page 157
95. Kuntz, Albert: *The Autonomic Nervous System* — 4th Ed.: Philadelphia, Pa., 1949: Lea & Febiger: Page 22
96. Rasmussen, Andrew Theodore: *The Principal Nervous Pathways*— 3rd Ed.: New York, N.Y., The MacMillan Co.: Page 39
97. Kuntz, Albert: *The Autonomic Nervous System* — 3rd Ed.: Page 22
98. Plutchik, Robert: *The Role of Muscular Tension in Maladjustment: Mental Health & Chiropractic:* New Hyde Park, N.Y., 1973: Sessions Publishers: Page 71
99. Sherrington, Sir Charles: *The Integrative Action of the Nervous System:* Page 160
100. Kamieth H.: *Pathogenetic Importance of the Thoracic Portion of the*

*Vertebral Column:* Journal of Amer. Med. Assoc., Nov. 15, 1958
101. Palmer, D. D.: Page 57
102. Ibid.: Page 212
103. Alverez, Walter C.: *An Introduction to Gastro-Enterology* — 4th Ed.: New York, N.Y., 1948: Paul B. Hoeber, Inc.: Page 638
104. Pottenger, F. M.: Page 160
105. *Gray's Anatomy:* 28th U.S. Ed.: 29th British Ed.: Philadelphia, Pa., Lea & Febiger: Page 1206
106. *Cunningham's Textbook of Human Anatomy* — 8th Ed.: Page 974
107. Krieg, Wendell J. S.: *Functional Neuro-anatomy:* Page 247
108. Ibid: Page 247
109. *Gray's Anatomy:* 28th Ed.: Page 874
110. Speransky, A. D.: *A Basis for the Theory of Medicine:* New York, N.Y., 1943: International Publishers Co.: Page 313
111. Ibid: Page 310
112. Kuntz, Albert: *The Autonomic Nervous System* — 4th Ed.: Philadelphia, Pa., 1949: Lea & Febiger: Page 467
113. Gordienko, A. N.: *Control of Immunogenesis by the Nervous System:* Washington, D.C., 1958: U.S. Department of Commerce, Office of Technical Services: Page 2
114. Palmer, D. D.: Page 358
115. Ibid.: Page 359
116. Spain, David M.: *The Complications of Modern Medical Practices:* New York, N.Y., 1963: Grune & Stratton, Inc.: Page 4
117. Pottenger, F. M.: *Symptoms of Visceral Disease:* Page 160
118. Ibid.: Page 202
119. Feldenkrais, M.: *Body and Mature Behaviour:* New York, N.Y., 1949: International University Press: Page 20
120. Freeman, G. L.: *Physiological Psychology:* New York, N.Y., 1948: D. Van Nostrand Co.: Page 135
121. Abrahamson, E. M. and Pezet, A. W.: *Body, Mind and Sugar:* New York, N.Y., 1951: Henry Holt and Co.: Page 61
122. Wyke, Barry D.: *Principles of General Neurophysiology Relating to Anaesthesia and Surgery:* London, Eng., 1960: Butterworth and Co.: Page 27
123. Best, Chas. Herbert; Taylor, Norman B.: *The Physiological Basis of Medical Practice:* Baltimore, Md., 1943: The Williams & Wilkins Co.: Page 1336
124. Wyke, Barry D.: *Principles of General Neurophysiology Relating to Anaesthesia and Surgery:* Toronto, Ont., 1960: Butterworth and Co. (Canada)
125. Freeman, G. L.: *Physiological Psychology:* Page 371
126. Matzke, Howard A; Foltz, Floyd M.: *Synopsis of Neuroanatomy* — 2nd Ed.: New York, N.Y., 1972: Oxford University Press: Page 9
127. Palmer, D. D.: Page 674
128. Cohen's Committee: *Independent Practitioners Under Medicare:* U.S. Printing Office, 1968: Pages 153-4
129. Kevran, Louis: *Biological Transmutations:* Brooklyn, N.Y., 1972: Beekman Publishers: Page 6
130. Ibid.
131. Palmer, D. D.: Page 374
132. Schwartz, Herman S.: *The Foundations of Chiropractic Psychosomatics:* January 1954: The Journal of the National Chiropractic Assoc.
133. Guyton, Arthur C.: *Textbook of Medical Physiology:* 5th Ed.: Page 764
134. Sachs, Wulf: *The Vegetative Nervous System:* London, Eng., 1936: Cassell and Co., Ltd.: Page 22
135. Lowman, Chas. L.; Young, Carl, H.: *Postural Fitness:* Pages 58, 59 and 34

305

136. Feldenkrais, M.: *Body and Mature Behaviour:* Page 5
137. Ibid.: Page 35
138. Fahrni, W. Harry: *Backache Relieved:* Page 9
139. Feldenkrais, M.: *Body and Mature Behaviour:* Page 128
140. Lowen, Alexander: *Chiropractic and Mental Health:* Herman S. Schwartz: New Hyde Park, N.Y., 1973: Sessions Publishers: Page 55
141. Curtis, Brian A.; Jacobson, Stanley; Marcus, Elliott M.: *An Introduction to the Neurosciences:* Toronto, Ont., 1972: W. B. Saunders Co.: Page 432
142. Palmer, D. D.: Page 216
143. Goldthwait, Joel E., et al: *Essentials of Body Mechanics in Health and Disease:* Page 99
144. Boyd, William: *An Introduction to the Study of Disease* — 6th Ed.: Philadelphia, Pa., 1971: Lea & Febiger: Page 329
145. Selye, Hans: *Stress:* Montreal, Que., 1950: Acta Inc.: Page 688
146. Rasmussen, A. T.: *Principal Nervous Pathways* — 3rd Ed.: New York, N.Y.: The MacMillan Co.: Page 39
147. Kamieth, H.: *Pathogenetic Importance of the Thoracic Portion of the Vertebral Column:* Journal of Amer. Med. Assoc., Nov. 15, 1958: q.v.
148. Reich, Wilhelm: *The Cancer Biopathy:* New York, N.Y., 1973: Farrer, Straus & Giroux
149. Feldenkrais, M.: *Body and Mature Behaviour:* Page 130
150. Schwartz, Herman S.: *What is the Connection Between Nerves and Nervousness?:* April-May, 1949: The Journal of the National Chiropractic Assoc.: q.v.
151. Mennell, James: *The Science and Art of Joint Manipulation:* London, Eng., 1952: J. & A. Churchill Ltd.: Page 46
152. Cobb, Stanley: *Foundations of Neuropsychiatry* — 4th Ed.: Baltimore, Md., 1948: The Williams & Wilkins Co.: Page 235
153. Gordienko, A. N.: *Control of Immunogenesis by the Nervous System:* Pages 95-121
154. Palmer, D. D.: Page 861
155. Boyd, William: *An Introduction to the Study of Disease* — 6th Ed.: Philadelphia, Pa., 1971: Lea & Febiger: Page 10
156. Abrahamson, E. M.; Pezet, A. W.: *Body, Mind and Sugar:* Page 157
157. Palmer, D. D.: Page 67
158. Pottenger, F. M.: *Symptoms of Visceral Disease:* Page 143
159. Guyton, Arthur C.: *Textbook of Medical Physiology* — 5th Ed.: Page 498
160. Matzke, Howard A.; Foltz, Floyd M.: *Synopsis of Neuroanatomy* — 2nd Ed.: Page 18-19
161. Ibid.
162. Sherrington, Sir Charles: *Integrative Action of the Nervous System:* Page 156
163. Ibid.: Page 155
164. Pottenger, F. M.: *Symptoms of Visceral Disease:* Page 174
165. Freeman, G. L.: *Physiological Psychology:* Page 28
166. Minckler, Jeff: *Introduction to Neurosciences:* St. Louis, Mo., 1972: The C. V. Mosby Co.: Page 155
167. Freeman, G. L.: *Physiological Psychology:* Page 121
168. Curtis, Brian; Jacobson, Stanley; Marcus, Elliott M.: *An Introduction to the Neurosciences:* Philadelphia, Pa., 1972: W. B. Saunders Co.: Page 16
169. Abrahamson, E. M.; Pezet, A. W.: *Body, Mind and Sugar:* Pages 61, 62, 121
170. Freeman, E. M.: *Physiological Psychology:* Page 370
171. Alpers, Bernard J.: *Clinical Neurology:* Philadelphia, Pa., 1963: F. A.

Davis Co.: Page 729
172. Magoun, H. W.; Rhines, Ruth: *Spasticity* — 1st Ed.: Springfield, Ill., 1947: Charles C. Thomas: Page 26
173. Cobb, Stanley: *Foundation of Neuropsychiatry:* Page 108
174. Feldenkrais, M.: *Body and Mature Behaviour:* Page 20
175. Kuntz, Albert: *The Autonomic Nervous System:* 3rd Ed.: Philadelphia, Pa., 1947: Lea & Febiger: Page 46
176. Pottenger, F. M.: *Symptoms of Visceral Disease:* Page 202
177. Guyton, Arthur C.: *Textbook of Medical Physiology* — 5th Ed.: Page 624
178. Curtis, Brian, et al: *An Introduction to the Neurosciences:* Page 20
179. Guyton, Arthur C.: *Textbook of Medical Physiology* — 5th Ed.: Page 679
180. Minckler, Jeff: *Introduction to Neurosciences:* Page 7
181. Curtis, Brian; et al: *An Introduction to the Neurosciences:* Page 47
182. Guyton, Arthur C.: *Textbook of Medical Physiology* — 5th Ed.: Page 647
183. Ibid.: Page 665
184. Melzack, Ronald: *The Puzzle of Pain:* New York, N.Y., 1973: Basic Books, Inc.: Page 85
185. Swanberg, Harold: *The Intervertebral Foramina in Man:* Pages 36 and 39
186. Ibid.: Pages 36 and 39
187. Guyton, Arthur C.: *Textbook of Medical Physiology* — 5th Ed.: Page 652
188. Sherrington, Sir Charles: *The Integrative Action of the Nervous System:* Page 160
189. Ibid.: Page 7
190. Minckler, Jeff: *Introduction to Neuroscience:* St. Louis, Mo., 1972: The C. V. Mosby Co.: Page 206
191. *Cunningham's Textbook of Human Anatomy:* Pages 1229, 1234, 1251, 1260, 1262.
192. Gray, Henry: *Anatomy of the Human Body* — 23rd Ed.: Philadelphia, Pa., 1936: Lea & Febiger: Pages 603, 627, 641, 649
193. Ibid.: Pages 576, 598, 609, 617
194. Elliott, H. Chandler: *Textbook of Neuroanatomy* — 2nd Ed.: Philadelphia, Pa., 1969: Lippincott Co.: Pages 449, 450
195. Curtis, Brian, et al: *An Introduction to the Neurosciences:* Page 183
196. Elliott, H. Chandler: *Textbook of the Nervous System* — 2nd Ed.: Page 306
197. Tasaki, Ichiji: *Nervous Transmission:* Springfield, Ill., 1953: Chas. C. Thomas: Page 7
198. Maximow, Alexander A.; Bloom, Wm.: *A Textbook of Histology* — 4th Ed.: Philadelphia, Pa.: W. B. Saunders Co.: Page 196
199. Curtis, Brian, et al: *An Introduction to the Neurosciences:* Page 50
200. Feldenkrais, M.: *Body and Mature Behaviour:* Page 15
201. Crelin, Edmund S.: *Development of the Nervous System:* Ciba Clinical Symposia: Summit, N.Y., 1974: Volume 26, Number 2: Pages 27-28
202. Clark, W. E. LeGros: *Anatomical Pattern as the Essential Basis of Sensory Discrimination:* Page 4
203. Ibid.: Page 7
204. Minckler, Jeff: *Introduction to Neuroscience:* Page 386
205. Guyton, Arthur C.: *Textbook of Medical Physiology* — 5th Ed.: Page 679
206. Singer, Marcus: *The Regeneration of Body Parts:* 1958: Oct.: Scientific American
207. Sachs, Wulf: *The Vegetative Nervous System:* London, Eng., 1936: Cassell and Co., Ltd.: Page 138
208. Sherrington, Sir Charles: *The Integrative Action of the Nervous System:* Page 148

209. Ibid.: Page 160
210. Ibid.: Page 7
211. Ibid.: Page 18
212. Kuntz, Albert: *Autonomic Nervous System* — 4th Ed.: Page 21
213. Krieg, Wendell J. S.: *Functional Neuroanatomy* — 2nd Ed.: New York, N.Y., 1953: The Blakiston Co., Inc.: Page 36
214. Guyton, Arthur C.: *Textbook of Medical Physiology* — 5th Ed.: Page 144
215. Basmajian, J. V.: *Muscles Alive: Their Functions Revealed by Electromyography:* Baltimore, Md., 1962: The Williams & Wilkins Co.: Pages 41, 43
216. Ibid.: Page 43
217. Palmer, D. D.: Page 7
218. Krieg, Wendell J. S.: *Functional Neuroanatomy* — 2nd Ed.: Page 41
219. Ibid.: Page 41
220. Sherrington, Sir Charles: *The Integrative Action of the Nervous System:* Page 101
221. Guyton, Arthur C.: *Textbook of Medical Physiology* — 5th Ed.: Page 618
222. Curtis, Brian, et al: *An Introduction to the Neurosciences:* Page 137
223. Sherrington, Sir Charles: *The Integrative Action of the Nervous System:* Page 160
224. Ibid.: Page 207
225. Guyton, Arthur C.: *Textbook of Medical Physiology* — 5th Ed.: Page 634
226. Ibid.: Page 637
227. Sherrington, Sir Charles: *The Integrative Action of the Nervous System:* Page 342
228. Krieg, Wendell J. S.: *Functional Neuroanatomy* — 2nd Ed.: Page 307
229. Matzke, Howard A.; Foltz, Floyd M.: *Synopsis of Neuroanatomy* — 2nd Ed.: Page 45
230. Krieg, Wendell J. S.: *Functional Neuroanatomy* — 2nd Ed.: Page 47
231. Guyton, Arthur C.: *Textbook of Medical Physiology* — 5th Ed.: Page 692
232. Curtis, Brian, et al: *An Introduction to the Neurosciences:* Page 285
233. Krieg, Wendell J. S.: *Functional Neuroanatomy* — 2nd Ed.: Page 470
234. Basmajian, J. V.: *Muscles Alive:* Baltimore, Md., 1962: The Williams & Wilkins Co.: Page 91
235. Sachs, Wulf: *The Vegetative Nervous System:* Page 24
236. Kuntz, Albert: *The Autonomic Nervous System:* Page 22
237. Swanberg, Harold: *The Intervertebral Foramina in Man:* Pages 36, 39
238. Palmer, D. D.: Page 293
239. Swanberg, Harold: *The Intervertebral Foramina in Man:*
240. *Gray's Anatomy:* 28th Ed.: Page 309
241. Swanberg, Harold: *The Intervertebral Foramina in Man:* Page 54
242. Ibid.
243. Palmer, D. D.: Page 515
244. Ibid.: Page 39
245. Swanberg, Harold: *The Intervertebral Foramina in Man:* Pages 36, 39
246. Ibid.: Pages 36 and 39
247. Ibid.: Pages 36 and 39
248. Ibid.: Page 39
249. Burke, Gerald L.: *Backache from Occiput to Coccyx:* Vancouver, B.C., 1964: W. E. G. MacDonald: Page 30
250. *Gray's Anatomy:* 29th Br. Ed.: Page 1125; 28th U.S. Ed.: Page 954
251. Sherrington, Sir Charles: *The Integrative Action of the Nervous System:* Page 230
252. Palmer, D. D.: Page 109
253. Ibid.: Page 293

254. Pinkenburg, C. A.: Hoisington, Kan.: Personal correspondence
255. Pottenger, F. M.: *Symptoms of Visceral Disease:* Page 202
256. Burns, Louisa; Chandler, Louis C.; Rice, Ralph W.: *Pathogenesis of Visceral Disease Following Vertebral Lesions:* Chicago, Ill., 1948: The American Osteopathic Assoc.: Pages 30-31
257. Ibid.
258. Sherrington, Sir Charles: *The Integrative Action of the Nervous System:* Page 192
259. Curtis, Brian, et al: *An Introduction to the Neurosciences:* Pages 129,133-134
260. Guyton, Arthur C.: *Textbook of Medical Physiology* — 5th Ed.: Page 616
261. Best, Chas. H.; Taylor, Norman B.: *The Physiological Basis of Medical Practice* — 3rd Ed.: Baltimore, Md., 1943: The Williams & Wilkins Co.: Page 1042
262. Pottenger, F. M.: *Symptoms of Visceral Disease:* Page 355
263. Guyton, Arthur C.: *Textbook of Medical Physiology* — 5th Ed.: Page 371
264. Matsunaga, F.: *"Air-pocket" Phenomenon:* Japanese Journal of Gastroenterology: excerpt in Postgraduate Medicine
265. Hilton's Law — See No. 61
266. Guyton, Arthur C.: *Textbook of Medical Physiology* — 5th Ed.: Page 664
267. Ibid.: Page 371
268. Sherrington, Sir Charles: *The Integrative Action of the Nervous System:* Page 320
269. *Gray's Anatomy* — 29th Br. Ed.: Page 38; 28th U.S. Ed.: Page 889
270. Burns, Louisa, et al: *Pathogenesis of Visceral Disease:* Pages 29-37
271. Wyke, Barry: *Principles of General Neurophysiology Relating to Anaesthesia and Surgery:* Toronto, Ont., 1960: Butterworth and Co. (Canada) Ltd.: Page 15
272. Sherrington, Sir Charles: *The Integrative Action of the Nervous System:* Page 69
273. Ibid.: Page 80
274. Best, Chas. H.; Taylor, Norman B.: *The Physiological Basis of Medical Practice* — 3rd Ed.: Page 1321
275. Wyke, Barry: *Principles of General Neurophysiology Relating to Anaesthesia and Surgery:* Pages 18-22
276. Curtis, Brian, et al: *An Introduction to the Neurosciences:* Page 16
277. Sherrington, Sir Charles: *The Integrative Action of the Nervous System:* Page 80
278. Krieg, Wendell J. S.: *Functional Neuroanatomy:* Page 102
279. Boyd, Wm.: *An Introduction to the Study of Disease:* Philadelphia, Pa., 1971: Lea & Febiger: Page 19
280. Cobb, Stanley: *Foundations of Neuropsychiatry:* Baltimore, Md., 1948: The Williams & Wilkins Co.: Page 117
281. Ibid.: Page 141
282. Curtis, Brian, et al: *An Introduction to the Neurosciences:* Page 16
283. Magoun, H. W.; Rhines, Ruth: *Spasticity:* Page 26
284. Cobb, Stanley: *Foundations of Neuropsychiatry:* Page 108
285. Freeman, E. M.: *Physiological Psychology:* Page 195
286. Abrahamson, E. M.; Pezet, A. W.: *Body, Mind & Sugar:* Page 61
287. Cobb, Stanley: *Foundations of Neuropsychiatry:* Page 7
288. Ibid.: Page 114
289. Ibid.: Page 180
290. Burns, Louisa, et al: *Pathogenesis of Visceral Diseases:*
291. Cobb, Stanley: *Foundations of Neuropsychiatry:* Page 180

292. Ibid.: Page 178
293. Hilton's Law — See No. 61
294. Sherrington, Sir Charles: *The Integrative Action of the Nervous System:* Page 160
295. Ibid.: Page 215
296. Krieg, Wendell J. S.: *Functional Neuroanatomy:* Page 203
297. Guyton, Arthur C.: *Textbook of Medical Physiology* — 5th Ed.: Page 144
298. Kuntz, Albert: *The Autonomic Nervous System* — 4th Ed.: Page 372
299. Freeman, E. M.: *Physiological Psychology* · Page 21
300. Pottenger, F. M.: *Symptoms of Visceral Disease:* Page 21
301. Kuntz, Albert: *The Autonomic Nervous System* — 4th Ed.: Page 373
302. Sherrington, Sir Charles: *The Integrative Action of the Nervous System:* Page 46
303. Pottenger, F. M.: *Symptoms of Visceral Disease:* Page 224
304. Minckler, Jeff: *Introduction to Neuroscience:* Pages 155-254-253
305. Curtis, Brian, et al: *An Introduction to the Neurosciences:* Page 65
306. Ibid.: Pages 36-103
307. Palmer, D. D.: *The Science, Art and Philosophy of Chiropractic:* Page 202
308. *Gray's Anatomy:* 29th Br. Ed.: Page 932; 28th U.S. Ed.: Page 799
309. Ibid.: 29th Br. Ed.: Page 1080; 28th U.S. Ed.: Page 874
310. Minckler, Jeff: *Introduction to Neuroscience:* Page 275
311. Krieg, Wendell J. S.: *Functional Neuroanatomy:* Page 247
312. *Gray's Anatomy:* 28th U.S. Ed.: Page 922
313. Ibid.: Page 933
314. Ibid.: Page 927
315. Krieg, Wendell J. S.: *Functional Neuroanatomy:* Page 153
316. *Gray's Anatomy:* 28th U.S. Ed.: Page 929
317. Pflueger's Fourth Law: With associated spinal reflex centres the irradiation spreads more easily in the direction towards than in the direction away from the head.
318. Pflueger's First Law: If a stimulus applied to a sensory nerve provokes muscular movements solely on one side of the body, that movement occurs under all circumstances and without exception on the same side of the body as the seat of application of the stimulus.
319. Kuntz, Albert: *The Autonomic Nervous System* — 4th Ed.: Page 205
320. Favill, John: *Outline of Spinal Nerves* — 1st Ed.: Springfield, Ill., 1946: Chas. C. Thomas: Page 73
321. *Gray's Anatomy* — 29th British Ed.: Page 1135
322. Carver, Willard: *Carver's Chiropractic Analysis:* Page 143
323. Beatty, Homer G.: *Anatomical Adjustive Technic:* Page 71
324. Logan, Hugh B.: *Logan's Basic Methods:* St. Louis, Mo., 1950: Vinton F. Logan and Fern M. Murray: Page 96
325. Krieg, Wendell J. S.: *Functional Neuroanatomy:* Page 307
326. Ibid.: Page 305
327. Curtis, Brian, et al: *An Introduction to the Neurosciences:* Page 290
328. *Gray's Anatomy:* 28th U.S. Ed.: Page 927
329. Minckler, Jeff: *Introduction to Neuroscience:* Page 277
330. Krieg, Wendell J. S.: *Functional Neuroanatomy:* Page 216
331. Sherrington, Sir Charles: *The Integrative Action of the Nervous System:* Page 342
332. Krieg, Wendell J. S.: *Functional Neuroanatomy:* Page 117
333. Rasmussen, A. T.: *Principal Nervous Pathways:* Page 43
334. Krieg, Wendell J. S.: *Functional Neuroanatomy:* Page 234
335. Ibid.: Page 118

336. Pottenger, F. M.: *Symptoms of Visceral Disease:* Page 412
337. Guyton, Arthur C.: *Textbook of Medical Physiology* — 5th Ed.: Page 119
338. Wyke, Barry D.: *Principles of General Neurophysiology Relating to Anaesthesia and Surgery*
339. Oppenheimer, Albert: *The Swollen Atrophic Hand:* Journal of Surgery: Gynecology and Obstetrics: q.v.
340. Kuntz, Albert: *The Autonomic Nervous System:* Page 43
341. Palmer, D. D.: Page 749
342. Mennell, James: *The Science and Art of Joint Manipulation:* London, Eng., 1952: J. & A. Churchill Ltd.: Page 41
343. Kuntz, Albert: *The Autonomic Nervous System:* Page 486
344. Curtis, Brian, et al: *An Introduction to the Neurosciences:* Page 642
345. Kuntz, Albert: *The Autonomic Nervous System:* Page 486
346. Palmer, D. D.: Page 137
347. Ibid.: Page 195
348. Carver, Willard: *Carver's Chiropractic Analysis:* Page 21
349. Beatty, Homer G.: *Anatomical Adjustive Technic:* Page 96
350. *Gray's Anatomy:* 28th U.S. Ed.: Page 932
351. Crelin, Edmund S.: *Development of the Nervous System:* Page 21
352. *Gray's Anatomy:* 28th U.S. Ed.: Page 1184
353. Minckler, Jeff: *Introduction to Neuroscience:* Page 10
354. Curtis, Brian, et al: *An Introduction to the Neurosciences:* Pages 238-395
355. *Gray's Anatomy:* 28th U.S. Ed.: Page 1183
356. Ibid.: Page 1183
357. Ibid.: Page 1071
358. Ibid.: Page 1184
359. Ibid.: Page 1060
360. Ibid.: Page 1037
361. Sachs, Wulf: *The Vegetative Nervous System:* Page 27
362. Kuntz, Albert: *The Autonomic Nervous System:* Page 45
363. Ibid.: Page 485
364. Ibid.: Page 165
365. Ibid.: Page 43
366. Sachs, Wulf: *The Vegetative Nervous System:* Page 91
367. Ibid.: Page 194
368. *Gray's Anatomy:* 28th U.S. Ed.: Page 1190
369. Kuntz, Albert: *The Autonomic Nervous System:* Pages 152, 157
370. Ibid.: Page 193
371. Rasmussen, A. T.: *Principal Nervous Pathways:* Page 63
372. Kuntz, Albert: *The Autonomic Nervous System:* Page 148
373. Curtis, Brian, et al: *An Introduction to the Neurosciences:* Page 394
374. Kuntz, Albert: *The Autonomic Nervous System:* Page 144
375. Guyton, Arthur C.: *Textbook of Medical Physiology* — 5th Ed.: Page 322
376. Moser, Robert H.: *Diseases of Medical Progress:* Springfield, Ill., 1964: Charles C. Thomas: Page 133
377. Spain, David: *The Complications of Modern Medical Practices:* New York, N.Y., 1963: Grune & Stratton: Page 135
378. Kuntz, Albert: *The Autonomic Nervous System:* Page 151
379. Johnston, Lyman C : Toronto, Ont.
380. Kamieth, H.: *Pathogenetic Importance of the Thoracic Portion of the Vertebral Column:* Munich, Germany, 1958: Archives orthop. u. Unfall-Chir. 49: 585-606 (No. 6); J.A.M.A., Nov. 15, 1958
381. Kuntz, Albert: *The Autonomic Nervous System:* Page 248
382. *Gray's Anatomy:* 28th U.S. Ed.: Page 1194

383. Abrahamson, A. M.; Pezet, A. W.: *Body, Mind & Sugar:* q.v.
384. Kuntz, Albert: *The Autonomic Nervous System:* Page 248
385. Palmer, D. D.: Page 328
386. Kuntz, Albert: *The Autonomic Nervous System:* Page 255
387. Ibid.: Page 258
388. Guyton, Arthur C.: *Textbook of Medical Physiology* — 5th Ed.: Page 378
389. Kuntz, Albert: *The Autonomic Nervous System:* Pages 265-266
390. Selye, Hans: *Stress:* Page 106
391. Ibid.: Page 31
392. Ibid.: Page 36
393. Ibid.: Page 10
394. Palmer, D. D.: Pages 195 and 216
395. Ibid.: Page 870
396. Illi, Fred: *The Vertebral Column: Lifeline of the Body:* Chicago, Ill., 1951: National College of Chiropractic: q.v.
397. Beatty, Homer G.: *Anatomical Adjustive Technic:* Page 87
398. Kuntz, Albert: *The Autonomic Nervous System:* Pages 270, 275
399. Reich, Wilhelm: *The Cancer Biopathy:* New York, N.Y., 1948; Theorgon Institute Press: q.v.
400. *Gray's Anatomy:* 28th U.S. Ed.: Page 932
401. Curtis, Brian, et al: *An Introduction to the Neurosciences:* Page 393
402. *Gray's Anatomy:* 28th U.S. Ed.: Page 932
403. Kuntz, Albert: *The Autonomic Nervous System:* Page 278
404. Ibid.: Page 279
405. Curtis, Brian, et al: *An Introduction to the Neurosciences:* Page 394
406. Kuntz, Albert: *The Autonomic Nervous System:* Page 304
407. Guyton, Arthur C.: *Textbook of Medical Physiology* — 5th Ed.: Page 670
408. Alvarez, Walter C.: *An Introduction to Gastro-Enterology:* 4th Ed.: New York, N.Y., 1948: Paul B. Hoeber, Inc.: Page 125
409. *Gray's Anatomy:* 28th U.S. Ed.: Page 242
410. Hollingshead, W. Henry: *Functional Anatomy of the Limbs and Back:* Philadelphia, Pa., 1951: W. B. Saunders Co.: Page 179
411. Johnston, Lyman C.: Toronto, Ont.: q.v.
412. Judovich, Bernard; Bates, Wm.: *Segmental Neuralgia in Painful Syndromes:* Philadelphia, Pa., 1946: F. A. Davis Co.: Page 3
413. Goldthwait, Joel E., et al: *Essentials of Body Mechanics:* Page 1
414. Mennell, James: *The Science and Art of Joint Manipulation:* Page 180
415. Fahrni, W. Harry: *Backache Relieved Through New Concepts of Posture:* Springfield, Ill., 1966: Charles C. Thomas: Page 10
416. Judovich, Bernard; Bates, Wm.: *Segmental Neuralgia in Painful Syndromes:* Page 6
417. Lewis, Sir Thomas: *Pain:* New York, N.Y., 1946: The MacMillan Co.: Page 41
418. Ibid.: Page 153
419. Walshe, F. M. R.: *Critical Studies in Neurology:* Edinburgh, Scotland, 1948: E. & S. Livingstone Ltd.: Page 53
420. Judovich, Bernard; Bates, Wm.: *Segmental Neuralgia in Painful Syndromes:* Page 221
421. Wolff, Harold G.; Wolf, Stewart: *Pain:* Springfield, Ill., 1958: Charles C. Thomas: Page 32
422. Wyke, Barry D.: *Principles of General Neurophysiology Relating to Anaesthesia and Surgery:* Page 15
423. Lewis, Sir Thomas: *Pain:* Page 135
424. Rasmussen, A. T.: *The Principal Nervous Pathways:* Page 39

312

425. Burns, Louisa, et al: *Pathogenesis of Visceral Diseases Following Vertebral Lesions:* Page 38
426. Sachs, Wulf: *The Vegetative Nervous System:* Page 149
427. *Gray's Anatomy:* 29th Br. Ed.: Page 500
428. Illi, Fred W.: *The Vertebral Column — Life-Line of the Body:* Pages 17, 13
429. Ibid.: Page 13
430. *Gray's Anatomy:* 29th Br. Ed.: Page 500
431. Hackett, Geo. Stuart: *Joint Ligament Relaxation Treated by Fibro-osseous Proliferation:* Springfield, Ill., 1959: Charles C. Thomas: Page 59
432. Bourdillon, J. F.: *Spinal Manipulation:* New York, N.Y., 1970: Appleton-Century-Crofts: Page 41
433. Hilton's Law — See No. 61
434. Favill, John: *Outline of Spinal Nerves:* Springfield, Ill., 1946: Charles C. Thomas: Pages 35, 37.
435. *Gray's Anatomy:* 29th Br. Ed.: Page 1128
436. Hackett, Geo. Stuart: *Joint Ligament Relaxation Treated by Fibro-osseous Proliferation:* Page 61
437. *Gray's Anatomy:* 28th U.S. Ed.: Page 500
438. Hackett, Geo. Stuart: *Joint Ligament Relaxation Treated by Fibro-osseous Proliferation:* Page 61
439. Kuntz, Albert: *The Autonomic Nervous System:* Page 36
440. Palmer, Daniel David: *The Science, Art and Philosophy of Chiropractic:* Page 827
441. Crelin, Edmund S.: *Development of the Nervous System:* q.v.
442. Allan, Frank D.: *Essentials of Human Embryology — 2nd Ed.:* New York, N.Y., 1969: Oxford University Press: Page 233
443. Kuntz, Albert: *The Autonomic Nervous System:* Page 486
444. Pottenger, F. M.: *Symptoms of Visceral Disease:* Page 330
445. Ibid.: Pages 306-307
446. Davis' Law — See No. 72
447. Beatty, Homer G.: *Anatomical Adjustive Technic:* Pages 299-307 and 308-313
448. Chusid, J. G.: *Correlative Neuroanatomy & Functional Neurology — 16th Ed.:* Los Altos, Calif., 1976: Lange Medical Publications: Pages 199-205
449. Palmer, D. D.: *The Science, Art and Philosophy of Chiropractic:* Page 446
450. Ibid.: Page 56
451. Ibid.: Page 169
452. Ibid.: Page 426
453. Ibid.: Page 453
454. Ibid.: Page 491
455. Ibid.: Page 699
456. Ibid.: Page 498
457. Ibid.: Page 505
458. Ibid.: Page 552
459. Ibid.: Page 616
460. Freeman, G. L.: *Physiological Psychology:* Page 163
461. *Gray's Anatomy:* 28th U.S. Ed.: Page 1123
462. Cobb, Stanley: *Foundations of Neuropsychiatry:* Page 114
463. Kuntz, Albert: *The Autonomic Nervous System:* Page 37
464. Cunningham: *Textbook of Human Anatomy:* Page 965
465. Rasmussen, A. T.: *The Principal Nervous Pathways:* Page 38
466. *Gray's Anatomy:* 28th U.S. Ed.: Page 1110
467. Lewis, Sir Thomas: *Pain:* Page 25
468. Rasmussen, A. T.: *The Principal Nervous Pathways:* Page 39

313

469. Pottenger, F. M.: *Symptoms of Visceral Disease:* Page 169
470. Rasmussen, A. T.: *The Principal Nervous Pathways:* Page 39
471. Kuntz, Albert: *The Autonomic Nervous System:* Page 284
472. Rasmussen, A. T.: *The Principal Nervous Pathways:* Page 39
473. *Gray's Anatomy:* 28th U.S. Ed.: Page 1182
474. Rasmussen, A. T.: *The Principal Nervous Pathways:* Page 39
475. Alvarez, Walter C.: *Nervousness Indigestion and Pain:* New York, N.Y., 1947: Paul B. Hoeber, Inc.: Page 311
476. Rasmussen, A. T.: *The Principal Nervous Pathways:* Page 39
477. Kuntz, Albert: *The Autonomic Nervous System:* Page 284
478. Lockhart, R. D.; Hamilton, G. F.; Fyfe, F. W.: *Anatomy of the Human Body:* Philadelphia, Pa., 1969: J. B. Lippincott Co.: Page 342
479. Kuntz, Albert: *The Autonomic Nervous System:* Page 301
480. Rasmussen, A. T.: *The Principal Nervous Pathways:* Page 39
481. Kuntz, Albert: *The Autonomic Nervous System:* Page 301
482. Ibid.: Pages 299, 301
483. Rasmussen, A. T.: *The Principal Nervous Pathways:* Page 39
484. Ibid.: Page 39
485. Kuntz, Albert: *The Autonomic Nervous System:* Page 300
486. Lockhart, R. D., et al: *Anatomy of the Human Body:* Page 342
487. Rasmussen, A. T.: *The Principal Nervous Pathways:* Page 39
488. Kuntz, Albert: *The Autonomic Nervous System:* Page 289
489. Ibid.: Page 304
490. Rasmussen, A. T.: *The Principal Nervous Pathways:* Page 39
491. Palmer, D. D.: Page 827
492. Carver, Willard: Pages 60-61
493. Palmer, D. D.: Page 742
494. Sachs, Wulf: *The Vegetative Nervous System:* Page 140
495. Pottenger, F. M.: *Symptoms of Visceral Disease:* Page 180
496. Rasmussen, A. T.: *The Principal Nervous Pathways:* Page 39
497. Pottenger, F. M.: *Symptoms of Visceral Disease:* Page 183
498. Kuntz, Albert: *The Autonomic Nervous System:* Page 427
499. Ibid.: Page 428
500. Judovich, Bernard; Bates, Wm.: *Segmental Neuralgia in Painful Syndromes:* Page 6
501. Kuntz, Albert: *The Autonomic Nervous System:* Page 429
502. White, Jas. C.; Smithwick, Reginald: *The Autonomic Nervous System —* 2nd Ed.: New York, N.Y., 1952: The MacMillan Co.: Page 65
503. Wolff, Harold G.; Wolf, Stewart: *Pain:* Page 56
504. Pottenger, F. M.: *Symptoms of Visceral Disease:* Page 185
505. Ibid.: Page 157
506. Kuntz, Albert: *The Autonomic Nervous System:* Page 373
507. Ibid.: Page 231
508. Pottenger, F. M.: *Symptoms of Visceral Disease:* Page 253
509. Kuntz, Albert: *The Autonomic Nervous System:* Page 490
510. Pottenger, F. M.: *Symptoms of Visceral Disease:* Page 194
511. Sachs, Wulf: *The Vegetative Nervous System:* Page 138
512. Cobb, Stanley: *Foundations of Neuropsychiatry:* Page 100
513. Kuntz, Albert: *The Autonomic Nervous System:* Page 457
514. Freeman, G. L.: *Physiological Psychology:* Page 279
515. White, Jas. C.; Smithwick, Reginald H.; Simeone, Fiorindo A.: *The Autonomic Nervous System —* 3rd Ed.: Page 65
516. Sachs, Wulf: *The Vegetative Nervous System:* Page 140
517. Curtis, Brian, et al: *An Introduction to the Neurosciences:* Pages 429-436

518. Guyton, Arthur C.: *Textbook of Medical Physiology* — 5th Ed.: Page 880
519. Ibid.: Page 764
520. Singer, Marcus: *The Regeneration of Body Parts:* Scientific American, Oct. 1958: q.v.
521. Minckler, Jeff: *Introduction to Neuroscience:* Page 205
522. Sachs, Wulf: *The Vegetative Nervous System:* Page 120
523. Feldenkrais, M.: *Body and Mature Behaviour:* Pages 37-38
524. Kuntz, Albert: *The Autonomic Nervous System:* Page 55
525. Feldenkrais, M.: *Body and Mature Behaviour:* Pages 119 and 152
526. Ibid.: Page 156
527. Cobb, Stanley: *Foundations of Neuropsychiatry:* Page 18
528. Sachs, Wulf: *The Vegetative Nervous System:* Page 138
529. Sherrington, Sir Charles: *The Integrative Action of the Nervous System:* Page 339
530. Curtis, Brian, et al: *An Introduction to the Neurosciences:* Page 129
531. Pottenger, F. M.: *Symptoms of Visceral Disease:* Page 202
532. Ibid.: Page 160
533. Rasmussen, A. T.: *The Principal Nervous Pathways:* Page 34
534. Pottenger, F. M.: *Symptoms of Visceral Disease:* Page 160
535. Kuntz, Albert: *The Autonomic Nervous System:* Page 86
536. Boyd, Wm.: *An Introduction to the Study of Disease* — 6th Ed.: Philadelphia, Pa., 1971: Lea & Febiger: Page 19
537. Pottenger, F. M.: *Symptoms of Visceral Disease:* Page 171
538. Selye, Hans: *Stress:* Page 87
539. Speransky, A. D.: *A Basis for the Theory of Medicine:* Page 164
540. Ibid.: Page 167
541. Ibid.: Page 176
542. Pottenger, F. M.: *Symptoms of Visceral Disease:* Page 199
543. Ibid.: Page 202
544. Speransky, A. D.: *A Basis for the Theory of Medicine:* Page 199
545. Palmer, D. D.: *The Science, Art and Philosophy of Chiropractic:* Pages 617 and 709
546. Pottenger, F. M.: *Symptoms of Visceral Disease:* Page 213
547. Speransky, A. D.: *A Basis for the Theory of Medicine:* Page 213
548. Ibid.: Page 177
549. Dubos, Rene: *Biochemical Determinants of Microbial Diseases:* Cambridge, Mass., 1954: Harvard University Press: Pages 2-5-12
550. Palmer, D. D.: Page 142
551. Haggard, H. W.: *Devils, Drugs and Doctors:* New York, N.Y., 1946: Pocket Books, Inc.: Page 298
552. Selye, Hans: *Stress:* Page 21
553. Ibid.: Page 25
554. Ibid.: Page 38
555. Ibid.: Page 60
556. Gordienko, A.N.: (translation) Washington, D.C., 1958: U.S. Dept. of Commerce, Office of Technical Services: Pages 1-16-21-62-15-121
557. Zinsser, Hans: *Rats, Lice and History:* New York, N.Y., 1967: Bantam Science and Mathematics: Page 180
558. Selye, Hans: *Stress:* Page 61
559. Kuntz, Albert: *The Autonomic Nervous System:* Page 492
560. Speransky, A. D.: *A Basis for the Theory of Medicine:* Page 313
561. Ibid.: Page 321
562. Gordienko, A. N., et al: *Control of Immunogenesis by the Nervous System:* Page 123

563. Young, Clara Gene; Barger, James D.: *Introduction to Medical Science:* St. Louis, Mo., 1969: The C. V. Mosby Co.: Page 22

# Index

– NOTES –

# – NOTES –

– NOTES –

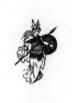